MW01679681

Recovery from Parkinson's

Dr. Janice Hadlock, DAOM

Illustrations by Ben Bateson

Recovery from Parkinson's
Dr. Janice Hadlock, DAOM, LAc
Illustrations by Ben Bateson

Other books by Janice Hadlock are available at www.JaniceHadlock.com:

Hacking Chinese Medicine
Tracking the Dragon *
Yin Tui Na: Hands-on Therapy for Traumatic Injury *
Stuck on Pause *
Medications of Parkinson's: Once Upon a Pill – Patient experiences with dopamine-enhancing medications and supplements * **

*Also available for free download at www.PDrecovery.org
** Not available in hard copy

Published by Raja Books, Santa Cruz, CA
www.JaniceHadlock.com
Fifth edition (heavily revised) 2020

Preface to *An Essay on The Shaking Palsy* by James Parkinson

It is hoped that the offering of the following pages to the attention of the medical public, will not be severely censured. He... [the writer] considered it to be a duty to submit his opinions to the examination of others, even in their present state of immaturity and imperfection.

James Parkinson
Member of the Royal College of Surgeons
1817

Preface to *Recovery from Parkinson's*

Dear reader, this book is written in a continuation of that spirit of hope of not being too severely censured and of that sense of duty, as well as a great sense of gratitude for being able to share my findings about Parkinson's disease not just with James Parkinson's "medical public" but with anyone wanting to learn more about this syndrome.

Dr. Charcot (1825-1893), considered by many to be the father of the modern science of neurology, named this syndrome Parkinson's disease in honor of James Parkinson's treatise on the subject. Parkinson himself had named the syndrome "the shaking palsy."

Janice Hadlock
DAOM (Doctor of Acupuncture and Oriental Medicine)
2020

Dedication and acknowledgements

This book is dedicated to those people who have idiopathic Parkinson's disease and especially to those who have been told that it is an incurable illness. It is not. To you, I offer this book.

It could not have been written without the insights and support of my patients, both in clinic and via email. I send all of you oceans of gratitude. Thank you Ben Bateson, ever-enthusiastic artist and cover designer; your artwork is so *clean*. Thanks also go out to my proofreaders: Linda Moyer, Laura Yeh, and Jim Elkin. And to my many teachers, from grade school up to the present, and especially Miss Connelly, Dr. Kenneth V. Thimann, PhD, Dr. Jeffery Pang, Dr. Sharon Feng, and Dr. Lucy Hu. Love and thanks to my supportive colleagues, especially Laura Walter, acupuncturist and craniosacral therapist supreme and Dr. Kevin Ryan, osteopath, naturopath, acupuncturist, and brilliant Chinese medicine theorist, always more than willing to discuss any point of theory with me and to serve as my muse.

My family, so loving, so supportive (alphabetically): Audrey, Clay, Cormac Laura, Maddy, Orion, Piper, and Simon, I could not have done this without you and the mint chocolate chip ice cream. I love you all so much. Thank you Steve, you taught me how to write and then edit, and then edit, again and again until it scans and makes sense.

Thank you Dr. James Parkinson and Dr. Charcot. Thank you St. Francis and St. Claire of Assisi. Thank you great saints and sages of every faith.

Denny West, thank you for your calming wisdom when you were diagnosed with Parkinson's disease, and for unintentionally igniting in me the rage and fire that drove me to the answers presented in this book.

Paramahansa Yogananda, your love has held me through every page.

⸙ Table of Contents ⸙

Sympathetic mode — fight or flight panic

Recovery from Parkinson's

Self-Induced Panic — Type I

"Although, at present, uninformed as to the precise nature of the disease, still it ought not to be considered as one against which there exists no countervailing remedy." [1]

– James Parkinson, 1817

Chapter One

A Curable Illness

Idiopathic Parkinson's disease is not – and never has been – an incurable illness.

I saw my first Parkinson's patient in 1996. I treated her for her foot problem, not her Parkinson's disease. After all, everyone in the field of medicine knows that Parkinson's is incurable. When she unexpectedly recovered, I logically assumed she had been misdiagnosed. When the next two recovered, questions began to fester.

This book tells what happened after that. More than twenty years have passed since those first patients recovered. I've worked closely with hundreds of Parkinson's patients. Hundreds more have conferred or contributed observations via emails. Almost from the start, I was obsessed with seeking answers to the mystery of Parkinson's disease.

I'll start this book with the answers.

What causes Parkinson's disease?

Parkinson's disease is a collection of symptoms. These symptoms are set in motion by the long-term use of a highly specific, rarely used set of bio-electric circuits. Non-neural (not in the nerves) currents flow constantly throughout the body's connective tissue and in the brain. The exact circuits used at any given instant depend on a person's thoughts and biological needs at that instant. The particular circuit configuration that causes the symptoms of Parkinson's should only run when a person is in near-death shock or coma. In people with Parkinson's, the non-neural currents flow in the near-death circuitry all the time. In many people with Parkinson's, their currents have been running this way since childhood.

In schools of Chinese medicine, the *main* pathways of the body's non-neural currents are referred to as channels. The electricity flowing through *all* the pathways, great and small, is called "channel qi." The word qi means "energy" and is pronounced chée-ee.

In this book, I sometimes refer to these currents as channel qi, sometimes as electrical currents. Feel free to call these currents whatever you want: electrical currents work the same way in English as they do in Chinese.

In a healthy person, these channels run in very specific patterns. When the channel flow becomes aberrant due to pathogens, injuries, toxins, and even subtle influences such as inclement weather or mood, the body might function poorly. Depending on the severity of the channel irregularities, health problems of corresponding severity can arise.

---

[1] Parkinson, James; *An Essay on the Shaking Palsy*; Sherwood, Neely, and Jones; London; 1817; page 56.

The flow of a patient's channel qi can easily be detected by hand. Most students can begin to feel these electrical currents by hand after a few weeks of training. Detection of the these currents is *objective*, not based on intuitional whims or personal opinions.

At Five Branches, the acupuncture college in Santa Cruz, California, I teach a class in feeling channel qi. For students' exams, they must correctly feel and write down for me the irregularities they detect, by hand, in a new patient's channels. Students are usually happily surprised, early on in the semester, when they realize that they have each detected the *same* channel behaviors, in the *same* locations, on a given patient. [1]

Very early on in my Parkinson's research, I noticed that the channel qi in people with Parkinson's was always running backwards in one of the channels on the leg: the Stomach channel. I assumed, incorrectly, that this backwards flow of current was an aberration, held in place by an injury, in *everyone* with Parkinson's. Several years later, I noticed that other currents in my Parkinson's patients were also behaving in a highly specific manner, a manner that conflicted with the healthy electrical patterns I had studied in school. Years passed before I learned that these electrical behaviors are related to the rarely used neurological mode that is only supposed to kick in when a person is on the verge of death or in a coma.

This near-death mode is *not* recognized in western medical theory, but it *is* in ancient Chinese medicine. The Chinese name for this neurological mode is "Cling to Life." I have taken the liberty of giving it a more brisk and more biologically descriptive English name: "pause mode." [2]

Early on, I observed that when the old, unhealed foot injuries of my first few Parkinson's patients recovered in response to the supportive hands-on therapy that I was using, the channel qi began flowing in the correct direction and stayed that way. The symptoms of Parkinson's ceased and never returned. This was before I knew about pause mode.

At that time, in the late 1990s, I naturally assumed that straightening out the aberrant channel qi by fixing the foot injury had gotten rid of the Parkinson's symptoms. Therefore, this would be an effective treatment for *everyone* with Parkinson's.

---

[1] I wrote a textbook for the class: *Tracking the Dragon*. The textbook can be used as a learn-on-your-own course by anyone wanting to learn how to feel the currents in the sub-dermal connective tissues. The book is addressed to the general public and does not presume any medical background.

The chapters with instructions on how to feel channel qi and the appendix with the maps of the channels are available for free download at www.PDrecovery.org, the website of the non-profit Parkinson's Recovery Project. Click on Publications, then click on *Tracking the Dragon*.

[2] Ancient Chinese medical theory recognized four neurological modes: sympathetic (fight or flight) and parasympathetic (hungry, happy, and curious) and modes that drive behaviors of sleep and of near-death. Western medicine still only recognizes two, and those two only relatively recently, in the last two hundred-plus years. In chapter thirteen of the ancient Chinese medical text *Huang Ti Nei Jing*, pause mode is called "Close to Life" and, in other translations, "Cling to Life."

– From the *Su Wen* portion of the *Nei Jing*, chapter 13-9, from *A Complete Translation of the Yellow Emperor's Classics of Internal Medicine and the Difficult Classic*; Henry C. Lu, PhD; published by the International College of Traditional Chinese Medicine; Vancouver, BC, Canada; 2004; p. 116.

I was wrong. My first few patients all had the same type of Parkinson's disease – the type set in motion by an incompletely healed injury. I soon met people with Parkinson's who did *not* respond to this type of therapy. I spent years working with hundreds of people with Parkinson's before I eventually figured out that there are four different ways to get locked into this electrical flow pattern. Each of the four ways of getting stuck in this flow pattern requires a different method for getting *un*stuck.

Happily, no matter which system was used for setting pause mode in motion, when pause turns off, the body resets itself back to a healthy flow pattern. When the pause-mode type currents are turned off, Parkinson's disease ceases.

Long term use of near-death mode

In healthy people, the near-death electrical pattern usually only kicks in for a very short duration. It can be triggered by excessive loss of blood, excessive perforation of the skin, concussion, or other *near-death* types of *severe* shock-inducing trauma or coma.

The symptoms of near-death trauma mode can include immobility due to inhibition of dopamine release for motor function, faint voice, lowered blood pressure, poor temperature regulation, inhibition of the swallow reflex, and even a sense of being outside the body – looking at oneself from outside the body – to name just a few. When attempting to come out of this mode, the body often exhibits tremor behaviors, also known as "shaking." These symptoms are also characteristic of Parkinson's disease.

The degree and type of immobility varies. In coma, a person is usually limp. In lesser degrees of pause, the body might manifest immobility with tension. Pause mode immobility with tension features automatic tightening up of certain muscles and relaxation of opposing muscles, leading to the body being curled into a somewhat fetal position.

As with the other neurological modes, all of the pause-mode physiology is activated and sustained via mode-specific electrical currents that run just under the skin and through the brain. Pause mode and the electrical circuitry associated with it are supposed to stop as soon as the body stabilizes and the risk of imminent death has ended. People with Parkinson's have typically been using the circuitry of this mode for decades – often since childhood. They have been able to override the immobility-with-tension symptoms of pause mode by using a brain-based emergency override that will be discussed later in this chapter. The symptoms of Parkinson's disease *appear* when a person stuck in pause mode can no longer summon up an adequate, self-convincing level of mental emergency, a level strong enough to fully activate the override.

Four ways to get stuck on pause

The unhealthy, *long-term* use (stopping only during sleep – maybe) of pause mode can be activated in four different ways. The *type* of mental event or injury that triggered the long-term use of this mode determines which therapy needs to be used to turn it off.

Two of the therapies involve altering some mental habits. Two of the therapies are physical and directed at old injuries. When, via these therapies, the electrical flow patterns of pause mode turn off, the currents automatically revert back to healthy flow patterns.

All of my hundreds of patients with Parkinson's disease had used one or *more* of the four triggers that activate pause mode.

People with Parkinson's completely recover after using the appropriate method to successfully turn off the electrical currents typical of pause mode.

One of the channel qi alterations seen during pause mode – and in Parkinson's

The following is a brief example of how one of the several pause-related circuitry shifts relates to symptoms of Parkinson's. In Chinese medical theory, each of the twelve "Primary" channels that flow just under the skin is named in honor of one of the organs. One of them, the Stomach channel, usually runs *from* the head *to* the toes.

When pause mode is activated, the Stomach channel qi flows *backwards*, from acupoint ST-42 on the foot up to ST-6 on the jaw.

Underlying muscles become rigid if the channel qi running over their surface is moving backwards.

In pause mode and in Parkinson's, the span from ST-42 up to ST-6 is one of the body sections along which muscles become rigid, pulling the neck and front torso forward, causing the back to hunch, and tightening the muscles on the sides of the legs: part of the muscle behaviors that create the characteristic Parkinson's posture.

When running backwards, the Stomach channel qi does *not* flow up to the center forehead. Instead, it flows from ST-6, on the jaw, up alongside the ear to ST-8, at the hairline, and then towards the back of the head. (See Fig. 1.2, page 5.)

If the Stomach channel qi runs backwards all the way up to the jaw, *no* backwards channel qi traverses the face portion of the Stomach channel.

When the Stomach channel qi runs *backwards*, there is no channel qi flowing between ST-42, at the center of the foot, to ST-45, at the tip of the 2nd and 3rd toes. An *absence* of channel qi makes the underlying muscles become numb, cold, and/or limp. An *absence* of channel qi somewhere can allow the growth of fungus in the affected skin and nails at that spot.

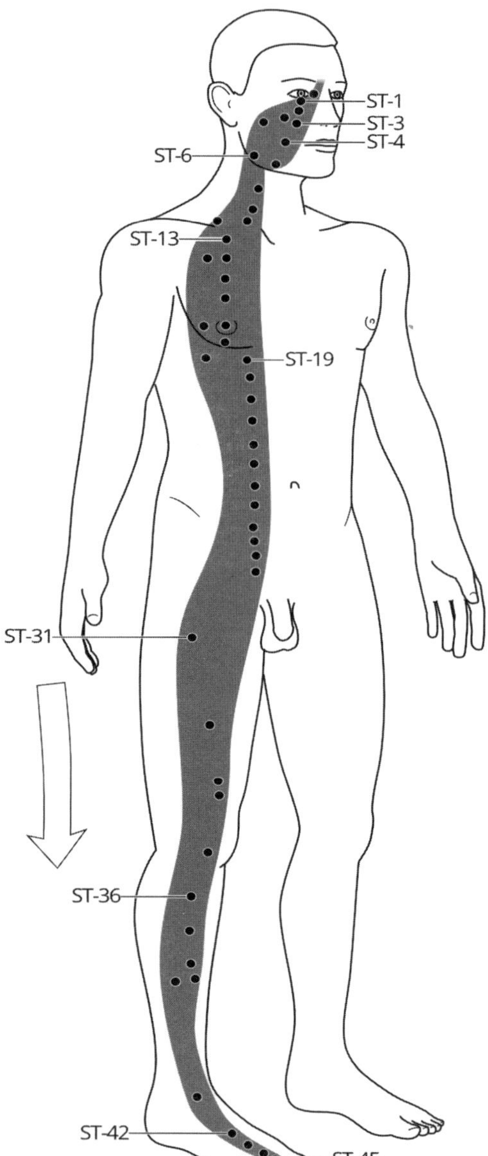

Fig. 1.1 The healthy, parasympathetic mode flow of the Stomach channel
Please note: All of the Primary channels (channels named in honor of organs, such as the Stomach channel) have symmetrical left- and right-side paths. In this book, the artwork shows all the Primary channels on one side of the body only, for a less cluttered look.

In people with Parkinson's, the *absence* of channel qi in the span from ST-1 to ST-6 on the face and from ST-42 to ST-45 on the foot causes the characteristic numbness and muscle limpness – *not* rigidity – that you might see in these areas.

The absence of channel qi on the face can contribute to the seborrhea (fungal growth in the skin) alongside the nose that is not uncommon in Parkinson's.

The absence of channel qi in the 2nd and 3rd toes contributes to the severe toenail fungus often seen in those toes, and sometimes in the first (the "big") toe, in people with Parkinson's.

In Parkinson's disease, people develop specific areas of muscle rigidity and *other* specific areas of limp, numb, or atrophied muscles. These areas correspond perfectly to the areas in which channel qi either flows backwards or is absent, respectively, during pause mode.

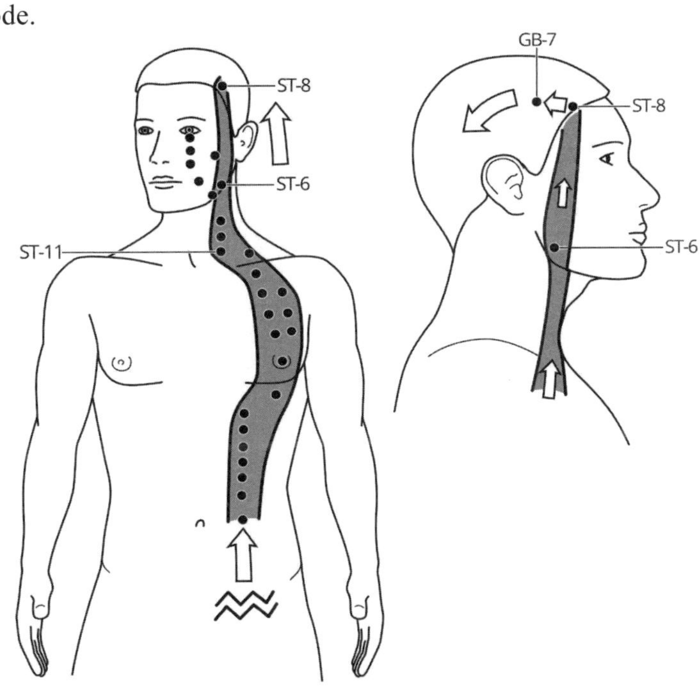

Fig.1.2 During pause, Stomach channel qi flows backwards and up to ST-6. When the channel qi arrives at ST-6, it is shunted up to ST-8 and then flows into the Gallbladder channel.

Compare the amount of energy flowing over the cheeks in Fig. 1.1 on the previous page and in Fig. 1.2 above. The absence of energy moving over the cheeks causes the expressionless "mask" face that can contribute to the characteristic look of Parkinson's disease.

When the electrical patterns of pause turn off, people recover from Parkinson's. Parasympathetic mode flow of channel qi resumes. The rigid muscles become soft. The inactive or atrophied muscles slowly resume tone.

When pause turns off, the toenail fungus and facial seborrhea, if any, very often clear up on their own over the course of six months to a year.

The above short section on the Stomach channel qi changes that occur during pause mode serves as the merest of introductions to the relevant Chinese channel theory and its relationship to PD that you'll get in this book. Other channels that are altered during pause – alterations that explain other symptoms of PD – are introduced in later chapters. [1]

The norepinephrine override

In the decades before Parkinson's symptoms appear, a person on pause is able to move around seemingly normally, or with even *more* strength and/or stamina than most people. How is this possible? This question takes us back to western medicine.

When a person or animal is on a high degree of pause, his release of brain-based dopamine for motor function *and* his release of adrenaline from the adrenal glands, located next to the kidneys, are both highly inhibited. He is nearly motionless.

However, if an animal or person on pause is still conscious and *needs* to move for some reason of extreme emergency such as the injuring predator now moving towards the victim's helpless offspring, the injured animal or person *will* be able to activate hyper-powerful emergency motor function. This motor function is very likely activated with norepinephrine. [2]

---

[1] New information is just starting to pour in from western medicine researchers on the subject of channel qi, or as they call it, "non-neural bioelectricity." "Non-neural" means not related to nerves or neurons.

A major researcher in the field, Dr. Michael Levin, professor at Tufts University and a visiting scholar at Harvard, has released on the internet an excellent video on his findings. He has bachelor's degrees in computer science and biology, a PhD in cell biology, and is a licensed acupuncturist. He refers to this non-neural bioelectricity, what the Chinese call "channel qi," as "the software of life." He explains that we can manipulate this physiological software layer. He defines this non-neural bioelectricity as "slow, steady ion fluxes, electric fields, and voltage gradients generated and sensed by all cell types." He goes on to explain, "This is not the rapid action potentials in classical excitable cells [nerve cells] nor effects of environmental electromagnetic exposure." He also says, "People might say that the cells are the hardware and the DNA is the software. But actually, the DNA only specifies the types of hardware, the types of components you might have. Bioelectric decision making [*which* components the DNA makes and how your cells use them] runs on the real-time physics [of bioelectric influences]...

He also mentions, "All these electrical processes disappear when the cell [or the animal] dies." This answers questions raised by the many western researchers who have failed to find evidence of channel qi in their cadaver explorations.

https://oshercenter.org/oc-event/grand-rounds-endogenous-bioelectric-networks-regenerative-medicine/

[2] "Norepinephrine loss produces more profound motor deficits than MPTP treatment in mice"; K.S. Rommelfanger, G.L. Edwards, K.G. Freeman, et al; *Proceedings of the National Academy of Sciences of the United States of America*; 2007 Aug 21; 104(34):13804-13809. Published online: 2007 Aug 16. Doi: 10.1073/pnas.0702753104.

In this study, mice brains' dopamine receptors were chemically inhibited using MPTP, a synthetic opioid. Instead of exhibiting the expected Parkinson's-like behaviors, the mice still had what appeared to be normal motor function. Only after the norepinephrine receptors were then chemically inhibited did the mice show the "poverty of movement" (extreme slowness and stiffness) also seen in people with Parkinson's disease.

More about norepinephrine: norepinephrine and adrenaline are structurally related. In the blood stream, norepinephrine, a neurotransmitter, is released continuously from certain nerves at low levels to maintain blood pressure, among other jobs. Adrenaline, the "fight or flight chemical,"

In nearly all of my PD patients, their symptoms began to appear when some life challenge that had long been consciously applied as a mental spur was finally laid to rest: the youngest child finished college; the mortgage was paid off; the predatory uncle died. With their fear motivator gone, they could no longer sustain a norepinephrine override strong enough to override the movement inhibitions of pause mode.

The reason their Parkinson's symptoms appeared is *not* that their dopamine levels had dropped. We now know that people have more than enough dopamine at the time they are first diagnosed with Parkinson's. The research supporting this statement is discussed in chapter three.

People with Parkinson's haven't *used* dopamine for motor function for decades – sometimes since childhood. When they recover, most of them are shocked and a bit giddy because of how utterly foreign it feels to use spontaneous (usually called "automatic") dopamine-based movement as opposed to the conscious (you might say "word-based" or "mental command-based"), norepinephrine-driven movement that they have used for decades – ever since their sub-dermal electrical currents started flowing in the pause patterns.

For example, one recovered patient recalled how, at age seven, a classmate asked her how she was able to run so fast. She had replied, "I tell my arms to move back and forth as fast as they can, and the legs have to follow at that speed."

Some forty years later, when she recovered from Parkinson's, this habitually stoic woman told me how she burst into tears the first time her body used dopamine-based movement to get up from the sofa. Her tremor had already mostly stopped some days earlier. She was sitting on the sofa when she had the thought, "I should go into the kitchen," and the next thing she knew she was standing up and moving towards the kitchen *without* having mentally instructed herself to stand up.

Sobbing, overwhelmed with relief and self-pity, she had exclaimed to the empty living room, "Is *this* how *easy* it's always been for everyone else?"

Based on patients' amazed reactions to using dopamine after turning off pause, it seems *very* probable that most of my patients with Type I Parkinson's have long used some alternative, non-dopamine neurotransmitter system for motor function. People with Type II and Type III Parkinson's have usually not been as surprised by the sensations that arise when they resume using dopamine for motor function.

---

is released from the adrenal glands, right next to the kidneys, during times of stress. Adrenaline increases heart rate and opens the bronchia (windpipes). Norepinephrine in the *body* maintains blood pressure. In the *brain*, norepinephrine increases alertness and wariness, sharply focuses attention, and can increase restlessness and anxiety: attributes of the medically recognized Parkinson's personality.

Neurotransmitters do not easily cross the selective, semi-permeable membrane known as the blood-brain barrier. The body supply and the brain supply of neurotransmitters are kept apart unless the bloodstream levels are *extremely*, unnaturally high, or there is a health problem affecting the integrity of the blood-brain barrier.

Brain-based norepinephrine and dopamine are produced and used in the brain. Blood-based norepinephrine and dopamine are produced and used throughout the body, and are kept *out* of the brain by the blood-brain barrier.

The four types of PD are detailed in the next chapter, but before discussing those four types we need to go through a bit more background and introduce some new vocabulary.

In the early years of my research, I wrongly assumed the neurotransmitter that people used instead of dopamine was adrenaline. That assumption was based on my use of the western medical hypothesis that there are only two neurological modes.

But during recovery, after turning off pause, some of my patients had to relearn how to activate their adrenal glands. The rush of adrenaline felt just as foreign ("Scary!" "Animal-like!") as did the use of dopamine.

Based on research studies such as the one with mice that was footnoted on page 6, I hypothesize that the brain's norepinephrine system is what my patients had been using for command-type motor function during all the years that they were stuck on pause.

Based on what I've heard from my PD patients, norepinephrine, if that's what they were using, enables a person to not only keep moving, but moving with abnormally heightened motor function. Many of my PD patients had been top athletes or ace pilots or captains of industry – roles that required an almost super-human ability to always be tireless, as well as stronger, smarter, and faster than everyone around them: emergency behavior. This doesn't apply to *all* my patients, but certainly a large majority.

During the pre-Parkinson's years, if a person who is stuck on pause can summon up a *constant* sense of emergency or intensity of purpose, he will be able to have what appears to be fairly normal or even *superior* motor function in spite of being on pause. However, this type of motor function is triggered by a mental-command process, a process very different from "automatic" or unself-conscious, dopamine-based movement.

Most healthy people are always using a blend of two types of movement: dopamine-driven and adrenaline/ norepinephrine-driven. At any given moment, the ratio of the blend depends on how relaxed or how uneasy they are.

I hypothesize, based on patient histories, that eventually, when the ability to concoct and sustain a mental sense of constant emergency *diminishes*, the ability to mentally activate the emergency norepinephrine override for pause also declines. *That's* when the long-hidden, pause-like symptoms that we call Parkinson's begin to manifest.

Adding to this hypothesis, people with Parkinson's, even those who are nearly immobile with *advanced* Parkinson's, can move perfectly normally during a true emergency. When fire is racing through the house, the vigorous norepinephrine override kicks in: emergency motor function is possible until the sense of emergency is over. (An exception: people who have brain damage from antiparkinson's medications might *not* be able to move normally during an emergency.)

Dopamine is present in the brains of people with PD in high enough quantities until the PD becomes quite advanced. In fact, even in people with advanced Parkinson's, dopamine levels are *higher* than normal in the right anterior cingulate part of the brain, an area used for risk-assessment, among other things. Dopamine use for *motor* function is inhibited during pause and during Parkinson's. Dopamine use for risk assessment is *increased* during pause and during Parkinson's. [1]

---

[1] "Personality traits and brain dopaminergic function in Parkinson's disease"; *Proceedings of the National Academy of Sciences USA* 98:13272-7*;* Valtteri Kaasinen, MD, PhD et al; 2001. This 2001 study, published in one of the most respected journals in American science, describes the

Clarification on the word "shock"

Some people refer to the near-death condition as "shock." I don't use the word shock much in this book because it has too many vague meanings. In the context of pause mode, the word "shock," if used, does *not* refer to surprise, fear, or the type of "shock" associated with post-traumatic stress disorder. Post-traumatic stress disorder occurs when a person is stuck in *sympathetic* mode, also known as "fight or flight" mode.

The normal sequence of steps for turning off near-death mode

1) When an otherwise healthy person's body has physically stabilized following a near-death trauma, when the likelihood of death is no longer *imminent* (meaning in the next *few minutes*), the body begins taking steps to turn off pause. When the *interior,* physiological functions of the body have stabilized, the body might begin to tremor, either visibly or internally.

A specific type of tremor can be a normal part of the process for coming out of pause mode. The tremoring performed while coming out of pause seems to serve as a query directed to the brain: "Hey brain! Internally, I'm on the verge of coming back to life! So tell me, is the coast clear?" or "Is it safe enough out there for me to come back to life?, to come out of the almost-paralysis of near-death trauma?"

2) The brain, using input from eyes, ears, smell, and touch, engages the risk assessment area of the brain to determine if the vicinity *outside* of the body is now safe, or at least safe enough to come out of the near-death mode.

When the *interior* of the body *and* the immediate vicinity *outside* of the body both seem stable and safe enough, the body will then perform three physical moves that turn off this mode and re-start the usual blend of the two more normal awake-time modes: sympathetic (fight or flight) and parasympathetic (curious and playful) modes. The moves include

3) taking a slow, deep, *audible* breath,

4) gently bobbling the head left and right at the very top of the neck, and then

5) allowing a shimmy to travel down the spine.

Five steps in all.

The latter two moves restart the vagus nerves and spinal nerves, respectively. This reinstitutes the normal, waking-hours blend of parasympathetic and sympathetic mode channel qi circuitries, which then trigger the release of neurotransmitters, thought patterns, and cellular and organ behaviors appropriate for these modes. The person's body resumes somatic awareness. "Somatic" refers to sensations inside the body, including *awareness* of being inside one's body. The physiological behaviors of pause mode then cease.

This five-step sequence for turning off pause mode is *not* all that unusual. You might have seen a dog do it, after being badly startled. You might have done it yourself.

A common example of turning off pause

If you have ever found yourself shaking or trembling after a swim in an icy mountain lake (which triggers a blend of pause and sympathetic modes) or following on the heels of some intense, pause-inducing trauma, you might recall this sequence as you

---

utterly unexpected discovery that people with Parkinson's have *elevated* levels of dopamine activity in the brain's anterior cingulate area, an area that manages risk assessment.

started to realize that you were warming back up or calming down, respectively. Your mind had an abrupt realization such as, "I don't *need* to be shaking anymore," and/or maybe "Hey, I'm gonna be OK, after all": some thought synonymous with "I'm safe!" or "The coast is clear!"

This thought is followed by a deep, audible breath like a sigh of relief, a subtle head wobble, and a shimmy or shiver up or down the spine that almost feels like hitting an internal reset button. This sequence might be familiar to you...if you don't have Parkinson's.

Most of the people I've casually asked about this sequence do recall performing it in response to the brief tremoring or shaking that might follow a trauma, severe chill, or full-body anesthesia. But most of my Parkinson's (PD) patients had no idea what I was talking about when I described the basic sequence for coming out of pause. Many even felt that it should be *impossible* for the brain *ever* to think that it's safe enough to come out of pause, a mode characterized by wariness and heightened risk assessment.

As so many of my PD patients put it, "Only an *idiot* could ever think he was *safe*."

People with Parkinson's, for various reasons, have become *stuck* in the electrical patterns of a neurological mode that can only be turned off when 1) the internal biological threat from the trauma has stabilized *and* 2) the person is willing and able to once again feel safe, or at least safe enough to turn off this mode.

My patients with Parkinson's either a) had an unhealed injury (most often at the foot or head) causing pause-like electrical flow *or* b) had *told* themselves to dissociate from a still unhealed injury *or* c) had gotten stuck on pause following a severe trauma and never healed fully enough to come out of pause *or* d) they gave themselves a pause-inducing command – often in childhood, often while staring into a mirror – a command something along the lines of "Feel no pain."

The body *does* have a neurological mode in which it is numb to several kinds of physical and emotional pain: pause mode – the mode associated with near-death trauma and coma. When a person using great mental focus and grim determination commands himself to feel no pain, his brain might very well obey. It might shift into the near-death neurological mode of relative numbness…and stay there.

I refer to pause mode that is triggered in *this* fashion as "self-induced pause."

PD from self-induced pause is by far the most common of the four types of Parkinson's disease, presenting in nearly ninety-five percent of my PD patients. I've named it Type I Parkinson's disease.

Many people with Type I Parkinson's do recall giving themselves some such command. Many who do *not recall* doing this nevertheless say that they embrace numbness, or something like "going into a dead place inside," or "a grey place" as their way of dealing with unpleasantness or negative emotions.

Type I Parkinson's has behavioral patterns not seen in the other types of PD. So even if a person with Type I PD doesn't *recall* any sort of self-instruction, this type is fairly easy to distinguish. This book has instructions for diagnosing the four types.

Whether or not a person *remembers* instructing himself to become numb or some other command that inadvertently induced pause mode, *if* this command is in place, the person will *not* be able to terminate the use of this mode until he changes some pause-related mental habits.

Again: in addition to Type I PD *self*-activation of pause mode, there are three other far less commonly used activation methods that can inadvertently lead to getting stuck with pause-like electrical patterns. As mentioned earlier, there are four ways to get *stuck* in the electrical patterns of near-death mode, and four ways to turn them off.

So if you or a loved one have been diagnosed with Parkinson's disease and are *not* taking dopamine-enhancing medications, be of good cheer. It is *not* an incurable illness.

Addendum to Chapter One

Please note: Before going any further, I want to make clear two things:

First, drug-induced and toxin-induced parkinson*ism* is not the same thing as Parkinson's disease. These two parkinson*ism* conditions have *some* symptoms in common with idiopathic Parkinson's, but they are recognized as being completely different disorders with different underlying causes. In cases of drug- or toxin-induced parkinson*ism*, the symptoms are the result of physical damage to brain cells. The treatments described in this book are not effective against drug- or toxin-induced parkinson*ism*. You will learn how to diagnose these "ism" syndromes in chapter fifteen.

Some MDs, if uncertain of a patient's diagnosis because the symptoms are still mild, will diagnose the patient as having "parkinsonism" rather than giving the more alarming but more accurate diagnosis of Parkinson's disease. This is a shame, because the incorrect diagnosis might cause a person with early-stage PD to delay treatment. The sooner a person with Parkinson's begins working on turning off pause, the easier it is. For the most common type of Parkinson's disease, Type I PD, the wary thought patterns triggered by the unceasing use of pause mode steadily increase. This in turn, fortifies the other mental behaviors that sustain pause and can make it increasingly harder to turn it off. This also contributes to the steady worsening of the symptoms of Parkinson's disease. The sooner the treatment begins, the easier it is to recover.

This book will explain how to make an earlier and far more accurate diagnosis for Parkinson's disease than is currently taught in western medical schools.

Also, Parkinson's disease is sometimes called "idiopathic Parkinson's disease." The two names mean the same thing. The word "idiopathic" means "cause unknown."

Second, modalities of Chinese medicine such as acupuncture, Chinese herbs, and moxa (smoking mugwort leaves) are *not* used in the treatment of Parkinson's disease. I'll discuss this more, later, but I want to mention this nice and early, before you rush off in search of the nearest acupuncturist in response to my references to Chinese medicine.

Your acupuncturist probably won't know anything about pause mode. We do *not* learn about pause mode in schools of Chinese medicine.

More than ten years into my Parkinson's research, I stumbled across this neurological mode in an English translation of one of the most important ancient tomes of Chinese medical theory, the *Huang Ti Nei Jing*.

The only reason I understood immediately what the garbled language was discussing was that it answered so many of the questions I had accumulated in my years of researching Parkinson's. I had acquired a *lot* of questions.[1]

---

[1] Here's an example of what I mean by "garbled language," followed by my translation using a more contemporary English. "Change of colors corresponds to pulses of the four seasons, which is valued by gods because it is in tune with the divine being and which enables us to flee

from death and stay close [cling] to life." That's from the *Su Wen*, chapter 13-9, from *A Complete Translation of the Yellow Emperor's Classics of Internal Medicine and the Difficult Classic*; Henry C. Lu, PhD; published by the International College of Traditional Chinese Medicine; Vancouver, BC, Canada; 2004; p. 116.

The word "colors" in the above quote is a very loose – and incorrect – translation from the Chinese characters for *Se Mai*, literally "pathways of light" or "currents of energy derived from lightwaves," or "energy from light waves" (electricity) and is a reference to channel qi, but is often incompletely translated into English simply as "colors."

The word translated as "pulses" in the above can also mean "rhythms" or "patterns." The word translated here as "seasons" is usually translated as "phases." However *if* preceded by the number four, it is often a reference to "the four seasons." In our case, it's a reference to the four neurological phases, or modes. The translator clearly doesn't know that.

A quick translation into medical English would read, "Changes in the electrical paths of the channel qi correspond to the physiological behaviors of the four modes. The first mode, parasympathetic, is 'in tune with the Divine being' [joy and ease]. The second, sympathetic, enables us to 'flee from death' [fight or flight]. [The third mode is not listed in this sentence, but it corresponds to sleep mode.] The fourth, pause mode, allows one to 'cling to life' while hovering on the edge of death."

The English- and Chinese-speaking practitioners of Chinese medicine that I've spoken to have had no idea that this section of the *Huang Ti Nei Jing* is discussing neurological modes because, since the mid-twentieth century, channel theory is no longer taught in schools of Chinese medicine. Current students and scholars alike no longer have a basis for translating this section. They have usually guessed that this sentence from the thousand-plus-years old medical tome is a random interjection about natural history, something along the lines of "Plants change color during the course of the four seasons."

The rest of the chapter that follows this introductory sentence makes no medical sense if this chapter is about leaves changing colors in the fall. The rest of the chapter makes stunning good sense if one recognizes from hands-on experience that the channel qi does flow differently in each of the four neurological modes.

Since the communist revolution in China, channel qi is regarded as an historical superstition, similar to religion and classical references to the Divine. Teaching channel qi as a medical reality has been illegal in China for more than half a century. You could be jailed for it: "sent to camp." For this reason, most acupucturists today are not taught about channel qi or how to feel it: the original essence of this field of medicine. This ban has led to some truly bizarre translations of the old medical books into modern, atheistic Chinese and thence into English. The political reasons for this legal ban are discussed in depth in some of my other books, including *Hacking Chinese Medicine* and *Tracking the Dragon*.

As with much of the classical Chinese literature, one needs to already know what is being discussed in order for the cryptic, terse language to be intelligible. The ancient medical writings were never meant as explicit guides for the general public. Rather, they were insider, very often metaphorical, references to a primarily oral, closely guarded tradition.

The modern English term "meridians" is sometimes used in place of the word "channels." The word "meridians" means "imaginary lines": lines used as a construct to help organize information. The channels are not imaginary. However, the use of the word meridian is in line with the modern Chinese political stance that channels do not actually exist.

Not only are the modalities of Chinese medicine not helpful in treating Parkinson's, professional help of *any* type is usually not necessary.

Acupuncture treatments by someone unclear on channel theory can accelerate the worsening of Parkinson's symptoms. Acupuncture treatments might temporarily calm the tremor, but over the course of months, the symptoms will worsen faster than the symptoms of a person with PD who does *not* receive acupuncture treatment. This was the finding of Dr. Ming Qing Zhu, the late, very famous Chinese neurology-specialist acupuncturist who developed the art of scalp acupuncture – with whom I once shared an office when he worked, briefly, in the late 1990s, in affiliation with Five Branches college of traditional Chinese medicine in Santa Cruz, California. For decades, in China, he had worked with hundreds of people with Parkinson's, and found that those who received acupuncture treatments experienced temporary relief and, over time, faster worsening of symptoms than those who simply let the syndrome follow its natural course.

In China, most people cannot afford to take antiparkinson's medications. This allowed Dr. Zhu to observe the natural progression of Parkinson's in people who *weren't* taking dopamine-enhancing drugs – something most American doctors never get a chance to see. After seeing the results that my patients were getting, he stopped working with people with Parkinson's and referred them to the clinic that I conducted up until 2003.

The following paragraph is intended for practitioners of Chinese medicine. It's included for that majority of acupuncturists who have not received much training in channel theory. Everyone else can skip the following paragraph.

Using the terminology of Chinese medicine, pause mode is an Excess condition. We never Tonify (strengthen) an Excess condition. Acupoints that purportedly "drain an Excess" do not actually reduce the amount of channel qi in the system, they merely break up some electrical blockage or area of high electrical resistance allowing for the dispersal of accumulated of channel qi, allowing the channel qi to resume flowing in its correct path. In the case of a person on pause mode, the insertion of needles will help the channel qi move better in its backwards direction – *increasing* the electrical signals of pause mode. Please don't do this.

If you have Parkinson's disease, please don't rush out to find an acupuncturist. Or a therapist. Recovering from Parkinson's is pretty much a do-it-yourself or a do-it-with-a-friend project.

This book will explain how to do it.

Chapter Two

Pressing Questions

The most pressing question for many people is: How long will it take for me or for my loved one to recover? The answer is, it varies. You'll have to learn what all the variables are and then see where your own case fits in. The most important variable is what type of Parkinson's a person has. So this chapter will start with that.

Then again, my readers who are doctors of any type of medicine usually have completely different questions: Can your hypotheses be proven? How can I help my own patients with Parkinson's? and How dare you give my patients false hope?

I'll try to answer as many questions as I can for all types of readers.

Four ways to develop idiopathic Parkinson's disease

I have found four reasons that people get stuck in the electrical configurations that are characteristic of pause mode. Of course, there might be more. I've numbered them in order of how common they have been in my experience.

Type I: self-induced pause.
Type II: being *stuck* in pause-like channel qi patterns due to unhealed or incompletely healed injury, surgery, or other tissue damaging events. Most often, these pause-like channel patterns are the result of a foot or ankle injury from which one has subconsciously dissociated – hence the incomplete healing. However, the pause-like channel patterns can also arise from surgery, spider and/or snake bites, severe burns, or any type of event that causes obstruction along the Stomach channels or the Du channel and then fails to completely heal.
Type III: self-induced dissociation from an injury or trauma, so that the injury ends up causing a pause-like flow of channel energy. This is different from Type II because of the mental component: the person *told* himself to not feel the specific injury.
Type IV: being *stuck* in normal, biological pause from a life-threatening injury that triggered pause but, for whatever reason, pause never got turned off. The syndrome referred to as "head-injury parkinsonism" is a form of Type IV PD.

Type I PD: self-induced pause

This type of pause is usually set in motion via a self-command, often given in childhood, to "feel no pain," "be spiritual: rise above pain," "I am not a part of this painful world" or some similar instruction commanding that one distance oneself from physical or emotional pain or trauma. The command was *not* a casual remark. A high level of intensity and determination was employed. As mentioned earlier, it was often performed while staring into a mirror. The instruction is often unremembered until *after* pause is turned off.

This type is by far the most common. Nearly ninety-five percent of my hundreds of PD patients had this type of Parkinson's disease.

This type does *not* respond to the five basic steps that turn off *normal*, or what you can call "biological", pause. A completely different set of techniques is involved in turning off self-induced pause. I repeat: Type I PD does *not* respond to the five basic steps. For that matter, most people on self-induced pause are not able to make themselves convincingly perform the last two steps: wobble the neck and let a shiver roll down the spine. Their brain will usually fight against or not *allow* these pause-ending movements to take place.

Recovery from Type I PD usually takes longer than recovery from the other three types. The time frame for recovery from this type ranges from a few hours to many years. Most people in my experience have needed a year or more.

The length of time is related to the degree to which a person has developed a steady habit of using a fear- or anxiety-based internal monologue and/or cultivated a habit of imagining himself to be separate from the rest of humanity, or even all alone in the universe. In general, the more a person has embraced pause-driven wary and/or judgmental thinking, the longer it might take him or her to recover.

I'll go into details about this type in later chapters, but first I want to give a quick overview of the other types. (If you notice that percentages vary slightly from previous editions of this book, it's because I've seen more patients since then.)

Type II PD: pause-like channel qi flow due to blockage in the Stomach and/or Du channels, also known as "pseudo pause"

This is the second most common cause for Parkinson's. People with this pattern have usually dissociated from a foot or ankle injury. The dissociation was *not* consciously activated. Instead, the normal, healthy dissociation that can occur *automatically*, subconsciously, in response to a significant injury, has never turned off. This type of automatic dissociation is supposed to automatically turn off when an injured person or animal finds itself in a safe place. In some people, the dissociation never turns off. This prevents complete healing of the injury or trauma.

An example of this automatic, healthy dissociation behavior, held in place until safety is attained, might be demonstrated by a small child or toddler who hurts himself and then wanders through the house looking for his mother or some other source of comfort. As soon as he sees someone who can help him, someone he trusts, he bursts into tears.

The mother or comforter might say, "It couldn't have been too bad; you didn't even start crying until you found me."

This statement reflects a lack of understanding. The injury might have been significant, but until the child knows that he is safe, he will be able to do what he needs to do – quietly look for mom or some other source of comfort and safety – with minimum awareness (automatic dissociation) of the pain.

I have seen more than a hundred *non*-Parkinson's patients who are still dissociated from some old injury or surgery: this inadvertent retention of automatic dissociation is a common reason for a chronic pain from injury, pain that doesn't respond to treatment, a "failure to heal" or, in the case of broken bones, "failure to knit."

In many cases, as soon as the patient's subconscious mind is brought to dwell on and re-associate with the problem area, the area begins to heal. Very often, when the long-sustained micro-muscle tension in the area finally loosens up in response to physical support and mental focus, the deep, *full* healing begins. Even if the injury was decades in the past, the injured area might not manifest its long-repressed swelling and/or bruising until the person turns his attention on it while mentally affirming that the area is, in fact, safe. Only then might the pain and damage become apparent.

Because of the specific electrical circuitries in the foot and ankle, a long-unhealed injury or an electrical blockage from scar tissue (which is non-conductive) in this area can cause the electrical disarray from the injury to grow larger over time. Eventually the disarray can create so much resistance in the foot that an electrical current – usually the Stomach channel current – begins to flow *backwards*, just as it does during pause.

This type of channel behavior can also be set in motion by just about anything that blocks the Stomach channel – not just accidental injuries. Surgeries that can cause this type of blockage range from surgeries on the leg (including knee, ankle, and foot), the groin (usually for hernia), appendectomies, C-sections, or even liposuction. If the surgery causes scarring, either visible on the skin *or* hidden under the skin (usually from laparoscopic damage) that blocks the flow of the Stomach channel, the channel qi can eventually start to get backed up and then set in motion the various channel qi and muscle behaviors that ordinarily should only occur during pause.

Other traumas that can block the Stomach channel include spider and snake bites. Usually, these types of bites will heal up on their own. However, if a person has multiple areas along the Stomach channel that are already almost blocked due to injury or surgery, the snake or spider bite might *not* flush out correctly. For example, if a person has an unhealed broken toe and still-displaced metatarsal bones from an old foot injury, a subsequent "insult" (either a bite, a surgery, or yet another injury) in the vicinity might not be able to heal correctly. The cumulative assortment of insults along the Stomach channel might eventually lead to complete blockage of the Stomach channel, setting in motion backwards, pause-type electrical flow.

Over time, usually decades, the domino effect of channel disturbances from unhealed injury(s) sets in motion electrical behaviors – and therefore physical symptoms – that are nearly indistinguishable from those caused by chronic use of pause mode.

In these types of cases the body might present *physical* symptoms similar to those of a person who is stuck on pause. However, the mental behaviors and brain functions in these cases might not be altered in the same way or to the same degree as in people who are locked into a near-death or want-to-be-numb mental posture. The pause-*like* channel qi behaviors and symptoms that are the result of unhealed injury, surgery, or other physical traumas, traumas that do *not* include the consciousness or sub-consciousness of impending death, can be referred to as "pseudo" pause.

Spontaneous recovery from Parkinson's

Type II PD is the type of Parkinson's disease that might spontaneously, permanently disappear in response to Qi Gong or other mental and/or movement disciplines in which mental focus is used to direct energy throughout the body – even to areas that might unknowingly have long been dissociated.

When you read online about people whose Parkinson's went away in response to Qi Gong, visualizations, positive affirmations, or hands-on physical support therapies, these recoveries most likely occurred in people who *only* had Type II PD.

People with only Type II tend to turn off the Parkinson's behaviors fairly quickly, in a matter of a few weeks or a few months, in response to appropriate treatment.

This type of Parkinson's is the second most common. I have seen *only* Type II PD in nearly five percent of my patients.

The one-two combination

I have seen Type II *combined* with Type I in nearly ninety percent of my patients.

This combination, I hypothesize, might be so common because if a person is stuck on pause, whether the biological type or self-induced, most subsequent injuries will be dealt with via dissociation until such time as pause turns off.

To understand this, consider an animal that is on pause and appearing nearly lifeless due to some sort of attack. The animal should *not* be responsive to ongoing *or* subsequent injury or pain. Being responsive might cause the animal to give itself away to, or re-excite, a nearby predator. An animal on pause automatically dissociates from its injuries until 1) it turns off pause and then 2) gets to a safe place.

After pause turns off *and* the animal gets to a safe place, it will automatically become painfully aware of, you could say re-associated with, its injuries. Once in a safe place, the animal might tend to its injuries by licking or scratching them, coddling them, or allowing another animal to lick them. A human, when safe, might seek suitable comfort and treatment.

Being *stuck* on pause can cause a person to *stay* dissociated from his subsequent injuries. Add to this that nearly everyone bangs a foot at one time or another: as the old joke has it, "The function of the little toe is to make sure that the furniture is in the right place."

Also, some patients have recalled giving themselves the original pause-inducing instruction to feel no pain in direct response to a painful foot or ankle injury. So an injury might stay unhealed either because the person was *already* on pause *or* because the person *responded* to the injury by commanding himself to feel no pain: to go into self-induced pause.

As an aside, due to the layout of the foot bones, the bone most likely to be displaced during any ankle or foot injury is the intermediate cuneiform, right in the center of the foot, just under acupoint ST-42. This is the bone most often displaced in my Parkinson's patients with a foot injury component. ST-42 is also the foot location from which current flows backwards when a person is on pause. Therefore, finding dissociated, unhealed injuries – most often in the foot or ankle – contributing to the pause schematics in a person who also has self-induced pause is *not* surprising. [1]

---

[1] The word "schematics" refers to a generalized design or purpose for an electrical configuration. The word "circuit" refers to the exact flow path of a current. For example, in the human body, the general electrical schematic for the Stomach channel has current flowing from the forehead to the toes. The specific circuitry at any given moment depends on the exact biological needs of the moment. For example, in a high degree of parasympathetic mode, more current flows from mid-foot to the tip of the second toe. In a high degree of sympathetic mode, more current flows from mid-foot over to the medial side of the big toe. In a high degree of pause mode, the current doesn't flow to the toes at all: it flows backwards from the mid-foot.

When I use the word "schematics," I am referring to the *general* sense of where and why a given current is supposed to flow, as opposed to a *specific* circuit pattern being used by a specific person at a given moment.

Most of my patients with Type I PD also had Type II. In these cases, Type I is the deeper problem and **must** be dealt with first, before dealing with the foot or other injuries, in order to prevent the nightmare of partial recovery.

Partial recovery is *not* a good thing. Partial recovery is the name I use to describe the horrible condition that arises when a person who *used to* have a combination of Type I and Type II Parkinson's becomes stuck in the strange, very hard to treat mental limbo that can occur when the *physical* injuries that were contributing to Type II pause-mode circuitries have finally re-associated and then healed but the *mental* behaviors caused by Type I Parkinson's are still up and running. The mental distress, even psychosis, and the *rapidly* worsening PD symptoms that can be a part of partial recovery can be avoided by recovering from Type I PD *prior* to doing any sort of physical healing work on the injuries contributing to the Type II PD.

The phrase partial recovery only means that a person with two or more types of PD has recovered from one or more of them, but that Type I PD is still present and causing increased mental distress *because* of the physiological changes from the *healed* injury. These changes can include resumption of parasympathetic mode-type electrical circuitry in the immediate vicinity of the injury, even though the mindset is trying to keep the whole body in pause mode. While on pause, dissociated injuries are not *supposed* to re-associate, as all mental focus is supposed to be directed towards staying alive until the crisis is over. The word partial in this usage refers to one of the *types* of PD being gone. The word partial does *not* refer to symptoms of Parkinson's disease being partially gone.

Type III PD: self-induced dissociation from an injury

In some cases, a person has commanded himself to "ignore the injury," "pretend the injury never happened," or even, if it's, for example, a left foot injury, "I don't have a left foot." In these cases, the person commanded himself to not pay attention to the *specific* injury.

This is *very* different from a pause-inducing command in which a person tells himself to feel no physical or emotional pain, period. In self-induced dissociation from an injury, the person has commanded himself to no longer recognize a *specific* injury event or a *specific* body part.

I repeat: in self-induced *pause*, the person has commanded himself to be numb, period. The exact wording might vary, of course. Very often, the person did not use the word "numb" but instead used words like "rise above my feelings" or "be more spiritual: don't be affected by pain." But the intention was nevertheless to obtain a body-wide condition of being apart from the world, from the body, or impervious to physical and/or emotional pain.

In self-induced *dissociation*, the patient has only compartmentalized one or a few events or body parts away from normal consciousness.

I have seen self-induced dissociation from an injury in dozens of *non*-PD patients. I have seen it in one person with idiopathic Parkinson's disease.

He told me how twenty-five years earlier he had intentionally dissociated from a knee injury that wasn't healing up fast enough. He was in college at the time and "...couldn't be bothered with this pain," so he powerfully commanded himself to not feel his knee. After making this command several times over the course of one day, the pain abruptly ceased.

He gave a rueful chuckle, "I was so proud of myself."

Recovery from this type might take a few weeks longer than Type II because destroying the mental instruction for dissociation might take a week or two.

Type IV: stuck in biological pause.

Being stuck on pause mode is a *somewhat* uncommon condition for the general public, but over the years I have seen it in quite a few patients with chronic conditions. I share a sampling of these cases in my book *Stuck on Pause*. I have seen it in two people with idiopathic Parkinson's disease. Both had experienced *severe* blows to the head, blows strong enough to induce coma. In both cases, the blow had dislodged an articulation in the cranial bones – displacements that had not yet been corrected.

Neither of them had ever *commanded* themselves to be numb. Neither one had an unhealed foot injury. They both did have an unhealed cranial bone displacement.

Case study #1: normal, or "biological" pause

One of the two patients, twenty years before I met her, had experienced a severe concussion when a large armoire fell on her, hitting her on the side of the head and putting her into a three-day coma. After she regained consciousness, she quickly recovered her brilliant mental acuity. However, based on the pause-type flow of her subdermal electrical currents when I met her nearly twenty years later, her bio-electrics had *not* come out of the coma event.

Her PD symptoms had been slowly developing over the years. A few years before I met her, she had been diagnosed with idiopathic Parkinson's disease.

Although this is an introductory chapter, I will go into a few details regarding her case because they demonstrate how pause mode, even with *no* self-induced components, relates to causing Parkinson's disease. It also demonstrates how turning off pause also abruptly turns off the underlying *cause* of PD. Although the many PD symptoms caused by slow, long-term physical degradation in nerves and muscles might heal up gradually, the underlying *driver* of Parkinson's turns off instantly when the body stops using the electrical circuitry of pause.

When I met this patient, she had all the symptoms of idiopathic Parkinson's including rigidity in her arms and legs, cogwheeling in her wrists and ankles, poverty of movement (moved slowly, needed help getting out of a chair), micrographia, faint voice, the classic Parkinson's hunched posture, a blank facial expression that was worse on the right side of her face, and a slowly worsening pill-rolling tremor, also on the right side. She had never taken antiparkinson's medications.

I did an extensive intake history – more than an hour. I always did this with my new Parkinson's patients or with any patient that had what seemed like a complicated case. While asking about her medical history, I learned of her head injury.

Based on the head injury, I started her treatment by doing some craniosacral work on her head. Craniosacral therapy is a type of Yin Tui Na. Yin Tui Na is a generic Chinese term meaning firm, supportive holding. For people with Type II or Type IV Parkinson's,

Yin Tui Na can help people re-associate with and/or recover from any *physical* injuries that are keeping pause-type electrical patterns in place. [1]

I discovered that the edge of my patient's right-side parietal bone (on the upper side of the head) was jammed under her right temporal bone (the bone with the ear hole).

When I did the basic craniosacral protocol, one segment of which allows the parietal bones to move freely relative to the temporal bones and properly reposition themselves, she immediately – right there in my office – went through all the long-delayed behaviors that a person experiences when coming out of pause: the giddy realization that she was safe, the deep breath, the head bobble, the shimmy down the spine.

Many of her more acute Parkinson's symptoms were reduced within minutes. Some disappeared entirely. Her mood changed instantly.

Her very elderly mother, who had never been informed that her daughter had Parkinson's, was present at the therapy session in which the underlying cause of the Parkinson's stopped.

Her daughter, my patient, sprang to a sitting position on the side of the treatment table, exclaiming over and over, "I'm OK! I'm OK! Its *good*! Its so *good*!"

This gushing, radiant joy in a person who has just come out of a near-death experience can be absolutely normal – just ask any emergency room nurse.

As she was still exclaiming over how good everything was, her mother said to me, "Finally! She's smiling again. I've been telling her for years to put a smile on her face, but would she listen to me? No. I guess she'd rather smile for you than for me."

A few weeks after this session, her neurologist told her that not only had she been *mis*diagnosed with Parkinson's, but she must also have been neurotic for having *pretended* to have Parkinson's disease. Most of her colleagues at the university, who had previously been kind to her, were furious when she recovered. Most of them assumed that she had been pretending to have Parkinson's to be assured of receiving tenure, or other hostile accusations. She had to undergo an academic trial by her peers to determine if she could continue as a professor. The two sides were bitterly divided. She squeaked past, but for the rest of her years as a professor, many treated her with scorn. They could not believe that a person could recover from an officially incurable illness.

Hostile reactions to recovery

Many people have asked me why my recovered patients do not promote their stories far and wide. Their recovery stories often have bitter endings, filled with accusations and hostility. The potential "fame" from going public with recovery might be seen as just another reason that the person had pretended to have Parkinson's.

Except for the ones who never went back to a neurologist, every one of my patients who recovered was subsequently told by the neurologist that he or she had obviously been misdiagnosed or else had merely had "psychogenic parkinsonism."

---

[1] The book *Yin Tui Na: Hands-on Therapy for Traumatic Injury* is available for free download at PDrecovery.org. This book was originally written as a textbook for students at the acupuncture college where I teach. However, the book is completely accessible for a person with no medical background whatsoever. Yin Tui Na techniques are *extremely* simple to master. They have been described as "using your hands like a human Ace [elastic] bandage until the patient's injured area starts to relax."

"Psychogenic parkinsonism" is a syndrome that looks exactly like Parkinson's, but it often comes on suddenly, following a severe physical or emotional trauma, and then goes away when the severe shock ebbs. This is what extended use of pause mode looks like when a person *doesn't* use the norepinephrine override.

Because it eventually goes away by itself – as pause is supposed to do – in a fairly short time, a few days or a few months, the syndrome (collection of symptoms) of psychogenic parkinsonism is often dismissed by MDs as being a purely mental phenomenon and not related in any way to the presumed brain deficiencies of idiopathic Parkinson's. In fact, with the exception of the extremely rare Type IV PD, *all* cases of idiopathic Parkinson's disease are technically psychogenic, meaning that they have a significant mental component.

Some doctors who declared "misdiagnosis" when confronted with one of my recovered patients had then, because of *recovery* symptoms that can include severe, sudden onset of extreme softness and limpness in long-rigid muscles, whimsically changed the diagnosis to either multiple-system atrophy (MSA) or progressive supranuclear palsy (PSP) – two other movement disorders for which, like Parkinson's, there is no *conclusive* test other than autopsy. When the patient was fully recovered and was strong again, so that a diagnosis of MSA or PSP was no longer appropriate, a typical MD response was anger and accusations, a diagnosis of psychosis, or a conclusion that the patient had been pretending to have Parkinson's disease. [1]

According to current western medical theory that is based on the *long*-disproved late nineteenth-century idea that brain cells and brain behaviors cannot ever heal or even change, Parkinson's, being considered a brain disorder is, by definition, incurable.[2]

---

[1] In his book *Cured: The Life-Changing Science of Spontaneous Healing*, author Jeffery Rediger, MD, psychiatrist on the faculty at Harvard medical school, shares how doctors dismiss as "misdiagnosed" cases that include "spontaneous" (not medicine-driven) recovery from many incurable illnesses. The cases he cites include late stage pancreatic cancers, encroaching fibrous lung disease, late-stage lupus, and other "incurable" illnesses. The patients had excellent scans and bloodwork *proving* that they had their illnesses.

His point is not just that many people recover from all sorts of "incurable" illnesses. His point is that western medical doctors are trained to not believe that those recoveries are possible. In his book's examples of "spontaneous" recovery, each patient had rejected the western treatment option, treatment that only delays or suppresses the illness. Instead, the patients decided to change themselves. They experienced an epiphany, or a change in thinking, in diet, or in some other aspect of life – and recovered from the "incurable." In the introduction to his book, Rediger explains that "the very subject [of recovery from an incurable illness] is taboo in mainstream medicine." The only allowable response is "misdiagnosed." In cases of Parkinson's disease, where diagnosis is unprovable to begin with, the conclusion of misdiagnosis following a recovery is almost a given.

[2] Research over the last twenty years has shown that brain behaviors do change in response to usage or even create compensations in response to damage. As for the 19th century idea that one can never grow new brain cells, new research suggests that not only is the brain able to grow new cells (neurogenesis), but that "impaired neurogenesis might be a potentially relevant mechanism underlying memory deficits in Alzheimer's disease." This quote was taken from the article "Adult hippocampal neurogenesis is abundant in neurologically healthy subjects and drops sharply in patients with Alzheimer's disease"; *Nature Medicine*; March 25, 2019; www.nature.com/articles/s41591-019-0375-9. The point here is that constant growth of new brain

Getting back to the subject of Type IV PD, I have only seen two cases in which the patient was *biologically*, not mentally (self-induced), stuck on pause *and* was officially diagnosed with Parkinson's. They both recovered when as the cranial displacements and, in the second case, the other bone injuries and displacements were treated. In both cases, gentle, light-touch craniosacral therapy was used to treat the long-ago head injury.

The patient in the above case study above had never commanded herself to feel no pain. Her body was simply waiting for some help to dislodge the cranial-bone displacement that had put her into a three-day coma, a displacement that was still sitting there twenty years later. Also, she did *not* have the medically recognized "Parkinson's personality" seen in people with Type I PD. Chapter sixteen addresses this subject in depth.

The other person with Type IV PD, twenty years before I met him, had flown thirty feet out of a car during a bad accident. He had blacked out, but only for a few minutes. His response to craniosacral treatment was similar to that in the above case study: within minutes of his midbrain's occipital-sphenoid bones' articulation sliding back into place he went from the mental depression characteristic of PD to "What happened? I'm blissed out!"

However, his *body* still felt as if he was using pause mode even though his midbrain was once again experiencing dopamine release. He still could not perform Step 5 in turning off pause: allowing a shiver or shimmy to travel down the spine.

More craniosacral and Yin Tui Na work in subsequent treatment sessions found jammed vertebrae from T-5 to T-8, a compressed occiput/atlas, and displacements in a hip and a shoulder blade, both of which had been broken. The bone breaks had healed, but the bones were still displaced. As these areas were treated over the course of more than twenty sessions, using techniques described in the book *Yin Tui Na*, his whole body finally shifted into a relaxed, pleasant state that matched his mental feeling of being "blissed out."

Very likely, the reason that I have seen only two examples of people with somewhat *advanced* Parkinson's being *biologically* stuck on pause is because I have only seen a very limited number of people with Parkinson's: only a few hundred. I am certain that, if I were to see several thousand people with PD, I would meet several more who are biologically stuck on pause rather than having self-induced pause.

Pre-Parkinson's symptoms in people with pre-Type IV

Although I've seen only two patients with advanced Parkinson's from Type IV, I *have* seen *many* patients who were stuck on biological pause and running the electrical currents of pause, who did *not* overtly appear to have Parkinson's. Yet. These people *might* have ended up in the Type IV group if their underlying problems had not been addressed in a timely manner.

Many of my patients who were stuck on biological pause had some subtle and some not-so-subtle pre-Parkinson's symptoms, very often including an internal tremor that ceased when pause was turned off. Remember, the underlying circuitry of pause is usually

---

cells, neurogenesis, is now considered normal *but* an outmoded idea still persists: Parkinson's disease *must* be incurable because of the historic, incorrect presumptions that the brain *can't* grow new cells and that brain cells *cannot* change their behaviors.

present for many *decades* before the pause symptoms become obvious. Symptoms might not become obvious until the person is no longer able to summon up the mental sense of emergency that can temporarily override pause.

In *some* cases of people being stuck on biological pause, the injury was already healed. All that these people needed to do was initiate the normal steps for turning off pause: confirm that they are both internally stable *and* externally safe, take a deep audible breath, wobble the head high on the neck, and let a shiver run down the spine a few times, until they felt something shift inside. Others still had unhealed head or spinal injuries.

You can read about such cases and the *pre*-PD symptoms of many pause patients in my book *Stuck on Pause*, available for free download at www.PDrecovery.org.

The main point to be derived from the above is that very possibly there is a higher percentage of people with Type IV than was represented in my own patients. My sample size has been so small that my percentages of who has what type of PD are not to be viewed as representing everyone with Parkinson's. They only reflect my personal experience. Next, I'm going to veer away from the subject of pre-Parkinson's symptoms briefly, while I explain a bit more about the speed of recovery.

Variable-speed recovery

As for the almost instantaneous recovery in the above case study, that speed is not unusual. Although many people worked at turning off the circuitry of pause very slowly, having gradual results over months or even years, many people *did* turn off the pause pattern *very* quickly. Some even recovered quickly from *some* of their symptoms in less than a minute. For example, in the above case study, the patient's pause circuitry turned off as soon as her parietal bone went back into the correct place and a shiver went down her spine. She was suddenly smiling without making a conscious effort or using "override" brain behaviors.

However, her facial muscles weren't yet strong enough for her to *sustain* an automatic smile. Several weeks would pass before those muscles were tirelessly, effortlessly strong again. During that time she could say she was "in recovery." She could no longer say that she had Parkinson's. She *could* say that when pause mode turned off, her neurological *inhibition* of facial expression was gone *instantly*.

In the sense of turning off pause mode, she recovered instantly. In the sense of having fully restored muscle endurance, she was in recovery for months.

It's impossible to offer a specific number on how long it takes to turn off pause. Turning off the electrical patterns of biological pause or pseudo pause, patterns that cause Parkinson's, might take one treatment session or might take a dozen. In people with *only* Type II or Type IV PD, recovery pace mostly depends on how *many* dissociated foot/ankle or other injuries the person has. It might take several weeks or months of once-a-week treatments to track down all the injured places in a person's body that are dissociated and that are causing the person to be stuck on pause. If there's only one location of injury, one to three hour-long treatments might be enough to turn off the pause circuitry. If there are dozens of injuries, it might take several months to re-associate with or turn off pause in all of them, treating them one at a time.

With Type I PD, a few minutes or a few years might be needed before a person can train himself to fully activate the striatum and thalamus (brain areas that regulate joy, anticipation of joy, and allow for "automatic" (spontaneous) movement, as opposed to mental-command movement). When they are fully activated, self-induced pause can turn off.

Recovery is instant…recovery takes months

When I say a person "recovered from Parkinson's instantly," which is *not* unusual, I mean that the *driver* behind the symptoms of Parkinson's completely ceased and didn't ever return. The use of pause mode and the accompanying neurological inhibitions such as inhibition of dopamine release for motor function, an oppressive sense of joylessness, or even a sense of impending doom were instantly gone. When I say a person recovered instantly, I mean that the *circuitry of pause* turned off instantly. And it didn't come back.

Following that instant change, people are "in recovery." People in recovery still have to go through the recovery symptoms: weeks and even months of overcoming the new, infantile softness and limpness in muscles that had long been *tight* and *rigid*; pins and needles in body parts that had long been numb or disconnected from proprioception; achy soreness in muscles that had been un-usable and atrophied and which were once again *automatically*, *unstoppably* being used for movements such as arm swing and holding the back straight. These recovery symptoms are *not* symptoms of PD. They are the *opposite* of the symptoms of PD.

People whose underlying *cause* of Parkinson's had ended could *not* suddenly move as easily as they had twenty years earlier. There were repercussions from their years, maybe decades, of having been on pause mode.

Being on pause is like being in a war. People with Parkinson's are in a relentless, long-term war. Their muscles, brain behaviors, joints and skeletal structure are under constant attack in the sense that they are no longer receiving their normal support and supplies of energy. Some of their body and brain parts are essentially being starved and being allowed to fall apart. Muscles have atrophied; nerves have gone dormant. The brain's motor imagining area – a crucial area for automatic movement, has become dormant due to non-use.

When a war ends, life does not instantly return to normal. Rebuilding after a war might take some time. How much time it takes depends on how much damage was incurred. Still, the post-war peace is glorious. You can celebrate and declare "The war is over!" even if much rebuilding is necessary.

When pause mode turns off, which takes only an instant in many cases, the war on the body is over. There is no more inhibition of dopamine release for motor function or for imagining positive images, including imagining motor behaviors. *However*, after turning off pause, a person's body and brain now have a rebuilding job to do. The rebuilding might take months. How long the rebuilding takes depends on how severe the damage was.

When I say, "the Parkinson's ended," or "the underlying cause turned off," or "the person recovered," I mean that pause mode was turned off for good: the war was clearly, obviously, without a doubt, over.

Also, although many people turn off pause in a flash, many others turn off pause *gradually*. Some people turn off self-induced pause gradually, some even going two steps forward, one step back, for months or years. They might find at first that they have odd moments, now and then, during which they feel different – not on pause. In these moments, the mind is more relaxed and movement in some parts of the body feels more fluid. If a person keeps up or intensifies his mental self-therapy, these moments gradually increase in frequency and duration. Eventually, these people find that they are using self-induced pause mode only once in a while, usually when they are concerned about something. The people who recover gradually, who turn off pause in fits and starts instead of instantly, might have a harder time believing, at first, that something is changing for the better. Even when their use of self-induced pause mode occurs very infrequently, maybe once a week for a few hours, they tend to be terrified, each time, that their Parkinson's has returned as strong as ever. Even so, they can *eventually* recover fully and have no more relapses.

For these people, the brief "relapses" can help serve as a reminder to keep up the specific type of cognitive retraining exercises that are explained later in this book. Most people who recover gradually also have a greater tendency to be alarmed by their *recovery* symptoms instead of encouraged. Even though recovery symptoms are the opposite of PD symptoms, entrenched negative thought habits cause some people to think of almost any physical change as problematic or even a melodramatic omen of doom. This subject will be discussed in detail, later.

I'm going into this preliminary discussion about recovery rates here, early on in the book, because rate of recovery is one of the most frequently asked questions. Hopefully, the reader is starting to see that there is no one-size-fits-all answer. No two people with Parkinson's have the same symptoms or develop symptoms in the same order. No two people with Parkinson's experience recovery in the exact same way. Most cases of Parkinson's originate with thoughts – mental commands: the origin of the pause pattern was psychological. Each person experiences and recovers from self-induced psychological disorders in their own way.

Next, I want to resume the discussion of "pre-Parkinson's symptoms" that I saw in many people who were stuck on pause who did not *yet* have a diagnosis of Parkinson's disease even though they had many early symptoms and pre-symptoms.

Case study #2: a ten year old boy with internal tremor

For an example of a pre-PD symptom, I had a ten year-old patient with a recent shoulder injury from sports. I noticed his Stomach channel qi running backwards *and* an obvious displacement of bones in his foot that he could not account for. The displaced shoulder moved itself back into place very quickly. I asked his attending father if I might also work on the obviously displaced bones in his foot.

Because his Stomach channel qi was running backwards, before starting each session's treatment I always asked the boy about certain pre-PD symptoms, including any feelings of agitation, shaking, or tremoring inside his head or body. He said no to every query. He was an extremely articulate and intelligent lad, competed in league sports, played violin, and had just won a place on the student council in his grade school despite being younger than most of the also-rans. He struck me as having an intelligence and articulate, focused, and highly driven personality very similar to that of many of my PD patients. I have since come to suspect that this type of personality might be driven by the powerful norepinephrine override.

I treated him with Yin Tui Na over the course of several, one-hour, once a week sessions until his foot bones moved themselves back into place. The Stomach channel qi starting flowing correctly.

At the beginning of every treatment session I asked him if he had any internal tremoring. He always said no. During the session of foot holding in which his foot bones finally slid themselves back into place, he remarked, "I just remembered when I hurt that foot. I was five or six years old. My mother drove over my foot with the car. I couldn't tell her; she would have been devastated. So I pretended it never happened."

After a few moments he spoke up again. "You know how you always ask me if I'm shaky inside? Well, I must have been, because it just stopped! It feels *so* good. It was always there. I just thought it was normal. Ahh. It feels *so* good now. It's so *still* inside. The shaking inside my head is completely gone!"

Based on his pause-like electrical flow and his remarks about pretending that the specific injury didn't happen, he probably had Type I or Type III *pre*-Parkinson's.

Case study #3: dropped as a baby

A woman in her late twenties came to see me because one foot was starting to drag. Her posture was starting to hunch forward. Her left arm tended to stay crooked at the elbow. She had been very athletic, and felt that she was becoming "old before my time." She moved stiffly when she tried to turn over in bed. Her left hand tremored when she conducted music.

She had several displaced bones in her left foot and no memory of a recent foot injury. Her channels were flowing in the pause patterns.

I held her foot firmly, for an hour, once a week, over a period of several weeks. When her foot muscles finally relaxed and her foot bones moved themselves back into place, she remembered a very old injury that she had assumed was long since healed.

When she was around three months old, she was baptized in her parents' Greek Orthodox faith. As the priest was about to dip her into the font, he dropped her. Before she landed headfirst in the water, the priest snatched her by her left foot and jerked her back up to safety, and then proceeded to immerse her in the cold water: a painful foot injury, followed by a shock.

Her grandmother, who had attended the ceremony, had told her many times over the ensuing years, "You were never the same after that day. You had been a very easy-going baby. After that day, you were always agitated, always guarded."

After her foot injury healed up in response to several Yin Tui Na foot-holding treatments and her pre-Parkinson's symptoms evaporated, she had quite a few of the very specific recovery symptoms – short-term symptoms that are the *opposite* of Parkinson's – that occur in people who've recovered from full-blown Parkinson's disease.

Whether she was dissociated from her injury, was stuck on biological pause, or both I cannot say. At the time I worked with her, I had no idea that it made a difference. Either way, her pre-Parkinson's symptoms cleared up quickly when the foot healed. As for her developing fairly obvious (to me) pre-Parkinson's symptoms at such a young age, I wonder if this might be due to her having run pause mode in her body since early infancy. As for the recent appearance of symptoms, she had graduated college in a field that she loved and her youthful stresses were gone. Very possibly she could no longer sustain an emotional scenario with enough sense of emergency to keep her norepinephrine override going. When her internal sense of emergency dropped away, her underlying pause symptoms started to appear even though she was fairly young: in her twenties.

This case study and the one previous are provided in part to point out that a person can have many pre-Parkinson's symptoms and yet still not be diagnosable from a neurologist's standpoint. Remember, Parkinson's disease can take years, usually decades, to develop enough that a doctor can *see* the physical problems. Nearly all of my non-PD patients that were stuck in biological pause had *many* pre-Parkinson's symptoms. By "pre-Parkinson's symptom," I mean any symptom of PD that is still too mild or intermittent to catch a neurologist's attention. However, even if their symptoms were very mild, when their channel qi *stopped* running in the pause patterns, they usually went through some of the distinctive and counter-intuitive recovery symptoms that are the opposite of Parkinson's.

The recovery symptoms can include sensations of pins and needles in the extremities, face, and scalp, gentle come-and-go spasms lasting for about twenty minutes, several times a day, in muscles that are relearning automatic movement, and even falling into a limp, motionless, but mentally alert state between 7:00 a.m. and 9:00 a.m. each morning (the time of day when injuries along the Stomach channel engage in healing) for a few days, or longer, and many, many other symptoms. This book has eleven *chapters* about recovery symptoms. Many of the people who had been on biological pause and had only *pre*-Parkinson's symptoms still experienced many symptoms that are highly specific to recovering from PD. This told me the true story: they *had* been on the path to Parkinson's disease even though they were still able to override most of the obvious symptoms and were not *yet* diagnosable for PD.

If a patient did *not* have an official diagnosis of Parkinson's disease, I *never* mentioned the possibility that, by turning off pause or pseudo pause, he or she had dodged developing Parkinson's in the years to come. I merely did Yin Tui Na on the old, unhealed injury(s), helped the patient go through the steps that turn off biological pause, or taught the mental exercises for turning off self-induced pause. Even if the person had electric currents consistent with pause mode, even if the person had subtle pre-PD symptoms *or* a few *glaring* Parkinson's symptoms, I just treated the injuries or mental postures. I never mentioned Parkinson's disease.

If the patient was surprised at how many other mild problems cleared up at the same time as the dominant symptoms, I just casually suggested that lots of *seemingly* unrelated physical and mental behaviors might be connected to an old injury. [1]

---

[1] In 2020, new research showed a link between sprained ankles and a long-term effect on health. The study, led by Phillip Gribble, associate professor of rehabilitation sciences at University of Kentucky, found that people with a history of ankle injury have significantly higher rates of health problems later in life when compared with people having no history of ankle injury. Problems included arthritis, heart or respiratory issues, and other disabilities, or limitations in their daily activities. This study was presented at the 2020 annual meeting of the National Athletic Trainer's Association in Baltimore. https://uknow.uky.edu/research/research-links-ankle-injury-health-problems-later-life.

So many articles by western doctors and researchers, while superficially having nothing to do with Parkinson's disease, lend support to what I saw in my patients with PD.

This particular article helps refute comments such as "There is *no way* a foot injury can have anything to do with the rest of the body, let alone healing dead brain cells!" That was the

For me to act the prognosticator and tell these people who had been stuck on pause that, by turning it off, they probably prevented themselves from developing Parkinson's down the road would of course have been ethically wrong. Even so, I am fairly certain that this was the case.

As for rate of recovery, this early-stage, not-yet-diagnosed type of patient *always* recovered very quickly. I loved working with people who had only pre-Parkinson's symptoms or who had full-blown symptoms of Parkinson's *but* didn't yet have a diagnosis and didn't suspect one. (I always described my medical practice as focusing on "movement disorders," *not* on Parkinson's disease.)

Unlike my patients who had similar symptoms but who *had* received an official diagnosis, my un-diagnosed or pre-Parkinson's patients never went into the abject fear and negative mental loops that I saw in people who *had* been diagnosed. Unlike my patients with the terrifying diagnosis of "incurable Parkinson's," my *un*diagnosed patients had no voice in their heads telling them to disbelieve their healing because recovery was impossible. They didn't live in dread of a "relapse" into Parkinson's disease or re-invoke self-induced pause as a way to deal with their fear of Parkinson's coming back.

Idiopathic Parkinson's is, in most cases, a psychogenic condition. Once diagnosed, a person's symptoms of PD can be *increasingly* psychogenic: mind-driven. Ironically, "psychogenic parkinsonism" is *not* a psychogenic condition. It is the *healthy*, correct, biological use of pause mode in response to a horrible trauma: pause *without* activation of the mentally-activated norepinephrine override. This condition eventually clears up on its own when the person decides that they are safe enough to "come back to life," as pause is *supposed* to do.

Looking ahead, if doctors of every school learn to recognize the electrical behaviors of pause mode and can direct their patients with this situation towards information on turning those electrical behaviors *off*, then many or even most cases of Parkinson's disease might be *prevented*. Ideally, people with pre-PD symptoms might someday be able to avoid developing the more glaringly obvious symptoms of Parkinson's altogether if the injuries or attitudes that triggered their dissociation and/or pause are treated in a timely manner.

Now, having given very brief, very generalized answers to the most common question, "how long will it take to recover?" and promising to revisit the question later with more specifics, it's time to consider the second most common question: what about all those dead dopamine-producing cells in the brain?

I'm glad you asked.

---

angry position taken by a local neurologist when one of my recovered PD patients tried to explain to her, the neurologist, about the Yin Tui Na treatment on her foot that she had received from me. This neurologist dismissed the recovery as "misdiagnosis" and then set out to sue me for practicing medicine without a license. She dropped the case when she learned that in California, licensed acupuncturists are, in fact, authorized to diagnose, prescribe, and treat within the scope of practice of Chinese medicine: licensed to practice medicine.

Chapter Three

Allopathic (Western) Medicine Guesswork

"Allopathic medicine," sometimes referred to as "modern medicine" or "western medicine," refers to medicine that uses drugs or surgery to treat or suppress a health problem.

The theory of the dead dopamine cells

Researchers in the field of Parkinson's have repeatedly disproved the hypothesis that idiopathic Parkinson's is caused by the death of dopamine-producing brain cells. That wrong notion, dating back to the late 1960s and concomitant with early research on L-dopa (synthetic dopamine), was further developed in 1982 based on symptoms in a small group of illegal-drug users, a group labeled "the frozen addicts," They all developed a few symptoms of parkinson*ism overnight* because of presumed brain damage from a weekend binge using a type of synthetic heroin. [1]

Their symptoms were *not* actually a good match for idiopathic Parkinson's disease. For example, they'd suddenly lost their ability to speak. *And* despite tight hand cramping, one of them was able to write out for the doctor at the hospital that they'd been using synthetic heroin. Oppositely, people with PD can form words even as their voices get very soft in volume, and problems with small motor function in the fingers is from muscle weakness and unresponsiveness – *not* tension – especially in the index finger.

For these drug users, their large motor immobility from sudden brain damage responded favorably to a mind-swamping level of L-dopa – the pharmacological equivalent of dopamine – in a manner *similar* to the L-dopa response of people immobilized with Parkinson's. A small team of MDs blithely concluded that Parkinson's itself must similarly be caused by some unknown factor that, like the synthetic heroin, destroyed dopamine-producing brain cells. There was *never* hard evidence for this quickly adopted hypothesis.

At that time, dopamine was assumed to be a neurotransmitter that *relaxed* muscles. In order to make sense of observations that people with Parkinson's could move easily after receiving large doses of L-dopa, researchers assumed, wrongly, that the normal, passive state of muscles must be rigidity: dopamine was required to relax muscles, thus allowing for movement. Dopamine therefore was also wrongly assumed to induce sleep by creating a state of heightened relaxation.

Two corresponding wrong "facts" invented at that time were that dopamine levels in the brain were 1) lower in the daytime and 2) higher during sleep. [2]

---

[1] *The Case of the Frozen Addicts*; Dr. Langston; Pantheon Books; 1995.

[2] This is a lengthy footnote, but I hope you'll forgive me because it makes an important point about how hard it is to change a widely accepted, presumably "scientific," wrong hypothesis.

In the first article I ever submitted for publishing, I mentioned that human dopamine levels were *higher* during awake times and *lower* during sleep. This was based on my very new, (late

1990s) understanding of the role played by dopamine in response to certain stimulant drugs such as cocaine and methamphetamine – though this disagreed with what I'd learned about dopamine two decades earlier, in my undergraduate days. The editor choked on my brazen contradiction of the long-known "facts" about dopamine. She said I would need to show her at least one research article that showed dopamine levels being higher in the daytime than at night if she was going to consider running my article.

Of the one hundred articles that I pulled up in my search at the Stanford University medical library, there were ninety-eight articles in which the subjects had *higher* dopamine levels in the daytime than at night. In every one of these studies, the main subject of the research was not dopamine or Parkinson's disease, but was some other illness being studied. The night and day *blood* dopamine levels (not brain levels) had merely been checked as a part of the general blood work. In every case, the researchers had been surprised that, *contrary* to the pattern that was presumed to be normal, all of their human subjects had higher blood levels of dopamine in the daytime, lower levels at night. In each article, the researcher concluded that the unanticipated and *obviously* pathological reversed dopamine levels might be contributing to the illness that was being researched. The various illnesses being studied included PMS, narcolepsy, epilepsy, mood swings, muscle cramping, mental retardation – the list went on and on. In every case, the researcher for each article had suggested that maybe the cause of the illness at hand was the presumably "pathologically" elevated daytime levels of dopamine and decreased nighttime levels.

Since it was a "recognized fact" that dopamine is a relaxant (now recognized as wrong), and is therefore present in higher quantities at night (based on the excess acetylcholine/ insufficient dopamine imbalance = excess rigidity theory of Parkinson's disease, also now recognized as wrong), every one of these studies concluded that the cause of the illness in question might be this reversal of the officially-correct dopamine pattern.

In other words, if the patients were in the headache study, the report proposed that this presumably abnormal reversal of the correct dopamine levels was causing their headaches. Ninety-eight of the one hundred studies followed this pattern. It didn't matter what the researchers were looking at. The conclusion in *every case* was that the illness at hand might be related to the abnormal, reversed situation of blood dopamine levels being higher during the daytime and lower at night. It seemed no one had noticed that *everyone* has higher dopamine levels while awake and lower dopamine levels while sleeping.

But, to be fair, there were two studies that had the opposite result. In these two studies they measured not *blood* dopamine levels, but the actual brain levels of dopamine. This was done by chopping off the heads of the subjects, tossing the heads in a blender, and quickly assaying the results. This gave the most accurate possible reading of brain dopamine levels.

In these two studies, the dopamine levels were higher at night, thus confirming the fact of dopamine as a nighttime relaxant. There was only one detail that had evidently missed everyone's attention: the subjects in these two experiments were rats. Rats are nocturnal – they are more active in the evening and at night; they tend to sleep during the day.

Armed with these research abstracts, abstracts that suggested that 100% of the time human and rat dopamine levels are higher during awake, active time and lower during sleep, my editor agreed to run my article. She also said, about my PD research, "They're going to have to kill you."

This was in 1997. I'm not dead yet. And hopefully, this footnote illustrates just how hard it is to defy the established facts, even when the "known facts" are unproven and *every* study produces data that *opposes* those so-called "facts."

Most of the current western medicine "facts" about idiopathic Parkinson's were never more than guesses, hypothesized in the 1960s and '70s, when *very* little was known about brain chemistry and brain cell behaviors, and much of what we *thought* we knew was wrong.

Wrong "scientific facts" about dopamine from the 1960s were still in place in the 1990s, when I started my Parkinson's research. In year 2020, as I write up this book, we now know that, in the midbrain, in parasympathetic mode, dopamine is the neurotransmitter of *consciousness*, of expectations of joy, and of *automatic* motor activation. Not sleep. Not the relaxation of rigid muscles. Looking ahead, insufficient dopamine causes *limp* muscles, not rigid ones. *Pause* mode causes rigidity. Insufficient dopamine does *not*. During both sleep mode and pause mode, midbrain dopamine release for motor function is *supposed* to be greatly *inhibited.*

Nevertheless, based on the *wrong* idea that dopamine makes people sleep or relax, and the fact that people who were rigid with Parkinson's *could* move freely using automatic-type movement when they took mind-smashing levels of L-dopa, just like the synthetic heroin users with brain damage mentioned earlier, the researchers of the early 1980s claimed to have proof, however indirect, of their hypothesis that the death of dopamine-producing brain cells causes Parkinson's disease.

Since the early 1980s, patients' inexplicable responses to L-dopa and the related hypotheses about dead brain cells have served as the basis for nearly *all* Parkinson's drug research. L-dopa treatments, treatments based on the dead brain cell hypothesis, do *not* actually help with *all* the symptoms of Parkinson's. The dopamine insufficiency hypothesis *never* explained the tremor. The "frozen" drug addicts pointed to as "proof" did *not* actually have idiopathic Parkinson's disease. In fact, the drug addicts died fairly soon after they started using L-dopa, in a manner similar to the deaths from the patients taking L-dopa in Oliver Sacks' book *Awakenings*. L-dopa in high doses is much more dangerous, can even quickly become deadly, for a person who *doesn't* have idiopathic Parkinson's disease. [1]

Even though the hypothesis didn't make a lot of sense, the dead dopamine cell idea thrived, along with the development of what has become a multi-billion dollars a year antiparkinson's drug business. The current antiparkinson's drugs are all based on the dead dopamine cell idea.

In the mid-1990s, researchers studying dopamine outside the context of Parkinson's were discovering that dopamine was the neurotransmitter of addiction,

---

[1] Please read *Awakenings*; Oliver Sacks; Duckworth & Co; London; 1973.

The book *Awakenings* describes the almost unbelievably monstrous pathologies and fatalities resulting from sustained use of L-dopa in people who did *not* have Parkinson's disease.

The results that Dr. Sacks, MD, saw in his early experiments with L-dopa in the late 1960s on people with long-term symptoms from the type of "sleeping sickness" caused by Encephalitis lethargica were at first so delightful, and then turned so impossibly, so superhumanly violent, and then fatal, that many doctors declared his observations fraudulent. When he presented films of these patients at a conference, emotions ran high. The severest critic got up and left the room. Many doctors simply could not accept that any drug with a six-hour half-life could have such paradoxical, inconsistent, and sometimes deadly effects over the long term. In Sacks' study, "long-term" refers to weeks – not years.

If you read *Awakenings*, be sure to read the introduction, as well. It describes the hostile, even vicious reactions doctors had to Dr. Sacks's alarming findings about L-dopa, the new "miracle drug."

consciousness, and the "reward center" (feel-good area) of the brain. Around this time, many people were starting to seriously question the dead dopamine cell theory and even the long-term safety of the antiparkinson's medications. Researchers were just starting to make the connection between the dopamine-enhancing medications and the appearance of *new* "PD symptoms": mentally-hyper symptoms like hallucinations, dyskinesias, and bi-polar-like mental problems. These types of drug-induced symptoms had *never* presented in PD patients prior to the introduction of L-dopa based drugs. And yet, since the late 1990s these *drug*-related problems have been included in lists of "symptoms of Parkinson's disease."

Even so, even though the dead dopamine cell hypotheses about Parkinson's have been repeatedly disproven *and* even though we now know that idiopathic Parkinson's is *very* different from drug- or toxin-induced parkinsonism *and* we know that dopamine-enhancing drugs cause brain damage and addiction, even so, the dead dopamine cell hypothesis remains at the core of the drug industry's ongoing push for new, "improved" dopamine-based drug treatments – not cures – for people with Parkinson's.

Meanwhile, *research* doctors in the field of Parkinson's, often far removed from the interface with actual patients, have known for years that the dead dopamine cell model does not hold up.[1]

In retrospect, the dead dopamine cell hypothesis was an embarrassing series of wild guesses that were primary used to explain why L-dopa, in mind-blasting amounts, was able to temporarily override *some* – though *not* all – of the neurological inhibitions of Parkinson's. Many medical people of the day saw that these Parkinson's hypotheses were very shaky. Also, this new idea did not explain *many* of the characteristic symptoms of Parkinson's, such as some muscles being weak while others were rigid. It did not explain

---

[1] The articles cited below are just two that I plucked at random from my large collection of research articles that disprove the dead dopamine cell theory.

1) "Unexpected Findings in Parkinson's Research Show Cells May Not Be Dead"; *Biospace*; Mark Terry; Nov 12, 2019, (Review article based on "Loss of SATB1 Induces p21-Dependent Cellual Senescence in Post-mitotic Dopaminergic Neurons; *Cell Stem Cell*; 25, 514-530, Riesslan at al, Oct 3, 2019 Elsevier Inc.) This article discusses research that proves the dopaminergic cells that were long assumed to be dead in people with Parkinson's are not dead, but have "shut down without dying."

2) "Myth about Parkinson's disease debunked"; *ScienceDaily*, 9-16-2014, www.sciencedaily.com/release/2014/09/140916084909.htm, based on "Three mechanisms by which Striatal Denervation causes Breakdown of Dopamine Signaling"; J.K. Dreyer; *Journal of Neuroscience*; 2014; 34 (37): 12444 doi: 10.1523/JNEUROSCI; 1458-14.201.

This article, like others, points out that, at the time of diagnosis, people with Parkinson's have more than enough dopamine in the brain. This article's point is that, for some inexplicable reason, dopamine is present in the brain but isn't used to provide motor function in people with Parkinson's.

This is not actually inexplicable. Dopamine release for motor function is *supposed* to be inhibited when a person is sleeping or on pause. After decades of *not* using striatal neurons because of being on pause, the brain, ever efficient and thrifty, begins to modify some of the un-used striatal neurons. Based on resumption of normal motor function that I've seen in recovered patients, it seems as if the brain restores these neurons when pause is turned off and parasympathetic mode's dopamine-driven motor function is called for once again.

the tremor at all. However, the antiparkinson's medications industry is still a strong supporter of this hypothesis.

In 1998, one of my PD patients, a senior neurologist at a top, university-linked medical school confided in me, "We don't actually know anything about Parkinson's disease. We're just making stuff up. Your ideas make more sense." He also told me that he would probably lose his seat on the school's neurology board if his colleagues found out that he was seeing an acupuncturist.

Many if not most *clinical* doctors – general practitioners and neurologists who are working with patients and prescribing drugs – often have *no* idea that the dead dopamine cell theory is considered passé in the *research* realm. They merrily pass along to their patients the misinformation they were taught in medical school. They are well-meaning, and besides, they have nothing else to offer. They are supported in this misinformation by companies that make the various antiparkinson's medications and by companies that make deep-brain-stimulating implants.

By the way, the deep-brain implants do *not* elevate dopamine levels in the automatic movement parts of the brain. This is a well-known fact. They work by creating a sense of emergency in the brain: increasing the level of norepinephrine. Recent research suggests that the implants *do* cause increased dopamine release…in those parts of the brain that use dopamine for risk-assessment and certain other danger-driven and pause-driven brain behaviors – but *not* in the automatic motor area.

Mainly, the electrical stimulation from the implants creates enough sense of emergency that what I call the norepinephrine override is able to once again mask the symptoms of pause. However, the brain soon becomes accustomed to the implant's electrical bursts in the brain. This is why an implant's signals need to be regularly altered or put on a varying schedule so that the brain does not become accustomed to the stimulation and then stops treating the implant stimulation as an emergency.

More than enough dopamine

Research shows that people who have been recently diagnosed with Parkinson's not only have more than enough dopamine in their brains, but we have known, since 2001, that the risk-assessment areas in the brains of people with Parkinson's have *higher* levels of dopamine than people without Parkinson's.

The problem in Parkinson's is *not* the absence of dopamine. The problem is the chronic *inhibition* of brain-based dopamine release for *motor* function and for some types of mental processing such as visualization of positive images, as well as the *inhibition* of adrenaline release from the adrenal glands…the exact same life-saving inhibitions that occur, correctly, during near-death shock and coma: during pause mode.

Western "possible cures" for Parkinson's disease

Every year or so, a news release hits the media with a report that researchers have possibly found a cure for Parkinson's disease. Invariably, these researchers were using an "animal model." Animals do not get Parkinson's disease. They simply do not have the ability to corrupt their own consciousness into dissociating from an injury for the long term or telling themselves to constantly pretend they are numb to the world.

In order to create an animal model of Parkinson's, researchers give an animal some toxic chemical that damages or inhibits certain neurons (brain nerve-cells) associated with movement. This does *not* cause Parkinson's disease in the animal. It *does* cause poor mobility or even paralysis. The researchers insist that the toxin-induced immobility *looks similar* enough to Parkinson's to make it a valid comparison, a "Parkinson's model."

Then, the researchers work to develop a chemical that will protect the targeted neurons from that specific toxin. When they find a chemical that serves as a protection against that specific toxin, they release a report stating that they have found a possible cure for Parkinson's disease. These press releases might be coordinated with a request for donations to a research "non-profit" or with a request for a research grant or grant renewal. These news releases can be considered public relations gambits rather than actual research breakthroughs in the field of Parkinson's.

In 2020, I learned of new research showing that dopamine receptors in rodents work very differently than they do in humans. This research further invalidates the idea that paralyzing a mouse with poison creates an acceptable "animal model" of Parkinson's disease. If you read any report claiming to have found a possible cure for Parkinson's disease based on an "animal model," you can throw it away. [1]

"Lewy body" Parkinson's

When brain cells undergo changes, the ensuing debris and waste products must be safely stowed away. In the rest of the body, the constant debris from metabolic processes or cellular change is cleared out of the system via the liver and kidneys. When this inevitable debris from cellular change occurs in the *brain cells*, there are not as many ways to flush it out. Instead, the brain cells create little "trash cans," known as Lewy bodies, to contain these bits of waste – typically proteins such as alpha-synuclein. When a brain undergoes more changes than the average, one will find more Lewy bodies than average.

In one of the more charming traditions of science, dating back thousands of years, our conjectures often reverse cause and effect. For example, for years, scientists presumed that giraffes have long necks because they prefer the leaves at the tops of the trees. This type of thinking, in which a phenomenon is explained by the purpose it serves rather than by its underlying cause, is called teleology. We now know that giraffes *can* eat the top leaves *because* their genes cause them to grow long necks.

In cases of so-called "Lewy body dementia" and "Lewy body Parkinson's," researchers have observed that there are more Lewy bodies in brain cells of people with these syndromes. A few researchers have jumped to the teleological conclusion that high numbers of Lewy bodies *cause* the dementia or the Parkinson's.

---

[1] "Subtle Differences in Brain Cells Hint at Why Many Drugs Help Mice But Not People"; Lein, Koch (president Allen Institute for Brain Science in Seattle); from "All Things Considered" review of an article in *Nature*, Aug 21, 2019. The researchers discovered that genes and proteins responsible for brain responses to neurotransmitters are different enough in rodents and humans that neurotransmitter research on rodents might not apply to how those neurotransmitters behave in humans.

https://www.npr.org/sections/health-shots/2019/08/21/753121107/subtle-differences-in-brain-cells-hint-at-why-many-drugs-help-mice-but-not-peopl

However, based on everything we know about Lewy bodies, it is far more probable that the Lewy bodies are *not* the *cause* of the brain changes. They serve as evidence that cellular changes have occurred. They do not tell us *why* these changes occurred.

The genetic angle

Just one more point will wrap up this chapter on western hypotheses about Parkinson's. Western researchers have observed that Parkinson's seems to run in families. This has led to a search for a genetic cause for Parkinson's disease. However, outside of the Contoursi Family genes that cause a Parkinson's-like syndrome featuring irregularities in alpha-synuclein (a nerve protein) production, irregularities that are *not* found in *most* people with Parkinson's, researchers have found no genetic smoking gun.

Instead, if we look closely, we see that Parkinson's runs, not specifically in families, but in social groups. Social groups *or* families that emphasize suppression of pain or of negative emotions are more likely to see higher numbers of people with Parkinson's disease.

In the United States, the demographic group with the most Parkinson's per capita is the Mennonites, some of whom are also known as the Amish. Their religion's social requirements include *never* showing anger, resentment or other so-called "unChrist-like" emotions. A famous example is that if someone murders your daughter, you should lovingly invite them to dinner and forgive them because that is what Jesus would supposedly have done. As you can imagine, *powerful* suppression of emotions is rampant in this culture, in those people who are mentally *capable* of it.

If there *is* a genetic link to Parkinson's, and there may well be one, it will be related to the high level of word-based intelligence and focus that a person needs in order to activate self-induced pause. A scatter-brain can't do it. You will almost *never* meet a dull-witted, poorly focused, or inarticulate person with Type I Parkinson's – unless he got that way from taking antiparkinson's medications or having some other sort of brain trauma after already putting himself into pause.

Components of what is referred to as the Parkinson's personality include a tremendous intensity of purpose and will power and a high level of word-based, analytical intelligence. *These* attributes might have a genetic component. Even so, a genetically supported high capacity for mental focus and word-based intelligence doesn't *need* to be used to induce pause. The genetics might provide the skill set used for inducing pause mode in oneself, but the genetics does *not* require those skills to be used in this manner. A suppressive community ethos or a cold and/or dangerous family dynamic *might.*

Not everyone with PD has the Parkinson's personality. However, nearly all of my patients with Type I PD *did* have it to some degree.

The identical twin study

In the late 1990s, I received an email from an east coast university researcher on the team doing the largest ever – at that time – identical twin study. The study was designed to see if there was a genetic component to Parkinson's disease.

Back then, before we had DNA analysis and before epigenetics (variability of DNA expression based on mental and environmental events) was discovered, identical twin studies were considered the gold standard for proving the genetic basis of an illness.

The premise was this: if the syndrome is always present or always absent in *both* of a pair of identical twins, the syndrome is genetic. If the source of the syndrome is *not* genetic then, if one twin has the syndrome, the odds of the other twin having it should be about the same as the national average for that syndrome.

A researcher contacted me. He had a numbers problem. The research showed that if *one* of the identical twins had Parkinson's, the *other* twin was *far* less likely than the national average to have it. This made absolutely *no* sense to him. Even if Parkinson's *wasn't* genetic, the other twin should have PD as often as the national average.

I explained that Parkinson's has a sociological component. In cases of identical twins, even in families or cultures that promote stern suppression of emotion and discourage coddling and/or use frightening levels of physical and emotional punishment and abuse on children, the *subordinate* identical twin might have something that *most* people don't ever have: a life-long, bone deep, physical and emotional connection with an at-hand champion, protector, or comforter: the dominant twin. In the very special identical-twin relationship, the dominant twin could serve as a secret confidant, an emotional support for the subordinate twin.

The *dominant* twin might command himself or herself to not feel or show pain, and go on to develop Parkinson's disease. But the *subordinate* twin might always be able to secretly lean on and find *safety* in the love and strength of the dominant twin. Because of this life-long, exceptional level of emotional support, a subordinate twin *would* be far less likely than the national average to issue a powerful self-command to be stoic and/or apart from humanity, and then go on to develop Parkinson's – even if both twins live in a social setting that encourages emotional suppression.

The researcher and I exchanged several emails. He completely understood how my hypothesis would account for their findings. However, his final email said something like, "Thanks, but I can't use your information after all. My grant *requires* me to prove that Parkinson's *is* genetic." (Italics mine.)

Now let's leave the misleading "animal models," the disproven western hypotheses about dead dopamine-producing cells and Lewy bodies, and the failed genetics theories behind us. The next chapter will provide some information about basic brain physiology. After that we can return to the details regarding what actually does cause idiopathic Parkinson's disease and what's needed to turn it off.

Chapter Four

A Peek Inside the Brain

Quite a few people have asked me to explain about the chemicals and structures in the brain that come into play in Parkinson's. This seems like the right place for it.

This chapter gives a quick overview of one neurotransmitter plus three brain areas: dopamine plus the substantia nigra, the striatum, and the thalamus. After that comes a discussion of how electrical "static" in the thalamus contributes to the tremor and other Parkinson's-related information about these brain parts.

Dopamine

The nerve-like cells located in the brain are called neurons. The chemicals that activate nerves and neurons are called "neurotransmitters." Dopamine is produced in the body and in several areas in the brain. In the brain, dopamine behaves like a neurotransmitter, activating neurons. Dopamine produced outside the brain, where it behaves more like a hormone, affects blood vessels and various organ behaviors.

Blood dopamine and brain dopamine are, for the most part, kept apart by the blood-brain barrier. However, extremely high levels of blood dopamine will lead to a small amount crossing into the brain. (Most pharmaceutical preparations that use L-dopa for Parkinson's treatment combine it with carbidopa. Carbidopa, when added to L-dopa, allows L-dopa in the blood stream to pass easily through the blood-brain barrier and into the brain.

The substantia nigra

The substantia nigra is made up of two very small areas just above the brain stem, on the underside of the brain proper, just to the left and right sides of the midbrain. "The midbrain" refers to tissues located on or near the front-to-back centerline of the brain. The midbrain structures are located along an imaginary line going from front to back of the brain, as opposed to those brain structures that are located in large lobes on the left and right *sides* of the brain. Looking up at the two substantia nigra areas from the bottom of the brain, they look like two wispy eyebrows that are darker colored than the surrounding brain cells. This darker color is the source of the name substantia nigra, which translated loosely means "black stuff."

The neurons in the substantia nigra have long tendrils that send dopamine-triggered messages to the muscle-moving neurons on the sides of the brain. These neurons provide for automatic (not mental command-based) movements.

In autopsies of people with advanced Parkinson's, the substantia nigra area is less black than it should be. The number of specialized, black cells in this area is reduced.

An early theory from the 1960s declared that the dark cells in the substantia nigra must have *died*. That was the only option, based on western medical theory at that time. Back in those days, we were taught that brain cells could never change or re-grow. The brain was thought of as static: an inert switchboard of unchanging connectors.

We now know that to be completely wrong. Brain cells are constantly changing their connections and behaviors. In brain areas that are newly stimulated or have increased stimulation, the neurons show an increase in number and activity level. Neurons are re-assigned, or decrease in number and activity level in areas that are *not* being used or that are being *inhibited* over a long period.

The photographic slides that I looked at in the 1990s, slides of the substantia nigra from autopies of people with Parkinson's, showed that some of the dark cells had been replaced with normal colored brain cells. This suggested to me even at the time that these cells that were no longer being used to make and store dopamine had not *died*. They had converted (re-undifferentiated) back into a more basic type of cell.

This is just good, thrifty and efficient use of materials on the part of the brain. If an area isn't being used, the brain can let cells in that area become reassigned from their specialized jobs, reverting back to the more basic, less specialized, lower maintenance type of cells…until they are needed again.[1]

So even in people with *unmedicated* Parkinson's, are there eventually fewer of the black, dopamine-making cells in the substantia nigra area? Probably yes. Are the cells dead? Almost certainly no. Can they resume their role as "black cells" if they are once again called upon? Based on steadily increasing duration and eventual complete restoration of recovered patients' dopamine-based, automatic-type movement, it certainly appears that they can.

As an aside, no one, and I mean no one, has ever done an autopsy study of this area comparing people with Parkinson's who never took antiparkinson's medications and those who did, using brains of people who had the same *degree* of Parkinson's symptoms. So we have no way of knowing how *much* of the reduction in blackness might be due to drug use.

Even so, based on recovery symptoms, and despite recent research showing that people *newly* diagnosed with PD have sufficient dopamine levels, I hypothesize that people with Parkinson's *do* eventually develop an insufficiency of dopamine in *certain* brain areas: for example, they develop a decrease in available dopamine for automatic movement, positive imagination and visualization, and temperature regulation. But there is *no* dopamine deficiency in other areas, such as those that regulate fear-based (sides of the brain) brain functions such as risk assessment.

(I associate dopamine from this part of the brain with *temperature regulation* because, in a person who is recovering from advanced PD, in a sudden spell of *very* hot or *very* cold weather, the slowly burgeoning dopamine supply runs out a bit faster than usual. The temporary "running out" is actually helpful: it serves as a spur to accelerate dopamine production. More on this subject is provided in the chapters on recovery symptoms.)

---

[1] "In Parkinson's disease (PD)…although dopamine is depleted, the cells in the striatum are *preserved*. This is unlike the PD-*like* disorders [drug- and toxin-induced parkinsonism] where, in the striatum, the dopamine content is decreased and the cells are lost." [Italics are mine.] This quote is from "Curing Parkinson's Disease in Our Lifetime: part 3"; Abraham Lieberman, MD; *Parkinson's Report*; Fall 2000, Vol. XI, issue 3, Parkinson's Foundation, Inc.

Notice the date on the above. The above research is now more than twenty years old but the cell-death theory is *still* being handed out to PD patients by some neurologists.

I can hypothesize this dopamine insufficiency because, during recovery, people with somewhat *advanced* PD find that they have only a limited amount of dopamine for motor function at first...even if they never took antiparkinson's medications.

When, during recovery, the *midbrain* dopamine supply temporarily runs out, a person does *not* become rigid, as he used to do with Parkinson's disease. Nor does he tremor. Instead, he becomes very comfortable, although motionless and limp: more like a rag doll than a person with PD. During a spell like this, when dopamine is temporarily, mildly, insufficient and drops below the threshold for automatic motor function, the *body* behaves as if it is peacefully sleeping even though the *mind* can be cheerfully and peacefully alert. After some time, ranging from a few minutes to twenty minutes or so, when enough dopamine has gotten recycled back into the midbrain's dopamine-holding tanks (vesicles), the person suddenly, effortlessly, springs back to full movement.

If, say, during one week the recovering person was consistently able to move for an hour at a time before going limp, and then have ten to twenty minutes of downtime, by the next week they might be able to move effortlessly for two hours at a stretch. In a few more weeks, the person might be able to go six hours and the downtimes in between will be much shorter. The body recycles dopamine, so as it also generates more *and* probably even re-differentiates the dormant substantia nigra cells, the amount of a person's functional motor time quickly increases. And every time a person runs out of dopamine, that's a signal to the brain that it needs to bring still more dopamine-making cells out of retirement. Fairly quickly, usually within a few months, the person no longer runs out of dopamine for motor function, ever.

This running out of steam will *not* happen during an emergency, or while driving a car or performing an activity in which being motionless is not an option. During recovery, a person is once again able to access adrenaline from the adrenal glands. And they can still use the norepinephrine override if they need to, even though doing so will feel mildly unpleasant and a bit stressful – a symptoms-free reminder of the *mental* intensity of one's Parkinson's days. Have no fear: during recovery, if the dopamine runs out during some *critical* activity, adrenaline and/or norepinephrine will kick in. But if the dopamine runs out while the recovering person is just hanging out around the house, he will have several seconds of warning that he is starting to fade, and should sit down.

This fade out is exactly the same as the sensations a person might experience for a day or two after recovering from a nasty case of the flu: although the overt flu symptoms might have cleared up, a person might still be so temporarily dopamine-depleted from a recent bout with the flu that he feels weak and/or easily breaks into a sweat after a mildly strenuous event such as climbing the stairs, talking on the phone, or eating a heavy meal. While the body is still recovering from the very last side effects of the flu, a person might suddenly become listless, feel a need to lie down, or just sit and stare at the wall for a few minutes – or maybe half an hour – until the body recharges. This is actually what a shortage of dopamine for motor function feels like.

The rigidity of Parkinson's comes from being on *pause*, which disconnects the brain's motor imagining area. The tremor comes from unsuccessfully trying to come *out* of pause. Rigidity and tremor are *not* directly related to the pause-based inhibition of midbrain dopamine release.

This recovery symptom of short periods of profound, temporary weakness does not happen to everyone. If and when it *does*, is not a dangerous problem. However, some people who have Parkinson's, especially Type I PD, who read about this are horrified by the idea that they might lose even more control over their body, however temporary. After all, excessive worry and/or anxiety is a part of the medically recognized Parkinson's personality. This subject will be discussed in depth later on.

The high level of wariness and/or anxiety, the inhibition of dopamine release and of visualizing positive scenarios, as well as the inhibition of other positive thoughts, will go away almost *immediately* when pause turns off. Dopamine *supply*, on the other hand, might build back up *gradually*.

But the point is, even if a person never took antiparkinson's medications, the recovering person's body might show evidence of short periods of dopamine insufficiency *and* an ability to quickly re-build the dopamine supply after pause turns off. This suggests that the dopamine supply for automatic movement *had* been somewhat reduced prior to recovery. Most likely the dopamine supply in *only* the substantia nigra and striatal area had been reduced, not the dopamine supply in the other areas of the brain. It had been reduced in the automatic movement area of the brain *because* it wasn't ever being called on in that area. As soon as the person is once again *able* to mentally use dopamine for motor function, his body evidently – based on patient performance – starts to re-activate this area and restore the *midbrain* supply of dopamine back to adequate levels.

For now, I mention it merely to show that, yes, a person diagnosed with early-stage Parkinson's still has more than enough dopamine to move normally and yes, a decline in dopamine levels in *some* parts of the brain (probably the substantia nigra and striatum) does occur in people with advanced Parkinson's, even in people who *never* took antiparkinson's medications. And here's the most important point: substantia nigra and striatal dopamine levels, *if* insufficient, are apparently restored to a healthy, more than adequate amount when a person turns off pause, based on patient experiences.

The striatum

The striatum is a brain area that regulates automatic and voluntary motor function and the "reward system" (determines how good you feel.) It sits on the midline of the brain about halfway along the brain portion of the "Du" channel. This portion of the Du channel connects the brain stem area (at the top of the medulla oblongata) to the point between the eyebrows on the forehead, a point often called the Third Eye or, in Chinese medicine, Yin Tang. The striatum receives dopamine from various areas in the brain and distributes it to other areas in the basal ganglia. "Basal ganglia" refers to some of the lower, central midbrain areas, but *not* to the big, left- and right-side lobes).

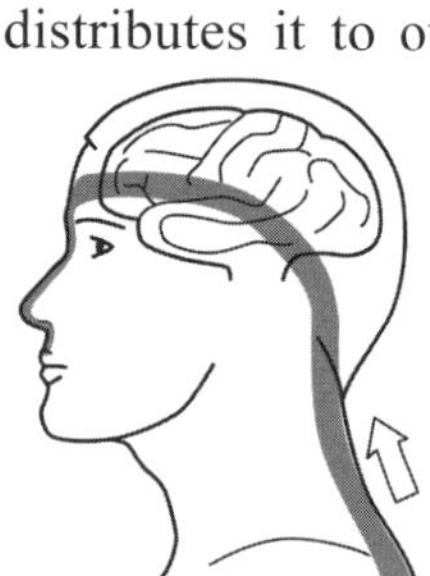

The Du channel's flow through the head is inhibited during sleep and during pause mode, thus inhibiting release of dopamine for movement at these times. The Du channel and its behavior when on pause is discussed in detail in chapter 13.

Fig. 4.1 The cranial path of the Du channel is a gently curving arc that passes from the brain stem and medulla oblongata, through the middle of the striatum, thalamus, and frontal lobe, and out to the forehead at the point between the eyebrows. For a more complete drawing of the entire Du channel, see Fig. 13.2, p.141.

The thalamus

The thalamus is like a little nut right in the center of the midbrain. It regulates internal sensory awareness, including the feeling that you are *inside* your body. The striatum is larger than the thalamus and wraps around the back, top, and front of the thalamus. The thalamus is the location of what western doctors refer to as electrical "static" in people with Parkinson's. This "static" has long been assumed to be the cause of the PD tremor.

As a side note, I hypothesize that the *origin* of the electrical "static" driving the tremor is in the sacrum (bone at the bottom of the spine), not the thalamus. I have seen that, in people with PD, when the pause-driven sacral tremor is temporarily turned off (using a type of visualization exercise described in the book *Stuck on Pause*), the *brain's* internal tremor also ceases. But during napping or deep calm, when the brains' internal tremor merely slows or seems to *temporarily* stop, the tremor in the sacrum continues.

The static in the thalamus seem to merely echo the electrical agitation in the sacrum. Whether or not the internal (sacrum and brain) tremoring also manifests visibly in the *physical* body depends on 1) the degree of alertness and the degree of concern the person is experiencing at the moment, as well as 2) the degree of atrophy and mental disconnect in the specific body areas that have become prone to tremoring.

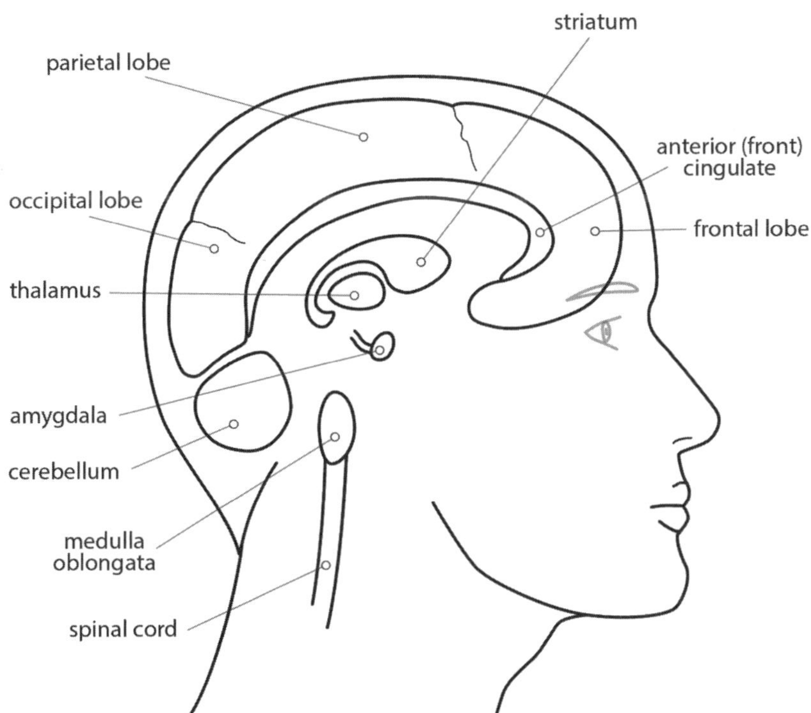

Fig. 4.2 A few brain areas

The assumption has long been that the problem in Parkinson's starts in the substantia nigra. This is due to visible changes in the substantia nigra seen in autopsies of people with Parkinson's. However, the recovery symptoms and behaviors I've seen when people recover from Parkinson's suggest that the actual brain sources of the movement inhibition and the visible, external tremor are the striatum and thalamus, respectively.

The decline in the number of *active* dark cells in the substantia nigra is very likely just a *side effect* of the brain being on pause over the long term, causing automatic motor function to be chronically inhibited. Again, the substantia nigra changes are probably *not* the underlying cause of Parkinson's. These changes are most likely a *side effect* of long-term use of pause mode – just as are all the other symptoms of PD.

When pause turns off, patients' recovery symptoms suggest that the long-unemployed substantia nigra cells once again produce and distribute that portion of the brain's dopamine that's used for automatic motor function and a few other brain jobs.

Channel theory intersecting with western medical thinking about the brain

Based on Chinese channel theory that says Du channel qi flow through the midbrain is significantly reduced during sleep and *extremely* reduced during pause, I propose that during sleep and during pause mode, activity in the striatum and thalamus, both smack in the middle of the Du channel's flow through the brain, is correspondingly decreased.

The striatum is recognized in western medicine as being the primary source of dopamine input for the rest of the lower midbrain area (the substantia nigra and basal ganglia) and is especially crucial for producing automatic movement. During sleep and pause modes, because electrical flow through the midbrain is reduced, flow through the striatum is reduced. Automatic movement is thereby inhibited. This is a good design: you don't want to be running around like a chicken with its head cut off when you are asleep or while trying to not die from a potentially mortal injury.

At the same time, decreased electrical flow through the midbrain when sleeping or on pause causes decreased electrical flow through the *thalamus*, causing inhibition of internal (not skin) sensory function. This is also all to the good while you are trying to sleep or focusing on not dying. This inhibition of the thalamus while on pause contributes to the inhibition of some types of pain, an inhibition that has long been associated with mortal injuries: as the old folklore tells us, "mortal injuries don't hurt." [1]

(Other neurological behaviors, such as the release of endorphins from the bases of the spinal nerves during pause, also contribute to the inhibition of pain from a potentially mortal injury.)

---

[1] The thalamus has recently been hypothesized to be a "location of consciousness" in the brain. Anesthetized, unconscious primates with electrodes at various locations in their brains became conscious when the electrodes at the thalamus were activated – overriding the anesthesia. They woke up. When the electrode stimulation was turned off, they dropped back into unconsciousness – once more under the influence of the anesthesia. Anesthesia works by putting a person into a high degree of pause mode.

The therapy for people with self-induced pause – therapy that consists of stimulating the thalamus and striatum by doing simple, mentally focused exercises and thus turning off pause – uses the exact same principles as in this experiment: the electrical stimulation of the primates' thalami temporarily turns off the effects of their channel qi running in pause (anesthesia) mode. But people with PD can learn to *lastingly* turn back on the currents that flow through the midbrain using visualization and other techniques – instead of using electrodes.

https://www.inverse.com/mind-body/tiny-area-of-the-brain-could-enable-consciousness

Striatum + thalamus
THERAPY

I propose that, while on pause, normal striatum and thalamus behavior is inhibited by the changes in channel qi flow that are characteristic of pause mode. *But* when the body has finally become physically stabilized following the trauma, that's when the sacrum and thalamus should begin their low-level, tremor-activating behavior. The low-level, nattering electrical signal in the thalamus can get your conscious attention: you begin to notice the internal agitation and maybe tremor in time with it, either visibly or internally.

The electrical current that drives the tremor can be thought of as a little starter motor, one that gives off a tiny, wobbly, static-y vibration. This vibration starts the mental processes that assess the safety of the *external* situation. This assessment determines whether or not it's now safe enough to turn parasympathetic and sympathetic modes back on. When parasympathetic mode and sympathetic mode do kick back in, the big electrical engines of these modes surge through the midbrain and sacrum. The brain "motor" purrs smoothly: the little "starter motor" current and its wobbly, tremor-inducing effects are turned off.

Allopathic doctors see the electrical "static" in the thalamus of people with Parkinson's as pathological. It is actually normal behavior following a steep drop-off in overall body amperage that occurs during life-threatening trauma or body-wide anesthesia. The "static" is the first sign that the body has *internally* stabilized enough and is ready to come out of pause…if the coast is now clear.

Based on how *non*-Parkinson's people respond to their trauma-related, short-term visible or internal tremors that occur just before coming out of pause, the tremor seems to be a helpful signal, not a pathology. The tremor says to the brain, "The body now feels biologically stable on the *inside* and we're starting to move a low-energy current through the body preparatory to turning on the high-energy current (the full-bore Du channel). Is the perimeter now safe?"

A somewhat common folk misconception holds that the Parkinson's tremor must be due to excessively high adrenaline levels. This is not the case. Many people with Parkinson's have greatly *lowered* levels of adrenaline. After recovering, some people have to learn how to re-start their adrenal glands if they don't start back up automatically.

– Fun with physics: the sacrum and the midbrain are located equidistantly from the two ends of the external Du channel. According to conservation of energy principles as taught in high school physics classes, changes that happen at distance x on one end of a closed electrical circuit will be replicated – in reverse – at distance x from the *other* end of the closed circuit. When detecting the flow of channel qi, one can often feel these "matching" or "paired" glitches: paired aberrant electrical behaviors along the path of a given channel.

This can be very helpful in medical diagnostics because very often a pain with no apparent cause at a particular location on some channel is being caused by a channel blockage at a matching distance from the *opposite* end of the same channel – a spot that might not hurt but might have an unhealed injury.

On the Du channel, because of their symmetrical locations, electrical phenomena in the sacrum and thalamus areas can behave as a pair: an oppositely-matched set.

One patient, after learning how to temporarily isolate and mentally turn off the sensation of low-energy, steady static (tremor) coming from her sacrum by visualizing a healthy, large surge of current flowing through the sacrum and coccyx and into the Du channel, said that the cessation of the static reminded her of getting back up to speed on her bicycle after having been at a full stop while balancing with her feet on the pedals. When stopped at a traffic light on her bicycle and keeping her feet on the pedals, the bike wobbles as she tries to stay upright. When the light changes to green, when she can power forward and resume the smooth, gyroscopic balance of a moving bicycle, the wobble from lack of forward momentum ceases to exist. The *low*-energy current causing electrical static (tremor) in the sacrum and its matching static in the thalamus feels sort of like the low-energy wobble from trying to maintain balance on an *almost* motionless bike.

The midbrain on pause

In order to turn off the pause-induced inhibition of dopamine release so that one can resume automatic (parasympathetic mode-type) motor function, a person must take specific steps to come out of pause. The brain isn't even allowed to *start* this process until the body *feels* physically stabilized: the blood pressure is stable; the person has stopped bleeding out; and so on. The internal *feeling* of stability is processed by the thalamus: the resumption of a feeling of biological stability then initiates the tremor.

If and when, in response to the query from the tremor, the conscious sensory functions of vision, hearing, smell, and/or touch confirm that the surroundings are now safe, the brain allows the resumption of the normal, awake-time flood of energy through the midbrain. The three physical moves (the deep breath, the head bobble, and the spinal shimmy) occur when the brain announces "All clear!" Following those three moves, pause turns off.

Then, the resumption of strong flow of energy in the most powerful current in the body, the spine- and brain-traversing Du channel, fully activates the striatum and thalamus. The weak, low-energy flow of starter current that caused the tremor-related vibrations then ceases.

In Type II, III, and IV Parkinson's disease, the channel qi flow is *physically* blocked or is stuck somewhere due to inertia. So pause-mode circuitries remain in place. The body is stuck between the first and second steps for coming out of pause: the tremor and the assessment process have started. However, because of some *physical injury* or inertia impeding the flow of channel qi, the body keeps running in the pause-mode electrical patterns. The body *cannot* turn off pause, *cannot* create the "we are safe now" large current that should flow through the sacrum and the midbrain after pause turns off. [1]

But in self-induced pause...

While in self-induced pause, the brain is evidently not able to respond correctly to the tremor because it has been *commanded* to be numb: to stay on pause. Based on patient responses and behaviors, the brain seems unable to respond positively to the tremor's question. The tremor is saying, "Hello! I'm feeling stable inside; are we safe on the outside?" And the brain, as per previous instruction, refuses to even consider the possibility that "the perimeter is now safe." Which means, I hypothesize, that the person is *mentally*, not physically, stuck in between the first and second steps of coming out of pause.

---

[1] Detailed information on how the channel qi schematics differ in the four neurological modes is provided in chapters 9 through 14 of *Tracking the Dragon*, available at JaniceHadlock.com.

In Type I PD from self-induced pause, the brain replies to the query with, "The perimeter can *never* be safe; we've been instructed to be numb to physical or emotional pain (be in pause mode: stay on the verge of death)."

The body tremor repeats the question, "Are we safe *now*?"

"Never."

"Now?"

"Never."

This mental impasse seems to be the underlying cause of Parkinson's from self-induced pause: Type I PD.

A person who has both Type I and Type II Parkinson's has both a physical blockage *and* a mental instruction preventing him from coming out of pause.

Again, in Type II, III, and IV PD, the channel qi in the body is *physically* stuck in pause circuits because of some unhealed injury *or* because the circuits have gotten *stuck* in the biological pause pattern due to a trauma and simply failed to go back to normal (turn off pause) when the trauma was resolved.

In Type I PD, the *mind* has been commanded to stay in the pause pattern. The relentless internal tremor and the urgency to come out of pause that it impels is countered by the brain's refusal to even *consider* that the world is once again safe.

So many people with Parkinson's have told me something along the lines of, "I'm always stepping on the gas and the brakes at the same time." Or that they are relentlessly commanding their body to "get going" but the brain *refuses* to make it happen or doesn't know *how* to make it happen.

With Types II, III, and IV PD, specific physical therapies restore the correct flow of channel qi. (Type III might require a small amount of mental re-training, but nothing as dramatic as the change required to turn off Type I PD). With Type I, the brain needs to learn how to activate the striatum and thalamus, the brain areas that run vigorously when a person feels safe. When currents run at healthy levels in these brain areas, a person automatically feels safe. The old mental instruction that initiated pause mode is neutralized. Pause can turn off. Oppositely, negative thoughts *diminish* the amount of current flowing through the midbrain even if a person is *not* on pause or sleeping. Negative thoughts *increase* the flow of energy in channels on the sides of the brain – channel qi that regulates behaviors in the in the left and right lobes of the brain.

When I write "sides of the brain," I'm writing in gross generalities. Some very *specific* electrical circuits drive the fear responses. For example, the brain areas just under the paths of the left and ride side Urinary Bladder (UB) channels, brain areas that include the amygdala, have increased activity in response to a surge in the UB channels. This surge occurs in response to fear, rage, or negative thoughts. "Negative thoughts" refers to attitudes such as pessimism, fear, and anger, and seeing the glass as half-empty as opposed to half-full. The *increase*, the fear-based surge, of the energy in the head portion of the UB channel simultaneously *reduces* the flow in the midbrain portion of the nearby *Du* channel, which flows in the opposite direction. The physics behind this paired, see-saw behavior will be addressed in the chapter about pause-mode biology.

The main point here is that, only when a person feels safe can they turn off the Type I PD self-instruction to "feel no pain" (be on pause mode). To feel safe, one needs to maximize the amount of current flowing through the midbrain, from the medulla oblongata, through the striatum, and on to the point between the eyebrows. Maximization of the Du current in the midbrain automatically diminishes the amount of current in the UB channel running along the *sides* of the head.

Turning off self-induced pause: a brain bypass

The brain scan research to be discussed in chapter twelve helped me devise exercises for people with Type I PD, mental exercises that vigorously stimulate activity in the striatum and thalamus directly.

Based on my patients' experiences, the mental exercises do an end run around Step 2 for turning off pause: sensory confirmation that the surroundings are safe. The exercises increase channel qi flow in the striatum and thalamus and can *bypass* the conscious, *sensory* (vision, hearing, smelling, touching) confirmation of safety and *directly* increase current flow in the striatum and thalamus.

This increase in current flow can eventually get enough stimulation going through these areas that the body and mind both *feel* as if they are safe again, and go on to activate the physical moves that complete the termination of pause – thus *overriding* the long-abiding instruction to "feel no physical and/or emotional pain." When this electrical override occurs, the old instruction is automatically turned off.

Again, the direct, mental activation of the striatum and thalamus, when powerful enough, seems to create the message "I'm safe now." This makes it possible for the last three steps for coming out of pause mode to kick in – a spontaneous deep breath, an automatic, spontaneous head bobble, and an automatic, spontaneous spinal shimmy.

Once the moves are complete and pause is turned off, the brain areas and body behaviors promptly go back to full, healthy function again; they "come back to life" – just as they are designed to do when a person is no longer hovering on the cusp of death. This set of movements can't be forced. They should occur automatically, spontaneously, when a person finally feels safe enough to turn off pause.

Going through the motions

Forced physical movements performed *without* feeling safe will *not* turn off pause. If the striatum is *not* anticipating feeling safe due to pause-type electrical circuitry from a still unhealed physical injury *or* from self-induced pause, just going through the last three physical steps for turning off pause will *not* work. Pause will *not* turn off. In fact, the body might physically resist attempts at wobbling the head and shivering along the spine. A person attempting these moves in spite of a brain message saying "I'm not safe yet" often finds that his body will refuse to obey his mental instructions to wobble the head or shake the spine. Even if he *can* force himself to make these movements, these moves will feel forced and unnatural, even *unsafe*.

Then again, if a person has actually healed from some pause-activating physical or emotional trauma and feels biologically safe *but* the channels never switched back to healthy flow patterns because of inertia in the channels, then in *that* case, prompting these movements *will* allow pause to turn off.

If you want to learn more about the various parts of the brain and their functions, excellent websites abound. For our purposes, the above is enough to be getting on with. Now, we can jump back into the subject of what actually causes Parkinson's and what is needed for recovery.

Chapter Five

Requirements for Recovery

Recovery from idiopathic Parkinson's disease requires three things: 1) correct diagnosis, 2) no brain damage from antiparkinson's medications and 3) in the case of *self-induced* dissociation or pause, the ability to understand the problem, and the desire and determination to mentally bring about changes in one's own thought patterns.

These next three chapters address these requirements.

Requirement 1: Correct Diagnosis

Starting with a good diagnosis is crucial. You will learn in upcoming chapters far more details than your neurologist ever learned in school regarding how to make an accurate diagnosis of idiopathic Parkinson's disease.

Having a solid diagnosis will also be of comfort to you when you recover and your doctor tells you that you never actually had PD: you were misdiagnosed.

My patients who have recovered have not *only* been told they were misdiagnosed, many have been accused of pretending to have Parkinson's in order to get early retirement, pity, or access to the mind-altering, euphoria-inducing (if you don't have idiopathic PD) medications. A cynical MD might also conclude that the presumably deceitful patient now wants to be lauded for their fake recovery.

I have learned that a patient doesn't stand a chance against a doctor with a frozen attitude. Also, many patients take their doctor's word for gospel.

One patient who attended the *free* clinic once a week for just over a year was thrilled when her dragging leg, tremor, bent arms, facial masking, slowness and rigidity slowly went away. Her symptoms had been worsening over two years and she had been diagnosed with Parkinson's. She had only Type II PD, and she'd been receiving Yin Tui Na at the free clinic for two semesters. However, after her victory visit to her neurologist, she was furious – with *me*.

"My MD said that, if my symptoms went away, my problems must have been caused by a pinched nerve. I spent all this time coming to Santa Cruz every week, and all I had wrong was a pinched nerve! I never had Parkinson's to begin with! I was just misdiagnosed! You should have noticed that from the start!"

Oppositely, a person who I never met emailed me a thank you after she recovered. She had been diagnosed six times. She had moved frequently due to work, and at each new location she had met with a new neurologist. Every one of them diagnosed or confirmed her diagnosis of Parkinson's. When she recovered, she didn't even bother to go back to her latest neurologist. She knew he would tell her she had been misdiagnosed. Still, she wanted me to know how *many* doctors had diagnosed her with PD prior to her complete recovery.

Misdiagnosis

In my clinic I saw many, many people who had been diagnosed with Parkinson's disease who clearly did *not* have PD. Usually, they had been very *obviously* misdiagnosed.

In many cases, these people had very *quickly* developed *one* or *two* symptoms similar to those of Parkinson's in *immediate* response to a surgery, injury, or a new medication.

For example, I saw a patient's post-surgical rigidity in the joint that was operated on then misdiagnosed as Parkinson's...in a person with *no* other symptoms of PD. I saw sudden-onset active tremor (as opposed to resting tremor) in response to a new heart medication that included tremor in its list of adverse effects that was misdiagnosed as Parkinson's in a person with *no* other symptoms of PD.

In so many of these obvious cases of misdiagnosis, the diagnosing MDs or surgeons had dismissed their own possible responsibility for the patient's new, sudden-onset symptom(s) by declaring that the new symptom was Parkinson's – a syndrome that cannot be confirmed with any test – thus clearing the MD from any responsibility for triggering the new symptom.

Based on autopsy studies, over thirty percent of people with a diagnosis of Parkinson's had none of the brain changes associated with PD and were presumed to have been misdiagnosed. Over thirty percent![1]

I saw an egregious misdiagnosis of Parkinson's based on an immediate-onset lack of arm swing due to a shoulder injury the night before. Her lack of arm swing wasn't Parkinson's-like. Her upper arm bone had become displaced from the shoulder socket and she literally could not swing the arm in a forward direction. The woman had *no* symptoms of Parkinson's, but had been given a diagnosis of PD by a qualified neurologist.

In the *many* cases of glaring misdiagnosis that I've seen, the patients' channels were *never* running in the pause circuits, although some of the channels, especially those in the immediate injury area, were often very obviously running incorrectly.

Oppositely, *all* of my correctly diagnosed Parkinson's patients were clearly running the electrical patterns that occur during pause.

---

[1] I regret that I can no longer put my finger on the several research papers that presented information on this subject. But I can say that in my own practice, at *least* twenty percent of the people who came to me because of a diagnosis of Parkinson's did not, in fact, have it. (I did not track these people and do not have exact numbers.)

Many of them had obvious misdiagnoses, as described above. Many others had some stuck or twisted joint that was preventing knee bending, wrist flexion or some other movement, and their grossly negligent neurologists had put the one or two symptoms down to Parkinson's.

If I could remove the one or two symptoms that had been misdiagnosed as PD in one or two hour-long sessions of physical therapy or acupuncture, I felt perfectly justified in telling the patient that they had been misdiagnosed.

Not one of these patients, to my knowledge, ever went back to inform the MD. They were just so tearfully glad to "get rid of the hopelessness of degenerative Parkinson's disease" that they didn't really care about follow-up. But then, they also didn't have the grim determination and drive of most people with Type I Parkinson's, necessary qualities for generating self-induced pause *or* for taking on an MD with really bad diagnostic skills.

Joke: What do you call a doctor or acupuncturist who graduates at the very bottom of their class? Answer: a doctor or acupuncturist.

For another example of uncertainty of diagnosis, consider the infamous Eldopa study of 2002. At the time, increasing numbers of research studies were proving that dopamine-enhancing drugs such as those used for treating PD are addictive and can cause lasting brain damage and drug-induced parkinsonism.

In response, a drug company-led study was cleverly designed to make it *appear* that dopamine-enhancing antiparkinson's drugs do *not* accelerate symptoms of Parkinson's. (Brain scans taken as a parallel part of this study proved that, in fact, the drugs *did* cause levels of damage that correlated to dosage levels, so the scan results were left out of the published conclusion.) For this study, six top-level Parkinson's research MDs were enlisted. The plan was to have unanimous confirmation that each of the two hundred plus participants did, in fact, have idiopathic Parkinson's. Why such attention to correct diagnosis? Because it's well known that there is abundant misdiagnosis for this syndrome.

My point here, with regard to the difficulty of diagnosing Parkinson's disease based on ambiguous western medicine criteria is that those top, PD specialist MDs were so conflicted over *who* actually had Parkinson's that they finally agreed that any person for whom three of the six doctors gave a diagnosis of idiopathic Parkinson's could be used in the study.

The misdiagnoses cut both ways: a study undertaken by the non-profit group Parkinson's UK found that over twenty-five percent of the people who ended up, eventually, with a diagnosis of Parkinson's had *first* received an inaccurate diagnosis of some other, non-Parkinson's syndrome. Most of these people had been prescribed medications, and some had even had surgeries – which of course didn't solve the problem – and were finally diagnosed with Parkinson's after the PD symptoms became more clear-cut.[1]

This is just to show you how hard it can be to make an accurate diagnosis of idiopathic Parkinson's using the vague western medicine standards.

Diagnosing idiopathic Parkinson's

You cannot trust your doctors to make an accurate diagnosis, nor should you blame them. The doctors are doing what they were taught in school.

So before you even try to decide which of the four *types* of idiopathic Parkinson's disease you have, you will first want to confirm that you actually have Parkinson's.

To qualify for a diagnosis of basic, idiopathic Parkinson's disease, a person must have a certain number of symptoms that fall under four categories: rigidity, poverty of movement (slowness, weakness, and difficulty in initiating certain movements), postural instability, and tremor. Details of these rules for an official western diagnosis are in chapter fifteen. Chapter fifteen will help you diagnose what you have and will go into this subject in *extreme* detail: far more detail than you will find in your neurologist's pamphlet on Parkinson's or on the internet.

Diagnosing becomes even more certain if one *also* uses the electrical currents running just under the skin as another confirmation for the diagnosis. If one has a sense of

---

[1] http://www.telegraph.co.uk/science/2019/12/30/one-quarter-people-parkinsons-disease-wrongly-diagnosed-survey

the electrical variations that occur during pause mode and has a friend who has learned to *feel* these variations, diagnosis becomes fairly straightforward.

If you think you or a loved one might have Parkinson's, go through the steps in chapter fifteen for confirming this syndrome. If you confirm the diagnosis is idiopathic Parkinson's, chapter seventeen will explain how to determine what *type*(*s*) of Parkinson's it is. In chapter eighteen, you will be directed to the appropriate treatment for that type.

If a person has more than one type of PD, instructions are provided that explain the safest *sequence* for treating the different types.

Chapter Six

Requirement 2: No Physical Brain Damage

Another requirement for recovery is not having brain damage caused by toxins or drugs, including antiparkinson's drugs. The symptoms from this type of damage are referred to as drug- or toxin-induced parkinsonism. Although these syndromes sport the name "parkinsonism," they have nothing to do with idiopathic Parkinson's disease.

The word idiopathic means "no known cause." The use of the word idiopathic to describe basic, or "classic," Parkinson's disease is no longer accurate since we now know what causes it. Even so, I still use the word now and then to mean "classic" Parkinson's when I need to differentiate between idiopathic PD and drug- and toxin-induced parkinson*ism*.

When *some* doctors refer to a syndrome as "parkinsonism" that might mean the patient has one or some symptoms *similar* to those of Parkinson's but they do not actually have idiopathic Parkinson's disease. Then again, some MDs, unsure of themselves, will give a diagnosis of parkinsonism to imply "might be early-stage PD." Other MDs use a diagnosis of essential tremor in the same way, to mean "might be early-stage PD, but I don't want to frighten the patient with a firm PD diagnosis."

These evasive diagnoses reflect wisdom and kindness on the part of the doctor. Many people with Type I Parkinson's go into an almost immediate tailspin with severe worsening of symptoms as soon as they receive the diagnosis of Parkinson's. To extend quality of life, many wise doctors who are silently thinking "It's Parkinson's disease" will nevertheless give the milder diagnosis of essential tremor or parkinsonism, thus giving the patient an extra year or two of mild symptoms before the slowly but steadily worsening symptoms call for changing the diagnosis to idiopathic Parkinson's, after which the symptoms might *rapidly* worsen.

For an example of what can happen to a patient upon receiving a diagnosis of Parkinson's disease, I had one middle-aged patient who, after his diagnosis with PD, went from very mild symptoms to barely able to move over the *very* short period of six months. When he discovered the Parkinson's Recovery Project information on the internet and learned that Parkinson's was curable, even *before* he started working on recovery his symptoms *immediately* went back to approximately the mild level he'd had six months earlier. This rapid worsening of symptoms in response to bad news, including a diagnosis of Parkinson's disease, is *very* common in people with Type I PD.

Back in the days when there was no effective treatment for Parkinson's disease, giving the patient a relatively milder diagnosis such as essential tremor or parkinsonism was an intelligent and compassionate approach, because this prevented an immediate, mentally-based, rapid worsening of symptoms. Today, however, not only is there an effective treatment, but the sooner it is implemented, the easier and faster is the recovery process. There is no longer a need for doctors to hide the diagnosis for as long as possible. Just the reverse.

Channel diagnostics

If a person is told he has essential tremor or parkinsonism *but* is running the electrical circuitry of pause, then he *does* in fact have the underlying cause of idiopathic Parkinson's disease, no matter what the diagnosing MD has declared.

In my limited experience, *every* patient with idiopathic Parkinson's disease was running all or most of the very distinctive electrical schematics of pause. There are four different ways to get there. But in every case, the resultant schematics will be very similar. And, although no two patients will have the exact same combination of symptoms, the symptoms that do manifest *will* all conform with what might happen when the channel qi is running in pause mode.

People with *only* drug- or toxin-induced parkinsonism do *not* have these circuits of pause mode running body-wide. Their symptoms do *not* create the same overall "look" as the symptoms of Parkinson's. They *do* have brain damage. I do *not* have any suggestions for people with this type of brain damage. This book does *not* address the treatment of drug- or toxin-induced parkinsonism.

Parkinsonism from dopamine-enhancing drugs

Nor does this book address the problems of people who have taken dopamine-enhancing antiparkinson's drugs for more than a few weeks. These people might have started out with idiopathic, pause-based Parkinson's disease, but within a few weeks of using the dopamine-enhancing drugs, they might already have incurred enough brain damage from the drugs to create drug-induced parkinsonism. This means they now have two problems: whatever caused the pause-type symptoms of idiopathic Parkinson's *plus* the brain damage that causes drug-induced parkinsonism.

Even if they recover from idiopathic Parkinson's, they might still want to take the antiparkinson's medications because they might now have drug-created damage in some of the brain's several dopamine-producing and regulating systems. A person who *is* on pause is *less* susceptible to the cumulative, adverse effects of dopamine-enhancing medication. At manufacturer-suggested low dosage levels (rarely prescribed), the adverse effects will accumulate slowly, maybe over five to ten years.

But a person who is *not* or is *no longer* on pause and is taking antiparkinson's medications in order to help with symptoms of *drug-induced* parkinsonism might *more* rapidly develop the nightmarish adverse effects of the medication, within a few years, or a few months, or, in some cases, within a few weeks. For example, all the members of the group of illegal-drug users (*The Case of the Frozen Addicts, p.31*) who were the basis of the dead-dopamine cell theory, died in a short period of time after taking the high doses of L-dopa that afforded them some degree of motor function. People with idiopathic PD can tolerate L-dopa for years.

I have seen *rapid*, horrible, mental destruction and psychosis in people who continued their previously safe levels of dopamine-enhancing antiparkinson's medication after pause was turned off. A person who has turned off pause *but* who still has symptoms of drug-induced parkinsonism might feel he *needs* to use the medication because of his brain damage-induced movement problems. He might even be pressured to use the now more powerful drugs against his will by his doctors or loved ones – I've seen a lot of this.

In a way, being on pause acts as a brake on the adverse effects of the drugs. So if a person does have drug-induced parkinsonism because of taking antiparkinson's medications, in *addition* to having idiopathic PD, he might be better off *not* trying to recover and just keeping his doses as low as possible while staying the course. Since 2003, I have not worked with a person who has ever taken any dopamine-enhancing antiparkinson's drug for more than three weeks. The reasons are explained in great detail in my book *Medications of Parkinson's or Once Upon a Pill: Patient Experiences with dopamine-enhancing drugs and supplements*

The early days

None of my first six patients had ever taken antiparkinson's medications. They had recovered easily. After I'd seen these unexpected recoveries, I recruited volunteer patients from the local Parkinson's support group for free treatments. All the new patients from the support group *were* taking antiparkinson's drugs. When, instead of simply recovering, these new patients slid into what I inaptly named "partial recovery," a nightmarish condition described more fully in an upcoming chapter, my first thought was that this had something to do with the medications. I was only partly right.

All the patients in the free clinic (1998-2003) were asked to keep daily logs of their suddenly unpredictable, drug-related symptoms and their attempts to moderate their drug doses. In patients who started showing symptoms of recovery while still taking their meds, the end results were uniformly disastrous, leading either to death, or excruciating, super-human dyskinetic spasms and/or severe, irreversible psychosis. [1]

Scope-of-practice laws

When it came to dose changes, I insisted that patients work with their prescribing physicians. I am a licensed acupuncturist (LAc). In California, a licensed acupuncturist has earned at *least* a bachelor's degree and has a Master's degree in Chinese medicine

---

[1] *Before* I read Dr. Sacks' book *Awakening* (footnoted on page 33), I saw the exact same unbelievable, violent, even fatal phenomena in my patients who recovered while they were still taking L-dopa. I was deeply relieved when I read his descriptions of his patients' responses to L-dopa because they confirmed what my patients and I were having trouble believing.

But at least, in the early days of L-dopa research, after Dr. Sacks' findings, MDs dosed with caution. Today, more than fifty years later, the very real dangers of quickly increasing or decreasing dopamine-enhancing medications are evidently no longer emphasized in medical schools. For example, one of my patients was told by his neurologist, "If you want an extra boost for going to a party or something, just double your dose" [of Sinemet, the standard dopamine-enhancing drug for Parkinson's in the USA for many decades now].

The manufacturer's instructions explicitly state that a person should *never* double the dose of Sinemet, even if a previous dose was skipped. Also, the manufacturers emphasize that people should be started at a low dose and *stay* at that low dose for ten weeks, by which point the full benefit of the drug will begin to manifest. However, most of the doctors that prescribed for my patients had irresponsibly told their patients at the outset to "increase your dose by one pill per day until you are seeing a benefit." This leads to grossly excessive dosages, with many patients taking three to six times as much L-dopa as is recommended by the manufacturer. This, in turn, leads to *much* earlier onset of the painful adverse effects and the ineffectiveness of the medication.

In the 1990s, when I started my research on Parkinson's, the literature reported that patients typically had five to ten years before the drugs were no longer effective. Today, in 2020, because of much higher starting doses, the readily available literature reports that the average effective span is now only two to five years.

which includes at least four years of medical schooling (the more recent licensees have five and a half years) including interning, and in California is legally considered to be a primary care medical provider, licensed to diagnose, prescribe, and treat *within* the scope of practice of Chinese medicine. We are required to study western pharmacology in school, but we are *not* legally able to give prescriptive advice about pharmaceutical medications. As an LAc, giving prescriptive advice or even *commentary* to a patient *or* to an MD regarding an *individual's* prescription medications is illegal.

Some of the recovering patients told their doctors about their symptom changes and asked what they should do about their increased adverse effects due to now-excessive medication levels. In *every* case, the doctor assured the patient with some grossly incorrect statement such as, "If you recover from Parkinson's, you can just stop taking the medications at that time."

Most of the patients' attempts to modify their suddenly over-strong drugs were tragically unsuccessful. Some patients became violently exuberant. Though determined to *reduce* their meds, they found themselves helplessly and joyously doubling and then tripling their doses over a matter of days. Others became paranoid and/or psychotic, complete with wild hallucinations. These behaviors were *far* more extreme than anything I ever saw in later years in un-medicated PD patients with mere partial recovery.

Over the course of that project, the *only* patients who died of neuroleptic malignant syndrome from over-fast drug reduction were the ones who followed their doctors' recommendations. Neuroleptic malignant syndrome is a sudden inability to regulate core life processes such as heart rate, breathing, and temperature regulation: the same syndrome that can kill a person going through withdrawal from other types of highly addictive drugs. Their doctors had invariably advised them to come off their drugs "slowly: over a few days" or "...over a week." A safer span would have been more like ten weeks to eighteen months, depending on a host of factors. [1]

For over fifty years it has been well known that over-fast reduction of L-dopa-based drugs can be fatal. But since the early, careful days of exploration with these drugs in the 1960s, many doctors have become cavalier and now treat these mind-altering drugs that have long-term adverse effects and which accumulate and disperse in the brain over months, not hours, as if they were similar to aspirin or antacids.

Overmedication can also be fatal. Two of my patients died when they became grossly overmedicated because of recovery. Their massive brain injuries were incurred during violent, super-human dyskinetic spasms. One patient was flung headfirst into the edge of a countertop. The other was flung onto a doorframe and then to the floor. One of these patients had wanted to reduce her suddenly over-strong medications. The Mother

[1] When some of my recovering patients had stroke-like symptoms after making a modest decrease in their recently (1997) approved dopamine-*agonist* drug, I wrote to the manufacturers asking what the dose reductions should be because their warning only said: "Reduce slowly." They wrote back, "Reduce slowly." I wrote again, and listed the symptoms my patients had experienced after making what seemed like very small decreases. They wrote back again: "Reduce slowly." However, they did take notice: the next year's edition of the *Physician's Drug Handbook* included new information: they quoted in my exact wording the details that I had sent to them about the adverse effects of making reductions from these drugs. There was still no specification of what they meant by "Reduce slowly."

Superior of her order forbid it, saying the nun had to follow her doctor's orders. The other was a neurologist who was recovering from PD. Despite his intellectual desire to reduce his medications, after turning off pause he could *not* reduce them: his cravings for the drugs grew daily stronger, as did his violent spasms.

Another patient who was a psychiatrist was shocked by his inability to reduce his medications even though he became grossly overmedicated. "I know all about these drugs! I'm a doctor, for God's sake! So why can't I reduce my dosage?"

According to the scope of practice laws for acupuncturists, I could not say a word to my patients *or* to their doctors about their medications or dosages. Doing so would be one of the easiest ways to lose my license. Legally, I *could* direct my patients to publicly available, generalized, written information about these drugs. So I wrote a quick booklet describing what I was learning about the drugs and posted it on the Parkinson's Recovery Project website for free download. Even today, anyone who asks me for advice about medications is directed to my free book, *Medications of Parkinson's: Once Upon a Pill*.

Over the next few years, the patients' drug-dose/ symptom logs proved to be a treasure trove. Poring through every detail of the patients' reports, I was eventually able to piece together logical answers for *why* the patient reactions to dosage changes of L-dopa-related drugs, as well as other dopamine-enhancing drugs, were highly predictable even though they have long been officially considered "unpredictable."

One glaringly obvious reason they are considered unpredictable is that researchers have wrongly assumed that the short, six-hour half-life of these drugs in the bloodstream means that half the drug is out of the patient's *system* within six hours. Ignored is the fact that these drugs cross the blood-brain barrier and very *slowly* accumulate in the brain, coming to equilibrium with the blood surges of the drug over *months*. The *brain* is where the drugs do their *work*.

Based on my collected data, I hypothesized that after the drugs pass the blood-brain barrier, they then slowly accumulate in the brain. Once in the brain, they are not subject to the half-life clearance that occurs in the liver and kidneys. Based on an almost five-year study that I ran from 1998 through 2002, it appears that approximately ten weeks are required for the *brain* levels of dopamine to come to equilibrium with the dose-related surges of L-dopa that have been going on two or three times a day in the *bloodstream*.

The drug manufacturers have known *something* about this right along, although they probably do not understand the full implications for dosage change. After all, many wrote in their pamphlets and drug literature that the drugs should be maintained at a low dose so the drugs can slowly accumulate in the brain to the point that effectiveness begins, usually around ten weeks *or*, with certain drugs such as the dopamine agonists, the patients should be brought up to full dosage very slowly and carefully: over a period of ten weeks – or as some of them put it, two to three months. The manufacturer of the most common antiparkinson's medication in the USA, Sinemet (levodopa/carbidopa), writes in its literature that *ten weeks* at the lowest, safest dose are required to slowly and safely attain the expected antiparkinson benefits of the drug.

Another of my hypotheses based on patient logs holds that the drugs also break down and disperse very slowly from their holding tanks in the brain. This hypothesis is what allowed long-term dose-related symptom changes to be highly predictable, once I figured out the breakdown rate. The very slow breakdown rate also means that a person who rapidly decreases or abruptly stops taking his medication won't get the full result of that decrease or stoppage for nearly ten weeks. During that time, if his body goes into failure when it crosses over the line into not enough brain dopamine to sustain core functions, usually about twelve to twenty days after abruptly stopping or excessively decreasing the medication, it is too late to do anything about it: no matter how much dopamine you shove into the *bloodstream* of a person whose brain is shutting down, it will take more than a week of high bloodstream levels to slowly restore enough dopamine in the various *brain* structures to keep the patient alive. And this one-week restoration scenario is physically impossible: by the end of the one week of pumping up the blood with dopamine, the patient who started having the *immediately* lethal symptoms of neuroleptic malignant syndrome will already have been dead for about six days.

A second reason that the drugs have long been wrongly considered "unpredictable" is that they are hideously addictive and cause long-lasting *alterations* in the brain's dopamine processing *throughout* the brain – not just in the motor-regulating areas of the midbrain. So a person with Parkinson's, one who had poor motor function but had enough dopamine to have stability in *core* brain function (breathing, heart rate, and temperature regulation) *prior* to starting the medications might have a highly altered brain following his drug use: he might no longer have enough *core* brain stability to survive *withdrawal* from the drugs.

Thirdly, the drugs cause lasting brain *damage* in the neurons that stimulate the motor areas of the brain – damage that causes drug-induced parkinsonism. So a person who has used the drugs long enough to see a benefit might also already have developed some degree of drug-induced parkinsonism, in *addition* to having idiopathic Parkinson's disease. This means that, even if such a person recovers from idiopathic PD, he might still need the medications to counter his motor symptoms of *drug*-induced parkinsonism.

But here's another problem: as mentioned earlier, the drugs are far more powerful, damaging, and mind-altering in a person who no longer has Parkinson's. The drugs behave differently, and much more powerfully, in a person who has *only* drug-induced parkinsonism. In our free clinic, we saw that when a *moderately* medicated patient's pause-type electrical patterns suddenly turned off, that's when the drug-based psychoses and hallucinations characteristic of severe *over*-medication suddenly showed up. We learned the hard way that a person with PD who was taking dopamine-enhancing antiparkinson's medications had about three days after the circuitry of pause turned off before the severe psychoses and hallucinations began…unless they got off their medication within three days. And if, on their MD's advice, they got off their medication in just three days, they died twelve to twenty days later of neuroleptic malignant syndrome from over-fast drug withdrawal. These people now had normal *potential* for dopamine release for motor function because they'd turned off pause *but* it seemed as if dopamine levels and other parts of the dopamine system had become altered in the *core* brain areas, as well – not just the movement areas. The depletion in the *core* areas when they reduced their medications too rapidly is what killed them.

If patients slowly, over a year or more, reduced their medication and finally got off of it, and only then did either the mind re-training exercises and/or hands-on therapy for self-induced pause, pseudo-pause from injury, or both, and *then* recovered from idiopathic Parkinson's, they might still be *somewhat* immobilized or tremoring mildly due to the brain damage of drug-induced parkinsonism. But at least the latter syndrome doesn't necessarily have the same internal sense of doom as Parkinson's from self-induced pause. And these people usually had painless, "soft" muscle slowness or immobility as opposed to the *painful* rigid-muscle slowness or immobility of PD.

I had one patient who slowly, over more than eighteen months, got off all three types of his antiparkinson's medications (an anticholinergic, Sinemet, and Requip, a dopamine-agonist drug). He then recovered from his very advanced case of Type II Parkinson's that had developed in the twenty years since his diagnosis. After recovering, his tremor was gone. He had a beautiful smile again. His motor function was very slow due to his drug-induced parkinsonism, to the point that he could not walk. Eventually his wife, now in her seventies, moved him into a nursing home. He too was in his early 70s.

However, he was very comfortable in bed and no longer had the painful rigidity of Parkinson's. He could even *slowly* but smoothly move his deeply relaxed arms and use his hands and fingers a little, which previously he had not been able to do, even with his antiparkinson's medications. When I first met him, his unbendable fingers stuck straight out and his hands flapped constantly, all fingers moving as a group, like flippers, from excess muscle tension from the medications. His bent arms had been as if glued to his sides. His face had been utterly expressionless.

Although, years later, he was in a nursing home, he felt he was far better off having the mere slowness and limpness of residual drug-induced parkinsonism than he had been from having Parkinson's. The last time I visited him he showed this off, with a big post-Parkinson's grin when, from his bed, he bid me farewell with a graceful "pranam" (raised his hands, placed them palm to palm, raised them to his forehead, and then bowed at the waist). There was no way he could have performed this smooth gesture back when I first met him. But though fluid, he was still weak, in a nursing home, unable to walk or care for himself.

When he was still living at home and finally got off the last of his medications, he was shocked that he basically had no knowledge of himself during the twenty years in which he'd been taking the drugs. His loyal, loving, very intelligent and sweetly dignified wife remarked, "His very last, once-a-week fraction of a pill of Sinemet was taken just over a week ago and yesterday, for the first time since he started taking it, he asked me how I was doing and expressed concern for my financial situation, asking if I was going to be OK given that he hadn't worked in nearly fifteen years. This was the first time he'd shown any awareness of me or my concerns since he started taking those damned drugs."

So neither he nor his wife wanted him to go back on dopamine-enhancing drugs even though they might have given him a bit of mobility…at a very high cost. They both had seen what had happened to other people in the clinic: that the psychoses and insanity from those drugs comes on a lot faster – maybe in days, not years – if the person taking the drugs has *only* drug-induced parkinsonism and no longer has idiopathic PD.

At the end of 2002, because of the medication-related tragedies, I ended the free clinic I'd led at the acupuncture college. At the same time, I announced that the Parkinson's Treatment team (another PD clinical project that I ran from the late 1990s to 2013 with four licensed acupuncturists, including me, all doing Yin Tui Na, not acupuncture) would *not* work with a person who had *ever* taken dopamine-enhancing drugs for more than three weeks, total.

The next year, in 2003, I wrote a much more complete version of the online Parkinson's medication booklet. This new book shared everything I'd learned about the medications *plus* the caveat that anyone who had ever taken dopamine-enhancing medications for more than three weeks might not be a good candidate for recovery. Again, the book is titled *Medications of Parkinson's: Once Upon a Pill.* It is available for free download at the Parkinson's Recovery Project website: www.PDrecovery.org.

One of the most important findings explained in the book, based on all those patient logs, was that no one died or underwent *severe*, life-threatening withdrawal symptoms *if* they never reduced the dose by more than ten percent at a time and then waited up to ten weeks, contingent upon symptom changes, before making the next reduction. This slow rate meant that most people with long-term (a year or more) drug use needed a year to a year and a half to safely get off their drugs.[1]

Because I am often asked about "natural" supplements like Macuna prupriens, please note that *anything* that elevates brain dopamine levels, whether pharmaceutical or herbal, is going to cause problems. This is discussed in the medications book.

This book also explicitly teaches how to safely decrease antiparkinson's drug dosages in order to reduce adverse effects from over-medication while not dying in the process. Drug reductions can often reduce or completely get rid of some of the more painful and distressing adverse effects of dopamine-enhancing medications, including the dyskinesias (uncontrollable muscle movements and powerful, excruciating spasms), sleepwalking, and the so-called "dementia of Parkinson's," which includes hallucinations. This book has been helpful to countless people, literally countless: we don't keep a counter on the Parkinson's Recovery Project website. But I've gotten thank-you emails from *many* people who've successfully used the information.

The "dementia of Parkinson's"

Prior to the introduction of dopamine-enhancing drugs for the treatment of Parkinson's, there was no such thing as the "dementia of Parkinson's." Just the opposite. Idiopathic Parkinson's was known as a syndrome in which the person, despite becoming mute and immobile, *never* lost his crisp cognitive function. Right up to the end, which was most often death from aspiration pneumonia, most people with Parkinson's retained their

[1] Nearly twenty years after I first published my findings on rate of change of brain dopamine levels from medications, findings that suggested safe withdrawal rates of a year to a year and a half, researchers in 2019 announced that people taking seratonin- and dopamine-enhancing anti-depressant medications should probably take a year to a year and a half to come off of them.

I know that the information I put on the internet has propagated – I have had new patients recite to me information "from the internet" explaining how a person will be safest if he never reduces his addictive drugs by more than ten percent at a time, and then waits while his body goes through the various stages of moderate withdrawal before making the next ten percent reduction – quoting *exactly* the information published in my book and *not* replicated in any study other than mine, that I know of. (You don't see a lot of research on how to *reduce* or *get off* of drugs. There is *not* a lot of grant money in the field of pharmaceutical-drug *reduction*. Not at *all*.) These patients have had no idea that I was the one who first put that information out there. I get a kick out of them telling me how to safely decrease dopamine-enhancing drugs in my own words. Now, twenty years later, this information, long available on the PDrecovery.org website and evidently also splashing around – unattributed – on various locations on the internet, is finally being tested and touted as surprising, *new* medical research.

As you can see, if there is not a significant *profit* motive for new information, change might come about very, very slowly in the research part of the medical world.

high intellect and alertness. Only after the dopamine-enhancing antiparkinson's drugs were introduced did the "dementia of Parkinson's" become a symptom PD.

The hallucinations and other mental aberrations that arise because of the medications are an absolutely logical side effect: taking these drugs is comparable to taking cocaine or methamphetamine several times a day, every day, for years. In fact, some of the MAO inhibitor drugs for Parkinson's do have methamphetamine in them. If a person takes this level of mind-altering stimulant drug(s) every day, three or more times a day, he will all too soon develop hallucinations, sleepwalking, and psychoses.

The healthy brain is supposed to *inhibit* the release of dopamine for movement during sleep. Not realizing this, many MDs have their Parkinson's patients space out their medications around the clock, presumably for "twenty-four hour coverage": coverage that is biologically inappropriate and even dangerous, as it increases the risk of sleep-walking, psychosis, and hallucinations. To better understand how each of the antiparkinson's drugs and the dopamine supplements such as Macuna pruriens works in the brain and why they cause the well-known adverse effects, please see *Medications of Parkinson's: Once Upon a Pill*. This book also explains *which* of the antiparkinson's drugs and supplements are dopamine-enhancing. This book is only available as a download at this time.

Please note: If you have ever taken dopamine-enhancing antiparkinson's drugs or supplements for more than a few weeks, you might not be a safe candidate for recovery. Please read *Medications of Parkinson's: Once Upon a Pill* to understand why.

People who are taking dopamine-enhancing drugs can have a hard time being objective about their own situation, due to the mind-altering effects of the drugs. The drugs can make a person be unrealistically, even blindly, optimistic. After all, the drugs work by making a person *temporarily* feel overwhelmingly safe – even invincible. That's also why these last few paragraphs have been highly redundant. I have a lot of experience trying to get through to a person who is taking antiparkinson's medications. As their spouses will attest, this is not always easy. Therefore, I highly recommend that a person taking these drugs who is considering trying to recover ask a friend or loved one to *also* read the medications book. The friend or loved one, after they've perused the literature, can consult with the patient as to how he might most safely proceed.

I am not your prescribing physician. I legally *cannot* and I *will not* advise you about any aspect of your medications, including whether or not your drug usage is problematic in terms of recovery.

The many tragedies detailed in my book on Parkinson's medications, including deaths from neuroleptic malignant syndrome from over-fast drug withdrawal and my inability to help ease symptoms of drug-induced parkinsonism, serve to explain why I will *not* work with a person who has ever taken the medications for more than a few weeks.

As a gentle side note, *please* do not send me hate mail because you are already taking medications or because I have not pushed harder to make my work more quickly acknowledged. My heart goes out to you. Please know that I am working as hard and as fast I can, while being careful to be as accurate as possible with every word I write. My observations and warnings about the medications have been available online, for free, since 1999.

As for those who send me accusations that my work must be bogus because "everyone who gets a diagnosis of Parkinson's automatically takes the medications," this statement is wrong. In much of the world, people are encouraged to stay off the medications for as long as possible because the dopamine-enhancing drugs have a *short* period of effectiveness (two to ten years). The higher the dose, the sooner the onset of ineffectiveness and the sooner the adverse effects show up. The adverse effects, especially the dyskinetic spasms, can be worse, far more excruciatingly painful, than the symptoms of Parkinson's.

In the USA, where doctors must stay wary of lawsuit-happy patients, people with PD are *encouraged* to start medications immediately despite the dangers and the well-proven *fact* that the drugs accelerate the worsening of PD symptoms. Even so, many people in the USA do their research and choose to delay taking the medications for as long as possible. [1]

---

[1] See: "Levodopa and the Progression of Parkinson's Disease," *New England Journal of Medicine*, Janice Walton-Hadlock, Vol. 352 No. 13, March 31, 2005 p. 1380.

The above, my commentary on the Eldopa study, was the first piece by a non-MD acupuncturist ever published in the *New England Journal of Medicine*. In addition to my own, very small five-year research project on antiparkinson's medications that gave me the information presented in *Once Upon a Pill*, research proof *abounds* that pharmaceutical dopamine is addictive and causes brain damage – brain damage of the type that accelerates symptoms of drug-induced parkinsonism.

These days, youth learn about brain damage from dopamine-enhancing drugs in their high school health class. They learn that a list of dopamine-enhancing drugs can include cocaine, methamphetamine, nicotine, alcohol, and the opiates, including heroin, in addition to nearly all of the antiparkinson's drugs, many anti-depression and anti-anxiety drugs, and many prescription pain-killers. You can do a search online for terms such as "brain damage, dopamine, L-dopa."

Any drug that elevates dopamine will 1) be addictive and 2) cause brain changes, including changes that can eventually lead to drug-induced parkinsonism...no matter what your well-meaning and maybe under-informed MD or neurologist tells you. If your doctor says that the drugs have no lasting side-effects, are safe or even, incorrectly, that the drugs *slow* the progression of Parkinson's, your doctor is wrong. Research this online.

Make sure you are visiting websites that share unbiased research reports, *not* sites supported by pharmaceutical companies or programs that *present* themselves as big-name, non-profit organizations while actually shilling or testing for drug companies. If a website or program consistently presents "research" showing that the drugs are safe or do not have dangerous side effects, and especially if the site presents "research" claiming that people with Parkinson's should start taking the medications as soon as possible after diagnosis, you might do well to investigate the source of the "research" site's funding, even if it claims to be an altruistic, highly respected, national level, not-for-profit organization. Some drug-testing programs even certify and promote themselves as *non-profit* research companies and do not disclose that their main "donors" are drug companies. The drug companies can pay these "non-profit" companies big bucks to perform the nationally required tests for drug-approval. It's of course *possible* that these companies might even be paid or otherwise be tempted to skew the results of their research. The testing might even – again, I'm being careful with my wording and I'm not naming names – be done on unsuspecting patients who think they are participating in the "pure research" of a non-profit organization looking for a genuine cure when what the program is actually doing is fulfilling the federally mandated testing requirements of a pharmaceutical company.

Chapter Seven

Requirement 3: Being willing and able to turn off self-induced pause

The four methods for turning off the flow of pause-type electrical currents – and thus recovering from Parkinson's – are methods that can be done either by oneself or, in cases of *only* Type II, *only* Type III, or *only* Type IV from *only* an unhealed physical injury or trauma, by availing oneself of the help of a friend or family member. The friend need not have any training whatsoever in the field of medicine, but must have the patience to apply the very simple holding techniques of Yin Tui Na.

However, a person with Type I PD, one who put himself into self-induced pause, did so on his own, in private. In the cases I've seen, turning it off has usually also been a deeply personal, private process. It must be done consciously and willingly. Outside help has been ineffective or maybe even counter-productive, maybe because so long as the patient can anticipate the therapist somehow doing the work or even giving pleasant encouragement or advice, the patient tends to *not* destroy the attitudinal behaviors that created self-induced pause. Very often, the patient has to be desperate, has to "hit rock bottom," before he'll work hard enough and consistently enough to successfully turn off his pause-inducing mind-set.

Getting professional help

Professional help is not needed, nor is it helpful, so far as I have seen.[1]

---

[1] People often ask if professional help for turning off pause is similar to the professional help some people get for addressing post-traumatic stress disorder, or PTSD. No.

A person with PTSD is usually considered to be stuck in "shock," meaning sympathetic mode. Biologically speaking, his body is endlessly looping through the neurological mode of fight or flight: *sympathetic* mode, *not* pause mode. A person with PTSD *might* benefit from professional help to find his way out of being stuck in this shock-related mode. Then again, improvement is often elusive, even with professional guidance. This is because, in many cases, a person diagnosed with PTSD is actually stuck on pause mode, not sympathetic mode. And pause is a condition that most medical professionals have never even heard of.

A colleague of mine runs a free clinic for people with PTSD, teaching them how to turn off biological pause, not self-induced. The results have been so quick and transformative that doctors from the local Veterans Administration clinic have been visiting his clinic to see what he's doing. One therapist remarked, "In one hour, patients doing the techniques you've taught them have completely recovered. I've been working with them, unsuccessfully, for years!" However, until this neurological mode is more widely recognized, we will not see many doctors wanting to learn about it or evincing interest in how people can help themselves come out of it.

Most people who have a near-death injury or undergo total anesthesia (which, by the way, induces pause mode, not sleep) do *not* need professional help or counseling to come out of their temporary state of rigidity and/or immobility, or even coma.

Pause is an on-or–off mode. The body is *designed* to be able to turn off pause. The process *usually* works correctly. As for sympathetic mode, the body does *not* have a specific biological sequence for overcoming excessive use of sympathetic mode. Hence the need for coaching, meditation, and other aids in turning down the excess levels of fight-or-flight mode seen in some

Professional therapy for coming out of pause or self-induced pause does not exist. There is no profession that is trained in helping people do this *usually* automatic process.

Therapists, psychologists, acupuncturists and doctors are *not* taught about pause mode. They are *not* trained in the very simple steps that are necessary for coming out of biological pause if a person gets stuck in it. Nor are they trained in treating *self-induced* pause and *self-induced* dissociation. They aren't taught anything about pause mode because, from a western medical standpoint, there is no such thing. From a Chinese medical standpoint, channel qi is an historical superstition. The old books that alluded to channel qi *or* the four phases (modes) are considered to have no modern medical value.

Many, maybe most, people with Type I Parkinson's still have within *themselves* the mental focus and determination to do the work that turns off self-induced pause. If a person using self-induced pause or self-induced dissociation that is causing pause-like channel qi flow *wants* to turn it off, he *must* have within himself the ability for circumspection, strong mental focus, and the capacity for the emotional surrender that is needed to change some of his pause-driven thought patterns. And he has to do it on his own.

Then again, if a person has *only* Type II, Type III, or Type IV Parkinson's, he *might* be able to recover even if he *can't* understand the theory in this book. In these cases, a friend might be able to provide hands-on support for injury(s) by using simple Yin Tui Na or walking the patient through the five steps of recovery from biological pause, as needed. These therapies might help the patient re-associate with the long-forgotten injury or turn off biological pause *even if* the patient doesn't remember the injury or is somewhat oblivious to the underlying treatment theory.

Please fix my grampa

Many people have contacted me because a very elderly parent or loved one has been diagnosed with Parkinson's and probably has Type I but shows no interest in, or even any understanding of, changing his or her way of thinking by doing the self-directed mental exercises you will read about in upcoming chapters, let alone turning off the constant, wary, maybe even negative and judgmental internal monologue that has become a way of life.

I have received many emails saying something like, "Can you explain to my elderly father why he needs to work on recovering?"

My reply is always a respectful no.

Please do not be panicked by the idea that recovery is not for everyone. Very elderly people with recent onset Parkinson's disease who have no interest in recovering very likely will still be able to maintain a decent quality of life during the years until their passing. Even if they use the drugs, if the drugs are used very, very cautiously, the person might continue to have a high quality of life – although mentally he or she will no longer be the person you knew and loved because of the mind-altering nature of the drugs. After all, the drugs *work* by altering mental perceptions, motivations, and personality.

---

people with PTSD. And no, the techniques for "waking the tiger," as Dr. Peter Levine puts it, do not turn off pause. His work focuses on people who have gotten stuck in *pre*-sympathetic mode, what we call "a deer in the headlights": physical or emotional *pre-action* paralysis.

I recommend reading *Medications of Parkinson's: Once Upon a Pill* in order to understand what is meant by the word "cautiously" in the previous paragraph, and to learn how to determine if a person is over- or under-medicated, and what dose changes your loved one might need to make in order to have the highest possible quality of life without recovering. Your MD's training will almost certainly *not* have taught him how to safely help you with this.

Heal my husband

A local woman brought to my office her husband with relatively early-stage Parkinson's. She was adamant that I needed to "fix" him. She had heard of my work through the local grapevine. Neither of them had read the free online materials despite having been requested to do so when she booked the appointment.

I did a full assessment and easily agreed with his doctor's diagnosis of Parkinson's. I explained a little bit about what was involved in recovering and asked him to please go home and read the online material to see if he was interested in recovery.

He very calmly replied, "No. I am the only remaining person in my family-line. Everyone in my family dies by age seventy-five. I'm already seventy-nine. My parents have died; my siblings have died. I should have died already. I don't want to change. I'm ready to die. My wife made me come, but I'm fine with having Parkinson's."

His wife became furious…with me.

She demanded that I start treating him then and there.

She clearly did not understand anything I had said about him needing to do the work himself. The man, on the other hand, seemed to understand perfectly. He simply wasn't interested. She then changed her tune, explaining that *she* needed for him to not have Parkinson's.

I assured the man that I understood completely, and if he ever had any questions he could give me a call. I ushered them out.

Many times I have heard from distressed people that a loved one has looked over the PDrecovery.org website and quickly announced something like, "I was exposed to bad chemicals many years ago, so I probably have toxin-induced parkinsonism. I know I can't recover so I don't want to waste my time on this."

Please be aware that living on pause can eventually make a person wary and fearful of everything, including change, and even the possibility of recovery.

Also, some people have told me that they would prefer to be the innocent victim of a cruel and random syndrome such as toxin-induced parkinsonism than consider the possibility that their own mental actions, however understandable and even necessary at the time, might have played a part in their syndrome, or than to even *consider* that in their own case Parkinson's disease might have a mental component.

I have been told, in anger, that I have ruined people's lives with my hypotheses: "Parkinson's used to be a respectable illness. People felt sorry for me because I had Parkinson's for no reason at all. Now, you make it seem like it's all my fault for having Parkinson's because it's a mental disorder." And "My spouse is now blaming me for having caused my own Parkinson's disease."

I've also received angry emails from health practitioners stating that my work "blames the victim."

And then there are the people who let me know, after I reply to their question-packed emails, that they've decided they don't want to try to recover. They plan to take medications instead because they need to hide their symptoms in a hurry. "It sounds like recovery might take too long. I can't let anyone at work know that I have a degenerative illness." Sometimes they add something like, "If people know I have a degenerative illness, they

"...won't trust me anymore."

"...won't believe in me."

"...won't admire me."

These might be wrong assumptions, based on a lifetime of wariness and the false idea, common in people with Type I PD, that a person has to be near perfect or at least not show "weakness" in order to stay safe, to not let others down, or to be considered a "good person."

Then again, if a person knows he will lose his job if the boss suspects a degenerative illness, then the person must do what is best for him.

Again, I will never pressure anyone to attempt recovery.

If a person with Type I Parkinson's disease from self-induced pause is not interested in or mentally not able to work steadily on creating some new, very specific thought habits, habits that will directly stimulate the striatum and thalamus and eventually lead to turning off pause, he probably will *not* be able to recover from Type I Parkinson's.

As for recovering from the other three types, *so long as* the possibility of Type I PD has been ruled out, it should not hurt to do Yin Tui Na, craniosacral therapy, or the five steps, whichever is needed, with a person even if he *doesn't* understand the theory.

Chapter Eight

Searching for Answers

To answer some of the next-most common questions, this chapter will share the approach I took, the questions *I* had, and the hypotheses I developed after my *first* few patients recovered easily but the symptoms in the next group of patients seemed to respond differently to the same treatment.

After I'd seen a few dozen Parkinson's patients, my own biggest question was: "Why have *some* of my patients recovered from Parkinson's in response to a simple, supportive holding therapy for old, unhealed injuries, while *most* of my patients with Parkinson's have become distinctly *altered*, both mentally and physically, in response to the same therapy, but have *not* recovered?"

Let me back up a bit.

The late 1990s

Shortly after my first Parkinson's patient unexpectedly recovered, two more PD patients recovered in response to the same, very simple, anyone-can-do-it treatment I'd used on my first recovered patient. I had used on their obviously injured feet a technique called Yin Tui Na, a Chinese medicine holding treatment that should be used for a dissociated, unhealed injury.[1]

At the time, I didn't suspect that there were four types of Parkinson's.

As it turns out, this type of treatment works for people with *only* Type II and *might* be part of the treatment for people with Type IV Parkinson's. I had no idea, at that time, that my patients who recovered so easily were either Type II or Type IV. As mentioned earlier, most people with Parkinson's have *both* Type I and Type II.

After I'd seen three people recover from a supposedly incurable illness, I was completely baffled and uneasy. Had *all* three of these PD patients been misdiagnosed? If not, was I morally responsible for announcing I'd found an effective treatment for Parkinson's disease…even though I didn't know how or why the treatment worked?

---

[1] Most acupuncturists do *not* learn Yin Tui Na in school. Tui Na classes are usually non-required, elective classes. Not only that, if a school offers a Tui Na class, it's almost always *Yang* Tui Na, a strong-arm type of physical manipulation that, in terms of force and intention, is nearly the opposite of *Yin* Tui Na.

For example, *Yang* Tui Na is used for forcefully popping a painful, recently dislocated arm bone back into its shoulder socket. *Yin* Tui Na is very subtle. It is used for injuries that are, "old, forgotten, and painless," as it says in the classic Chinese book on Tui Na – injuries that we might refer to in English today as "dissociated." The Yin Tui Na treatment might consist of firmly holding a displaced joint or injured body part until the body relaxes in the area so that the damaged or displaced bits can nestle back in or realign themselves.

In my limited experience, I've seen that many acupuncturists from China are disinclined to do *any* sort of Tui Na or hands-on therapy even if they studied it in school. In China, acupuncture is considered more highbrow than the lowly hands-on techniques. And if a doctor only inserts needles and uses *no* hands-on techniques, he can treat - and charge – more patients per hour.

By chance and by word of mouth, several more people with Parkinson's happened to contact me for appointments. After I'd seen these people also recover from Parkinson's, my distress level soared. They couldn't *all* have been misdiagnosed. I had to do something with this information. [1]

At that time, I was a painfully private person. I abhorred controversy. Still, I forced myself to attend the local Parkinson's support group, where I made a very short announcement of what I'd seen. I offered the attendees with PD a few free weekly treatments in exchange for letting me examine their feet, looking for unhealed injuries, and do Chinese holding therapy if it was appropriate.

Twelve people from the support group volunteered. When each of them met with me in my office and I physically examined their feet, they all had evidence of significant foot injury. Many only remembered the incident, or details of the incident, following some Yin Tui Na treatments.

Their degree of dissociation was astonishing. For example, I might be able to feel a severe bone displacement in the left foot. If I asked something like, "Was it the *left* foot that was hurt in the railroad-tie incident?" the reply was usually something like, "I don't know." The rest of the dialogue might go like this:

"Was it the *right* foot?"

"No!"

"Was it the *left* foot?"

"I don't know."

Was it the right foot?"

No, I'm certain it wasn't the *right* foot."

"So was it the left foot?"

"I told you, I have no idea which foot it was."

---

[1] The disproportionate number of people who recovered quickly and easily in my first few years of PD research and who in retrospect had only Type II PD might be explained by the fact that, in the early years of my acupuncture practice, many if not most of my clients were in the music department at the local university or were their friends and fellow musicians around the bay area.

At one point, I even hypothesized that maybe people who are classical music performers have an advantage in recovering from Parkinson's. I suspect now that I was confusing cause and effect. A person who is on pause might not be able to become a top level, expressive musician because being on pause inhibits the ability to feel one's heart-feelings, let alone convey them. Performing music via a higher degree of soul-expressing "automantic" movements as opposed to using a higher degree of command-based movements is what *makes* a great performer.

A person using self-induced pause might be able to cerebrally compose or perform music. A musician using self-induced pause might have good technical skills but find it increasingly difficult to perform empathetically *heart*-stirring music. For that matter, he might not *understand* that there is a difference between a *technically* correct music performance and the type of musical performance that vibrates the listeners' heart strings or causes the listeners to experience tears of joy. Therefore, my first PD patients, who also happened to be old school, classically trained, highly successful, *heart-stirring* musicians, were unlikely to be on self-induced pause. This lucky coincidence meant that I first worked with people who had easy-to-treat Type II and Type IV PD. If I had started out with people with Type I, I would *never* have seen recoveries. I would never have obsessively embarked on what became the Parkinson's Recovery Project.

The above, highly illogical type of dialogue is not unusual when trying to get information about an injury from which a person has dissociated. This is *not* a problem of intelligence. Most people with Parkinson's disease come across as disproportionately high on the intelligence scale. I'll include more on that subject in chapter sixteen.

For another example of the extreme dissociation from injury in my patients, when trying to ascertain if the primary dissociated injury was on the left side or right side and I suspected it was, for example's sake, on the left, I would ask the patient to raise his *left* arm. Inevitably, the patient would look at the mentally healthy, *right-side* arm, because that was the arm he knew existed. Then he would slowly shake the head as if to say, "No, not that one," and then hesitatingly raise "the other one," the one with the injury.

If I asked him, thirty minutes later, to raise the *right* arm, the arm on the side of the body that he *wasn't* dissociated from, the right arm would simply shoot up in the air. With regard to the whole side of the body that had the dissociation, it's as if the patient didn't really know it was there, so he could only figure out how to raise the arm on the dissociated side by looking at the one arm that *was* consciously part of his body, recognize that this wasn't the one I had asked him to raise, and then go for the only remaining option: the other arm, the arm he didn't really know about because he didn't really know about that whole side of his body. This was a *consistently* useful tool for quickly figuring out which side of a PD patient's body had the more severe dissociation.

A project is born

Around the same time that I recruited volunteers, some colleagues and friends helped me set up the non-profit Parkinson's Recovery Project, the website of which is www.PDrecovery.org. The website was originally a place to share my observations with other practitioners of Chinese medicine and ask if they could replicate my findings: a "call for replication."

A few could. Most could not. Again, I had no idea at this time that there were four types of Parkinson's, each of which has to be treated in a specific way.

I also had to post instructions for the fairly obscure art of Yin Tui Na on the website. This was the earliest version of what is now a book: *Yin Tui Na: Hands-on Therapy for Traumatic Injury*. As noted earlier, since the beginning of my research, all my writing related to recovering from Parkinson's is available for free download at this website.

A call for replication

I've been asked many times if I have any background in "real" medicine, if my research is "scientific," and/or do I know what constitutes legitimate research. I have also been asked if acupuncturists need to attend a class or two before they start poking people with needles. Good questions, all.

First, in the USA, acupuncture has been regulated state by state. However, this is changing. Starting in 2019, licensing has been moving slowly towards a national model. For example, in 2020 an acupuncturist must have a California license to practice in California but must *also* have a national license if doing work for the national system of Medicare (medical insurance for people over age 65).

In California, an acupuncturist spends as many years in post-graduate education as an MD. We study Chinese medicine as well as western medical theory, red flags, and western pharmacology. We are required to spend nearly a thousand hours interning and must pass a rigorous board exam before we are allowed to practice medicine. As mentioned in the previous chapter, in California a licensed acupuncturist (LAc) is considered a primary care provider: licensed to diagnose, prescribe, and treat, according to the scope of practice of Chinese medicine, and we are qualified to refer out to western specialists. Currently, an LAc's degree in most states is at the "Master's" level. However, this is changing even as this book goes to print. In future, an acupuncturist will be a "doctor" of Traditional Chinese Medicine, not a "master" and will have even more hours of study under his belt.

Both an acupuncturist and an MD have what is called a "*practical* Master's degree," sometimes called a "technical" master's degree, meaning some hands-on skill has been learned. An "academic" master's degree means that some academic question was pursued. A "doctoral" degree (PhD) implies that research has been pursued *and* written up and approved by a committee of peers. An allopathic doctor who also has a doctoral degree is an MD, PhD. An acupuncturist with a doctoral degree in acupuncture and oriental medicine in California might have the letters DAOM or DTCM after their name, as well as LAc. However, the lettering is changing, as several boards of study are working on new formats for standardizing acupuncture credentialing across the USA.

As an aside, students in most European medical schools are usually required to try their hand at a research project, though not at the doctoral level. Medical schools in the USA do *not* require students to participate in research. I think this might lead to the USA doctors' tendency to be less critical regarding research and more likely to accept it at face value. *Doing* actual research tends to make a person appreciate how often research results aren't accurate or meaningful, and how easily the published results can be skewed in favor of the desired outcome.

Returning to the subject of my education, after I got a master's degree in "traditional" (modern) Chinese medicine and my license, I continued my studies and earned a doctoral degree, as well.

Second, regarding research, my writing in this book is directed mostly towards people with Parkinson's, including those who might *not* have a strong background in science/research. Therefore, I'm going to include some bits of information on the subject of research and the "scientific method" over the next few chapters, to answer questions I've received.

A "call for replication" is an important part of *qualitative* research: What happens in response to a treatment? Can the result be replicated? Can we isolate the variables? This research phase must precede the *quantitative* studies: big studies that focus on how *many* subjects are examined or treated by how *many* doctors. For example, an individual might claim thousands of successful outcomes with some medical therapy, but if *no one else* can replicate his results, his research is worthless, even suspect.

In the early stages of any paradigm-shifting research, the most important question after a seeming medical cure is found for an "incurable illness" is: Can another doctor/therapist replicate this result? Ideally, the "cleanest" replication occurs in a separate setting, even a different country, and with the replicating researchers working only from printed instructions without ever having met or spoken with the original researcher and without having a financial or vested interest in the success of the research.

Controlled studies: single-blind and double-blind studies

A controlled study in one in which some patients receive treatment while others do not, or are given placebo treatments.

A double-blind is a study in which neither the patients nor the doctors know who is getting the real therapy and who is getting a sham treatment or a placebo. Although some people feel that the highest level of qualitative scientific proof for *all* medical research has to be the double-blind study, double-blind studies are more often used for testing drug safety and drug effectiveness or testing for surgical interventions than for doing research on physical pathologies or psychological disorders.

Many studies in which sham surgeries or other sham procedures are performed are single-blind: the patient doesn't know if he's receiving the real treatment or not, but some doctor within the system has to know. For example, the doctor who did the procedure knows what he did. Sometimes, the doctor doing the sham surgery is not the same doctor who is doing the assessment, making the process closer to a double-blind. But even in these cases there might not be a perfect double-blind.

The point of a double-blind study is to *isolate* a chemical, mechanical, or biological process and remove any potential influence from the patients' or doctors' mental attitudes. In cases where a mental attitude *is* the predominant problem, a double-blind study might be meaningless. It might even result in the person with the *sham* treatment having a *superior* response compared with people who got the real treatment, as is often the case in research studies on people with Parkinson's disease.

Cohort studies

Some people assume that cohort studies (studies with hundreds or even thousands of subjects with more or less the same problem) are of the greatest value.

Many very useful cohort studies do *not* necessarily show that everyone gets the same result. For example, in cohort studies for some cancer drugs, an improvement in outcome for even a very small percentage of the subjects – four or five percent – might be enough to qualify a drug to be approved as potentially useful.

But for any given individual, what matters most is his own outcome. The fact that a benefit appears in five percent of people in a cohort, or in ninety-five percent, doesn't necessarily mean anything predictive for any one individual.

For syndromes such as migraine headaches, diabetes, or Parkinson's, where the researchers sometimes fail to account for the fact that people can have similar symptoms but have different underlying *causes*, results from cohort studies can be meaningless, and even *mis*leading.

Psychological and physical therapies

Sometimes, double-blind and even single-blind studies are not possible. With psychological retraining therapies or hands-on therapies such as Tui Na, both the doctor or therapist and the patient need to be cognizant of what's happening.

This means that double-blind studies cannot be used in testing the effectiveness of a patient-participation psychological therapy: a person cannot perform mental exercises that help change the mindset without knowing that he's doing those exercises. Likewise, a doctor or therapist cannot teach a person new cognitive skills without knowing whether or not he's teaching cognitive skills. And although a final evaluator might not know who was taught the therapies and who was not, the patient knows what he has or hasn't done to himself.

The same goes for hands-on therapies.

And merely substituting a "sham" location for physical therapies doesn't work. Sometimes, the benefit of physical therapy might have as much to do with the psychological changes that come about through being touched, period, as it has to do with the *location* of the touch.

I repeat: in general, double- and single-blind studies are *not* much used for syndromes with a mental component, especially those that are treated via talk therapy or cognitive type therapies as opposed to drug therapy. Self-induced pause, dissociation, and self-induced dissociation all qualify as mental components.

One model that is now widely accepted for psychological research is the "single-case study." A later chapter will discuss the growing importance and acceptance of the single-case study for developing non-drug treatment strategies for problems that have a mental component.

Getting back to the subject of my budding research project, I started the website as a call for replication: the first step for the type of research I was getting into.

Doing more research

As mentioned earlier, in the late 1990s I started a small qualitative research project at the local acupuncture college where I teach. Free, weekly Yin Tui Na treatments were provided for people with Parkinson's by students working towards a Master's degree in Chinese medicine.

Soon, word of mouth and the website of the Parkinson's Recovery Project brought more people with Parkinson's to my personal office. By now, enough people had recovered that I thought I might be onto something, so I was charging my newest PD patients for their treatments. I was still keeping my prices as low as possible for them. My original twelve recruits and the patients at the acupuncture college's clinic were still being treated for free. My world was filling up with Parkinson's.

Nearly all of the patients *changed* in response to the Yin Tui Na treatments. But for most of them, the strange, even bizarre changes in symptoms and personality that I referred to as *partial* recovery were nowhere near complete recovery, not by a long shot.

Becoming obsessed

I spent *hours* interviewing every Parkinson's patient I worked with. I didn't just dwell on their symptoms.

At *every* patient's weekly, one-hour session, while treating the patient with Yin Tui Na, I continued my inquiries about childhood, hobbies, professions, food preferences, amusements, attitudes towards life, and spiritual paths, if any. I dug deeply into anything that seemed a little outside the norm. I started noticing uncanny similarities in the personalities and the *type* of intelligence of *most* of my patients.

These similarities squared with the observations of other twentieth century doctors dating back to the 1930s. These observations suggested that most people with Parkinson's are different, somehow, from the "ordinary Joe" or the hypothetical "man on the street."

Many studies through the years have examined and tried to define what western Parkinson's researchers refer to as the "Parkinson's personality." The list of traits can even vary a bit from one theorist to the next. No consensus exists as to whether or not the personality is related to the underlying *cause* of Parkinson's or is the *result* of the PD.

I also noticed many inexplicable mental behaviors. For example, most of my PD patients responded to traditional mind-calming or anti-depression self-therapies with the exact opposite response from the norm. Self-therapies such as meditation, Qi Gong, chanting, affirmations, or the various types of cognitive behavioral therapy are supposed to *reduce* the use of sympathetic mode and thereby *automatically increase* the use of parasympathetic mode.

As an aside, although some medical professionals speak as if a person is either in pure sympathetic mode or pure parasympathetic mode, people are nearly always using a blend of these two modes. At any given moment, a person is somewhere on a continuum. One end of the continuum is a high degree of parasympathetic mode and a low degree of sympathetic. The other end is a high degree of sympathetic and a low degree of parasympathetic. We constantly move back and forth along this continuum, depending on our stress levels and our thoughts at any given moment.

Most of my patients did *not* have the normal responses to these therapies. They did not move closer to parasympathetic mode, not by a long shot. Instead, these therapies made them more adept at sliding into a state of deep numbness. Again, they did *not* slide towards the expected joy, ease, and spontaneous automatic movement associated with parasympathetic mode. And in nearly all cases, even though the person *might* move more easily after a one-hour session of mildly calming techniques, the improvement would only last until the patient's next negative thought, which might be a few minutes or a few days later. And after that, the symptoms might even be distinctly *worse* than before.

Compared to the general public, what seemed like a disproportionately high percentage of my patients had spent a long time, maybe decades, practicing meditation, church-approved prayer, yoga, Tai Ji or Qi Gong. Nearly all of them said that they never or only rarely felt joy from it. It was more like a job or a duty, or something to help them feel either mentally virtuous or else "still" inside – meaning deathly still or numb. But the expansive joy and/or radiant inner peace of meditation or various other spiritual and/or energy practices had never made an appearance, or only a fleeting one.

Most of these patients usually felt that the deeply numb state was a good thing. Very often making themselves more numb *did* temporarily slow or stop their tremoring. But it was obvious that the numbness and *temporary* reduction of symptoms, if any, wasn't related to any long-term improvement. In fact, as my patients got better at doing my suggested exercises for turning off sympathetic mode (the typical goal for most self-calming therapies), they got better at going *deeper* into pause.

As it turns out, in a *deeper* degree of pause, moving closer to the state of coma or sleep, the tremor is stilled. After all, it's only when the body is saying, "I'm *alert* and stable now on the inside and therefore ready to come out of pause" does it ask the question, via the tremor, "So is the outside vicinity safe?"

Only when a person is wide awake and alert does his tremor become or resume being overt. For most of my patients, when their bodies slid into sleep *or* deeper numbness, the question-provoking tremor backed off. Then, even though the electrical agitation in the sacrum and thalamus might continue, the *physical* tremor was usually not visible.

Then again, according to their spouses, a very small percentage of my PD patients *did* tremor even in their sleep, usually while dreaming. But most do not.

Wrong assumptions

Early on I observed that all my Parkinson's and pause patients had channel qi running in a weird, *backwards* direction in their Stomach channels – and *none* of the other, non-Parkinson's, non-pause patients in my all-purpose acupuncture practice had backwards Stomach channel flow.

In Chinese medicine, backwards-flowing channels, though uncommon, are not unheard of. They are referred to as flowing "Rebelliously." This condition is considered to be incorrect and unhealthy. Except of course, in pause mode, when it *is* correct. But we don't learn about pause mode in school. [1]

This backwards electrical flow pattern in the Stomach channel that I observed in my PD patients actually *explained* many of the classic *symptoms* of Parkinson's. And *if*, in response to foot therapy, a person's channel qi started running the correct way, running in the path I'd learned in school, then the Parkinson's stopped and never returned. At least that's what happened in my first Parkinson's patients.

After seeing the first few recoveries from Parkinson's, I assumed that the trick to recovering from Parkinson's was correcting the backwards flow of these channels – flow that I referred to in the early days as an injury-triggered channel qi aberration.

Certainly, in all my patients who completely recovered, their channel qi had resumed running normally. I didn't suspect that, for most cases of PD, I was reversing the roles of cause and effect. As it turns out, backwards channel qi flow does indeed cause symptoms of PD *but* in most patients the channel qi is *not* behaving "aberrantly." In most people with Parkinson's, being on pause is what *correctly* causes the backwards flow. For most patients, the problem is being *stuck* in a neurological mode that isn't supposed to be used long term. The backwards channel qi flow *and* the resultant symptoms of Parkinson's are merely *side effects* of the long-term use of pause mode-type circuitry.

Most of my newer, recruited patients failed to recover in the same quick manner as my first six Parkinson's patients. I assumed it was because the new patients were all taking antiparkinson's medications. None of my earliest patients had ever taken the drugs.

In 2003, after I stopped working with patients who had ever taken antiparkinson's medications, for reasons mentioned in chapter six, I assumed that any new, un-medicated patients would recover in the same simple manner that my earliest Parkinson's patients had done.

---

[1] In some British publications, *Rebellious* channel qi is referred to as Counterflow or Retrograde channel qi. I prefer the term Rebellious, a more appropriate translation from the Chinese. For thousands of years, the Chinese political system has considered rebellion to be *the* single greatest threat to civic peace and harmony.

Using the word Rebellious to refer to channel qi running backwards suggests how *very* dire this condition can be. Rebellious channel qi doesn't merely prevent correct physiology in the immediate vicinity of the blockage that's causing backwards flow. Like political rebellion, backwards-flowing channel qi might eventually bring down the entire system.

But most of my new, medication-free patients did *not* completely recover. In response to healing from their foot injuries, most of them experienced distinct changes in their personalities and symptoms, as so many of the medicated patients had done. Some of the new symptoms and personality changes were bizarre. Weirdest of all, after the foot injury healed, their channel qi might still run backwards in their legs…sometimes. When a person has backwards-running currents because of a channel-blocking injury, the channel qi should run backwards *all* the time.

Overly optimistic, I named this baffling set of changes “partial recovery.”

In people with now-healed foot injuries, people who clearly were not recovered from Parkinson’s, people in what I called “partial recovery,” I found I could usually make their channel qi go one way or the other by something as innocuous as telling a joke. While telling the joke, their Stomach channel qi might run correctly. When I finished the joke, if I said something even mildly negative such as “Uh oh…”, the Stomach channel qi would immediately run backwards.

Chinese medical theory with regard to psychological components

From a Chinese medicine perspective, this quick variability in channel qi flow in response to thoughts should only occur if the syndrome has a mental / emotional component. Symptoms with a large and/or quick variability in location and severity are referred to as being caused by “*Qi* Stagnation.” Symptoms attributed to Qi stagnation are considered to have a mental / emotional component.

Although many western doctors dismiss mentally driven symptoms as being “merely” psychological, doctors of Chinese medicine recognize that many, if not most, illnesses do have some degree of mental component...and mental components are just as worthy and needful of treatment as physical components.

As an aside, Qi stagnation is sort of the opposite of “*Blood* Stagnation.” Blood stagnation refers to a *physical* trauma such as a broken bone, appendicitis, or a torn tendon. The pain from a physical trauma or physical “insult” tends to stay in one place. The pain only ebbs as the injury heals.

However, even a purely physical trauma can, in some people, cause enough anguish that a mental component such as dissociation arises. The mental component can slow the healing of the injury. Very often, a person with Blood Stagnation will also have some amount of Qi Stagnation that will also benefit from treatment.

Most people with idiopathic Parkinson’s disease have symptoms that come and go or at least worsen and ease up in immediate response to positive and negative thoughts. In these cases, “positive thoughts” refers to thoughts that are encouraging, grateful, hopeful and/or in the moment. “Negative thoughts” might be wary, resentful, self-pitying, angry, and so on – the types of thoughts that make one feel more fear or anger, and which tend to dwell on the past or negatively predict the future.

A person with a *physical* deficiency of dopamine should have fairly *constant* immobility problems. Those dopamine deficiency symptoms should be body-wide and distributed equally on the left and right sides – and should make a person limp, not rigid. This is *not* the case in idiopathic Parkinson’s disease: rigidity occurs in specific muscles and limpness and/or weakness occurs in other specific muscles, just as it does in pause mode. Also, in most cases of PD, the severity of symptoms comes and goes depending on the degree of fear or confidence that the patient has at any given moment: a psychological component.

An introduction to partial recovery

Partial recovery symptoms were the strongest suggestion to me that there *was* a psychological component in Parkinson's, despite the strong convictions of people with PD that there was none.

People who previously had Type I *and* Type II but who, following successful healing of their injury(s) still have Type I and *only* Type I, still have Parkinson's. They are in "partial recovery." Partial recovery can be a very strange type of come-and-go Parkinson's: When a person in partial recovery is wary, the channel qi in the Stomach channel runs backwards and other pause-like channel behaviors kick in. The Parkinson's symptoms might be drastically worse than they were *before* receiving treatments for the unhealed injury, when the person still had *both* Type I and Type II PD.

And yet, in partial recovery, after the foot injury has healed up, *if* the person is feeling temporarily safe, the channel qi *might* run normally. The symptoms of Parkinson's might subside or temporarily stop to a much higher degree and duration than they ever did *prior* to the healing of the injury.

As an aside, in people with PD, even if the *visible* tremor stops in response to feeling temporarily safe or "more deadened," the internal tremor does not stop. When the stopping of the *internal* tremor finally happens, it is permanent – and stunning. When the internal tremor truly stops, during *full* recovery, it's an event so profoundly peaceful and still that, for a few seconds, people sometimes think that they must have died, even though they are still breathing.

In partial recovery, when feeling safe, the external, visible tremor might diminish or stop. The patient might *say* "My tremor has stopped!" but he's only referring to his visible tremor. His internal tremor, the shaking in the midbrain and sacrum, continues. When the *internal* tremoring stops, it can be a glorious, life-changing, permanent experience.

Symptoms come and go

As an example of the come-and-go-symptoms of partial recovery, I had one Parkinson's patient who successfully re-associated with and healed from his childhood foot injury. Shortly after that, he bragged that, on a recent "good" day, he was once again able to playfully chase his wife around the dining room table.

He also told me that on the following day, a day that featured an appointment with the dentist, he spent the day curled on the living room floor in a fetal position, *painfully* rigid, tremoring, drooling, unable to speak or move…until his wife cancelled the appointment.

Prior to his receiving successful Yin Tui Na treatment for his dissociated foot injury, his Parkinson's symptoms were fairly mild. He could always walk and take care of himself, although his movements were becoming a bit stiff and slow. In partial recovery, in his *bad* hours or bad days, his symptoms were utterly debilitating: a high degree of pause mode. This patient no longer had Type I *and* Type II PD. He now had the come-and-go behaviors of *only* Type I *plus* the ability to access parasympathetic mode sometimes, with regard to the healed injury: a confusing combination.

Not accepting the idea of a mental component

The channel qi behaviors in my patients in partial recovery could switch from parasympathetic flow to pause flow – an *extreme* switch, biologically speaking – in the blink of an eye. This suggested to me, based on Chinese medicine theory, that a mental component was involved. But most of my patients with Parkinson's tended to think of themselves as extremely logical, and often considered themselves *not* susceptible to suggestion or mental influences. So after healing from the foot or ankle injury, *despite* the appearance of new, rapid, severe channel qi fluctuations in response to positive or negative thoughts, behaviors that suggested a significant mental component, I figured that the problem just *couldn't* be psychological. Certainly, my patients insisted that it wasn't.

Since those early days, I've collected research articles that show that most people with Parkinson's are *extremely* susceptible to suggestion and to the placebo effect. But of course I didn't know that in the beginning days of my research.[1]

---

[1] *Suggestible You*; Eric Vance; Penguin RandomHouse; USA; 2016. This book on suggestibility and the placebo effect leans heavily on studies that used people with Parkinson's as the test subjects. For decades now, people with Parkinson's disease have been used in placebo studies because it's so easy to tell if they are affected by placebos or not: if they are, they can go from rigid and immobile to moving somewhat normally after taking a mere sugar-pill: a pill that they have been *told* is a dopamine-enhancing drug. So the observers don't have to ask the patients' opinion or guess as to whether or not the placebo is working. They can *easily* see and *objectively* measure the response to the placebo.

If and *only* if a person with Parkinson's has already become accustomed to taking dopamine-enhancing medications and gets a predictable response from them, *and* if he thinks he is receiving his usual dopamine-enhancing dose of medication, then in response to a sugar pill he usually can move as if medicated. The benefit of the sugar pill lasts until the person assumes that it's time for the medication to wear off, as per usual. One placebo study showed that the effect of the placebo was even stronger in people with Parkinson's who were falsely told they were receiving a new, far more *expensive* brand of dopamine than the other patients in the study. They were still only receiving sugar pills, but their "On" time lasted longer than usual.

It's important to note that, within a few days, the placebo benefit ceases because the person starts down the dangerous road of over-fast drug withdrawal and possible death.

As another indication of how susceptible people with PD are to the placebo effect, the first test groups for fetal cell implants included people who got sham surgery and people who got actual implants. The sham surgery recipients got shallow incisions on the scalp that were sewn back over, and were then *told* that they'd received a fetal cell implant, even though they hadn't.

A very few of the people who got the implants did okay. The people who got the *sham* surgeries did far *better*. All of the participants were taking antiparkinson's medications at the time and continued to do so following the surgery. One qualifier for the experiment was that people had to have such advanced Parkinson's that their medications were no longer effective enough. A year after the test surgeries, participants in the study were told whether or not they'd had the implants or had the sham surgery. The people who'd done the very best, had even resumed skiing or doing their other favorite sports, had a hard time believing that they'd only had the sham surgery.

Sadly, *most* of the patients who *had* received actual fetal cell implants had disastrous results. The new cells in the brain had grown into all sorts of tissues. Some of the fetal cells grew into dental tissue, including teeth. Many people who received fetal cells developed bizarre movement problems including flailing dyskinesia so severe that some patients had to be kept sedated or permanently pinned down with physical restraints. A few years after this experiment, I met one of the researchers who'd been on the team doing the fetal cell implants. He had quit

The wrong modes

From the start, I mistakenly assumed that my patients with Parkinson's, since they obviously were not in a significant degree of parasympathetic mode (non-judgmental, curious, and joyful), *must* be primarily in sympathetic mode. Based on my western schooling, I incorrectly assumed that these were the only two possible modes. I was wrong.

My PD patients were using a blend of pause mode and sympathetic mode channel qi patterns – and both at *low* amplitude: *low* energy levels in terms of the amount of channel qi that is flowing in a healthy body. The brain might be releasing prodigious amounts of norepinephrine while on pause. This can allow a person to feel extremely focused and even physically powerful. However, to the degree that pause is being used, the actual *amount* of channel qi flowing throughout the body is reduced. Again: channel qi flows in lower *amounts* throughout the body to the extent that pause mode is being used.

---

practicing western medicine as a result of the disastrous tragedies inflicted on those who'd gotten the implants, and had become an herbalist. But many people who had the *placebo* surgery had significant and lasting improvements.

See "Parkinson's Research is Set Back By Failure of Fetal Cell Implants"; *The New York Times*; Gina Kolata; March 8, 2001.

Why did the people with *sham* surgery do so well? Maybe *all* the people in the study felt extra lucky and therefore relatively more *safe* because they had been selected for this study – a mental component. Possibly this positive feeling translated into a conviction in the sham patients that they'd had the real implants. *And* people with only sham surgery didn't have the same brain trauma, tissue damage, and fetal cell overgrowth as the people who'd gotten the actual implants. Maybe that's why the people with the sham surgeries had the best results, results suggesting lasting physical improvement.

Many of those who'd only had sham surgeries did not believe the doctors when they learned that they'd had the sham. And you can see why: if sham surgery had given them such improved quality of life, the obvious implication was that a significant aspect of their Parkinson's was psychological. And no one with PD, in my experience, has ever wanted to hear that, whether out loud or implied.

The placebo studies using subjects with PD discussed in the book *Suggestible You* are examples of research being done in western medicine that has powerful applications for *understanding* what is going on in people with Parkinson's. For example, high levels of suggestibility and high levels of expectation-dependant behaviors could be related to a high level of susceptibility to self-commands – including those that cause self-induced pause.

But no one doing these studies seems to be looking for applications to PD, specifically. In these studies, researchers have only been interested in learning about the placebo effect, not about PD. They did their placebo studies with PD patients based on the wrong idea that all people, with all syndromes, will respond to placebos in the same manner. The people with PD were used only because their responses were easy to observe and measure. In fact, the effectiveness of placebos very much depends on whether or not a health problem is expectation dependant: has a mental component. Dopamine release for motor function is *inherently* expectation dependent. But the researchers never asked what these studies might imply for Parkinson's itself – they just assumed – incorrectly – that a placebo works the same in *all* health scenarios. They often use people with Parkinson's for these studies because the results – whether or not the person can go from *not* moving to moving – are so easy to objectively assess. But then they extrapolate, wrongly concluding that the powerful placebo effects they see in people with Parkinson's must be universal across all or at least many, health syndromes, and not particularly associated with PD, per se.

When my patients *decreased* the use of sympathetic mode by using various calming techniques ranging from affirmations to Heartmath techniques to yoga, they temporarily decreased their use of sympathetic mode and therefore *increased* the use of pause. Remember, their bodies were a continuum with pause on one end and sympathetic on the other. Using pause *inhibits* the amount of wave energy streaming into the body at the back of the neck. As these people started using less sympathetic and more pause, the overall *amount* of channel qi flowing throughout the body decreased even more, reflecting an increased use of pause mode. These people felt a welcome, but temporary increase in internal stillness – moving in the direction of sleep or coma. They felt this was a good thing. But they sure as heck were not moving towards parasympathetic mode, which is what is *supposed* to happen in response to these types of exercises.

I had not yet heard of the other modes (sleep and pause modes). I thought sympathetic and parasympathetic were the only options. I was confused. I had a lot of questions. Fortunately, I also had a lot of varied resources thanks to my interests in many seemingly unrelated fields.

A bit about my academic background

I am often asked, "What books or articles did you read that led you to your conclusions?" as well as "Have you ever heard of the scientific method" and "Do you know what *real* research is?" So I'll mention here that, while getting a BA in biology at the University of California, I also studied history of western science, ancient and modern. This field of study quickly dispels the notion that scientific breakthroughs flow out of the so-called "scientific method."

The scientific method uses measurements, observations, and proven repeatability, combined with previously "proven hypotheses" (theories) as building blocks to further advance or refine a theory. It is a way to bolster and further the status quo. The scientific method *cannot* create a paradigm shift. In fact, due to the premise that one cannot prove a negative, the scientific method often cannot even be used to *conclusively* prove that a previous theory is *wrong*: only that another theory might be *more right*.

Few of the great paradigm shifts in science, since the days of the ancient Greeks up to the present day Nobel prize winners in science, have come about via the scientific method. Rather the opposite: when we come up against something where the conflicting outliers and exceptions start to predominate over a current theory, people on the leading edge of research have to *throw away* the existing theory – not build on it by using the so-called "scientific method." *Very* often, it's a dream or a hunch from out of left field that can account for the outliers and conflicts and provide entirely new solutions.

The idea that a scientific method drives research is scorned by a large percentage of actual researchers.

Please go online to learn more about how the neat and tidy, fairly recent, concept of an orderly "scientific method" came about, and why it is mostly disregarded, if not openly laughed at, by people who are doing actual science research. And yet, scientists tend to be fairly conservative. They tend to resist shifts in the current paradigm. Despite the observed facts fitting better with a new hypothesis, overcoming the comfort of a previous theory, however inadequate or outright wrong, is often a slog.

As Mark Twain, a beloved 19th century American humorist noted, there are three stages in the acceptance of a new idea: First it is mocked. Then it is despised. Finally, it is accepted as *self-evident*. (The italics in the quote are my addition. "Self-evident" mean *obvious*.)

One of my first advisors on my Parkinson's project, a former professor of medical research theory, helped me understand that my work was *not* going to use the so-called scientific method to build on work that had gone on before, at least not western medical work in the field of Parkinson's. He explained that, when a new concept was as far off the accepted norm as mine was, a researcher had to "bootstrap himself up." This means getting small "Observation" articles and "New Hypothesis" articles published in top ranked, peer-reviewed journals.

He said I wasn't going to start out with a large, quantitative study. Instead, I would start with publishing short "hypothesis" articles that people in my own profession could agree with even if they said to themselves something like, "I hadn't thought of it that way before, but it makes sense." Or "It does give answers to questions that were inexplicable using the current paradigm." Then, when I had published enough hypothesis-type articles, I would be able to write bolder articles, and then books, and support my statements with citations from articles I had already published in *peer-reviewed* journals. This is one way to grow research that 1) is based on radically new ideas and 2) has no potential for significant profit.

After reading my first article published in the peer-reviewed *American Journal of Acupuncture*, in 1998, proposing my radical thoughts on the cause of Parkinson's symptoms, he semi-jokingly told me, "They're going to have to kill you…"

– For a light aside, not only did my main advisor and an editor both tell me that "they're going to have to kill you," I actually *was* killed in response to my Parkinson's research in a short book titled *Strong Medicine* by Richard MacAndrew. (Cambridge University Press, 2006.) The character based on me is named Deborah Spencer, an acupuncturist in Santa Cruz who finds a cure for Parkinson's. A fictitious, nearby pharmaceutical company that makes antiparkinson's drugs contracts for her successful murder.This book gives me peace of mind: if I *was* destined and willing to die on behalf of my research, I have now done so, on the pages of fiction. This 56-page book is part of a series for adult students of English as a Second Language. Mr. MacAndrew generously donated the ongoing proceeds from this book's sales to the Parkinson's Recovery Project.

Getting back to fielding questions about my academic background, I will add that despite getting a BA in biology in 1974 and being fascinated with the field of medicine, I lost all interest in applying to medical school during my second year of college. I felt that most of the very kind, highly intelligent, even brilliant pre-med students in my classes had very narrowly focused interests: med school applications and science "facts" rather than the vast cosmos of subjects outside the lab. I was questioning everything. My friends planning to go to med school, for the most part, regarded *current* biology facts as if they were Ultimate Truths rather than posits on a historical continuum of ever-changing hypotheses. They were *so* sure that the current "scientific facts" were right and true. I feared that a profession made up of students and teachers like this would *not* be a good fit for me. And so *many* of those modern facts about biology that I memorized in college have turned out to be wrong. For example, the fact that dopamine causes muscle relaxation and leads to sleep.

Upon graduating, I started a small deli and continued to voraciously study books on *western* medicine on my own. *Chinese* medicine was a subject that didn't even exist in the USA. Acupuncture wasn't revealed to my narrow world-view until President Nixon's historic trip "opening up China" in 1974.

In the 1980-90s, impelled by curiosity, I got a master's degree in traditional Chinese medicine, but had no plans to become licensed. In the early 1990s, I got licensed after all. In 2009 I earned a doctoral degree in acupuncture and oriental medicine (DAOM). Now, in 2020, I am a professor of Chinese medical theory and have been since 1998. I also am a professor of psychology and counseling since 2010.

This combination of studying western medicine, Chinese medicine, counseling, and abnormal psychology, plus a life-long interest in Newtonian and quantum physics, ancient physics, world history, history of science, metaphysics, and various languages, all contributed to my unanticipated conclusions regarding Parkinson's disease and to my other researches in Chinese medicine. So in answer to the frequent question, there is no particular book that led me to my conclusions. Rather, my academic training showed me why and how to question those aspects of the scientific status quo that lead to dead-ends, and how to compile and analyze data. My spiritual teachers have taught me to be philosophically adventurous.

A breakthrough

I don't remember exactly when it happened, but after at least ten, maybe even fifteen years of struggling with the limitations and implications of the western two-neurological-modes system while trying to understand Parkinson's, I came across pause mode while poring over a baffling English translation of a revered Chinese medical text, as mentioned in chapter one. This Chinese medical theory helped me figure out that my patients were in pause mode, not in sympathetic mode. That freed me from the prison of having to fit my findings into the incorrect western framework.

Only at that point did I began to suspect that backwards-flowing channel qi was not a channel aberration that *causes* Parkinson's – although when it ran non-stop, it accounted for *all* the *symptoms* of Parkinson's. Instead, being on pause *correctly* causes the channel qi to flow backwards in the Stomach and Large Intestine channels as well as flowing in weird, highly specific patterns in many of the *other* channels, and thus triggers the physiology of Parkinson's disease.

From a research standpoint, this changed everything. For people with Type I or with Type IV Parkinson's, the channel qi *wasn't* aberrant; the long-term use of pause mode in a non-emergency situation *was*. I still didn't know that there were four different ways to get stuck on pause, that there were four kinds of idiopathic Parkinson's disease. That understanding was still a few years in the future.

As I was later to figure out, all of my first six patients had either Type II or Type IV Parkinson's, the easiest types to treat: the types that respond to Yin Tui Na or that respond to the steps for coming out of normal, biological pause.

Fortunately, right along, while I was busy being confused by what was happening to my patients who slid into partial recovery, new research on brain behaviors from a wide spectrum of western medical fields steadily poured in – research that was going to help me enormously.

Helpful research

For example, new research in the field of hypnosis showed that a hypnotic command to inhibit motor function works by inhibiting the ability to *imagine* motor function. [1]

As it turns out, the specific brain locations of inhibition of motor function in hypnotic immobility are *identical* to the brain locations of inhibition in people with Parkinson's disease. Movement is inhibited in both hypnosis and in Parkinson's because the locations where *imagination* and/or *visualization* of movement are supposed to occur are turned off. These brain behaviors are a crucial step in the performance of automatic movement.[2]

Matching the findings of the articles cited above, most of my patients with Parkinson's have assured me that they cannot visualize, in general, let alone imagine images or somatic sensations of themselves performing motor functions. Many of them are even aware that they use silent, *word*-based thoughts and/or mental commands to initiate movement. Many don't know that there's any *other* way of generating movement.

Learning that the same exact brain mechanism is used in hypnotic immobility and in Parkinson's immobility didn't help me at the time, but I remembered the connection when I discovered the phenomenon of self-induced pause. Then I had to wonder, could the

---

[1] "The Brain under Self-control: Modulation of Inhibitory and Monitoring Cortical Networks during Hypnotic Paralysis"; Cojan, Waber, Schwartz et al; *Neuron*, Vol 62, iss 6;862-875, 25 June, 2009.

The gist of this article is that, following successful hypnotic suggestions for left-side paralysis, they saw in brain scans that "...Preparatory activation arose in right motor cortex despite left hypnotic paralysis, indicating preserved motor intentions, but with concomitant increases in precuneus regions that normally meditate [inhibit] imagery and self-awareness [proprioception].

In other words, the brain *tried* to activate movement but was stymied because it was unable to *imagine* the arm moving. "Imagine" in this context can mean "visualize or imagine the sensations of." Imagining is an important step in what is called "automatic" (dopamine-based) movement, as opposed to command-based (norepinephrine-based) movement. The "concomitant increases in precuneus regions" refers to increased activity in the part of the brain that drives wariness.

[2] "A dissociation between real and simulated movements in Parkinson's disease"; Cohen, Pourcher; *Neuroreport*; June 28, 2004; 15(9):1489-92. Based on brain scan results, "...in individuals with Parkinson's disease motor imagery is impaired...execution of overt movements is spared." In other words, the *potential* ability to move is there ("execution is spared"), but it is blocked because the person cannot mentally *imagine* the movement. People who are on pause cannot *imagine* self-movement, either the sensations of or visual images of self-movement.

Also, from a few years earlier, "Motor imagery in normal subject and in asymmetrical Parkinson's disease"; Thoois, Dominey, Decety, et al; *Neurology*; Oct 10, 2000; 996-1002. This article reports, "Previous work in PD has shown that bradykinesia (motor slowness) is associated with slowness of motor imagery."..."Conclusions: In patients with PD, brain activation during motor imagery is abnormal."

And I'll add, it's abnormal in the same manner as with people whose immobility was hypnotically induced.

powerful self-commands to "feel no pain" have acted on the brain in a manner similar to how the brain responds to hypnotic commands?[1]

For another example, I discovered in Dr. Temple Grandin's book *Animals in Translation*, a book on animal behavior and its relationship with human brain behavior, research showing that people with a logic and word-based intellect ("left-brained") as opposed to sensory-dominant ("right-brained") were far less likely to develop post-traumatic stress disorder (PTSD) in response to a horrible trauma. Instead, people who were word-dominant often created a mental story line that put the trauma into a controllable mental compartment.

Most of my PD patients were extremely left-brained, at least in their own opinions and in the opinions of their friends and spouses. Most of them had some powerful physical or emotional trauma in their past. They had dealt with it either by staying dissociated from a specific injury or event *or* by commanding themselves to feel no pain in general. These two *very* different mental processes are both left-brain processes. People with PD tend to *not* be susceptible to PTSD. Possibly, the use of dissociation and/or going into pause mode is their alternative, left-brain way of dealing with trauma. [2]

Their mental ability to control and/or not consciously experience the results of trauma seemed to dovetail with some of the elements of the Parkinson's personality, as well as the idea of a person getting stuck in an unhealthy neurological mode.

I collected stacks of research articles that seemed related to some of the behaviors I'd seen in my patients, even if the research wasn't *overtly* linked to Parkinson's. Just as the article on movement-imagination inhibition in hypnosis and the book on placebo-research mentioned earlier were *not* directed at Parkinson's specifically, they n evertheless, they had *implications* for Parkinson's disease. Hundreds of research articles

---

[1]As a possibly related aside, research based on brain scans shows that the brain inherently has two personalities: one is the "narcissistic" or "boss" personality and the other is the "obedient" personality. When the boss is dominant, the obedient nature obeys without thinking.

The physical resonance between brains in *groups* of animals or people is what allows an alpha personality or a bully, a person with a *highly* developed boss personality to "take over" the group. The followers have a relatively weaker narcissistic area in the brain and a stronger "obedient" area. This is what facilitates the phenomenon of "alpha" personalities and the creation of blind followers. In animals, these paired, group-brain behaviors are extremely helpful in regulating herd and pack dynamics. In humans, this dynamic can be abused to the point that people using primarily the "follower" part of the brain might literally be unable to think for themselves.

In a bit of pure conjecture, I have to wonder if, in people with Type I Parkinson's, the boss aspect of the personality is the one that is stuck on pause. The "follower" personality might have an extremely difficult time turning off its blind following.

This might be why, as you will learn later, a therapy for Type I PD that develops a relationship with an "outside" or "someone else" personality is so much more helpful than trying to change your thought habits by just talking to yourself. "Neuroscience Explains How a Narcissist Can Control Our Brain"; *Neurology Today*; Lancer, Darlene, LMFT; 2019.

https://www.psychologytoday.com/us/blog/toxic-relationships/202004/neuroscience-explains-how-narcissist-can-control-our-brain

[2] "The Nature of Traumatic Memories: A 4-T fMRI Functional Connectivity Analysis"; Ruth Lanius et al; *American Journal of Psychiatry* 161, no. 1 (January 2004); 36-44.

on brain science or psychology that were *not* directly related to Parkinson's nevertheless contributed support for my paradigm-shifting hypotheses about PD.

I am *not* a born paradigm shifter. At the time I started my Parkinson's research I was extremely shy and my live-by rule was "Don't make waves." No one would have been happier than me if I could have found a way to explain my patients' recoveries while staying in the comfortable confines of western medical theory or even modern Chinese medical theory. But even while western research was frequently if indirectly providing proofs for my hypotheses, I was steadily moving further away from the western medicine dead-dopamine cell model for Parkinson's disease and away from the formulaic, one-size-fits-all protocols of modern, government-approved Chinese medicine.

I was moving closer to what is considered by some the fringe realm of ancient, channel qi-based Chinese medicine and ancient Vedic (from India) theories of biophysics and consciousness. These theories, though ancient, are often more in sync with our most *recent* breakthroughs in western physics than they are with the older Newtonian theories of physics. In western medicine, we are still very much caught up in the mechanistic, Newtonian idea that that human body is the sum of its chemistry and mechanics as worked upon by entropy: the old physics. In *modern* physics, we see that the vast universe is *first* a manifestation of *ideas*, and only later becomes a manifestation of atoms. The same can hold true on the small, human scale when it comes to sickness and health: in many cases, our *thoughts* can have a larger influence on our DNA expression and our neurological behaviors than our physical structure or chemistry at any given moment.

Even though so many unrelated fields in medicine and psychology were doing research that appeared to have *glaring* significance for the subject of Parkinson's, no one seemed to be connecting the dots. Slowly putting together ancient eastern medical theory and modern western research, I kept collecting widely scattered dots until a picture emerged: for *most* of my patients, their emotional traits and intellect, as well as their PD symptoms and their inexplicable recoveries – or failures to recover – all began to make sense…but only if I was willing to consider a psychological component. Eventually, hesitatingly, grudgingly, based on the newest western research as well as the older eastern theories, I headed off towards a new, radically different hypothesis for what causes Parkinson's disease.

Meanwhile, as for Parkinson's from dissociation, not pause…

At the same time, the methods I was developing to help my *non*-PD patients self-diagnose and heal from dissociation from long-injured body parts and chronic health problems were also causing me to notice that a small percent of my *Parkinson's* patients were manifesting symptoms of mental dissociation from injury and the *physical* symptoms of pause but were *not* exhibiting the *mental* behaviors associated with pause.

These patients appeared to have merely dissociated from injuries – usually ankle or foot injuries – which had then failed to fully heal. Due to the location of their injuries, failure to heal had, over decades, caused electrical aberrations upstream from the injury, including backwards flow in the Stomach channel. Eventually, the domino effect of these aberrations was an electrical flow pattern that very closely *resembled* that of pause mode...and which therefore caused the physical, but not necessarily the *mental*, symptoms of pause.

I realized in retrospect, years later, that those PD patients who had recovered easily in response to Yin Tui Na treatments had only had dissociated injuries – they had *never* told themselves to feel no pain or embrace numbness. Looking back at my notes about their self-described attitudes and personality traits helped confirm that they had *not* mentally or emotionally been using pause mode. Instead, their electrical circuits were running in the pause patterns because of injury *only*, causing the physical symptoms of pause but with no or few signs of the "Parkinson's personality." They'd had *only* Type II, *only* Type III, or *only* Type IV PD.

Yin Tui Na causing partial recovery

In people with *only* Type II, III, or IV PD, whose channels were flowing in the pause patterns *only* because of a dissociated, unhealed injury, the re-association with and the healing of the injury via Yin Tui Na caused the Parkinson's to cease.

On the other hand, most of my patients had self-induced pause or, more likely, self-induced pause *and* a dissociated injury.

In people with self-induced pause *and* an unhealed injury, Yin Tui Na therapy *did* allow their foot injuries to heal.

In people with self-induced pause *and* an unhealed injury, Yin Tui Na therapy did *not* turn off pause. The treatment helped heal the injury and only the injury. But because these people were still mentally using self-induced pause mode for the rest of the body, the bits of localized, small-area *healing* – which should *not* occur while a person is on pause – often triggered unexpected, even bizarre, physical, emotional, and mental behaviors: the symptoms of partial recovery.

Chapter Nine

Partial Recovery

This chapter shares a sampling of early-on case studies that baffled me. In these cases, people healed from injuries that were causing Type II or Type III Parkinson's *but* hadn't yet turned off the self-induced pause that was causing their Type I Parkinson's. I didn't know yet that Type I PD even existed. After their foot injuries healed, these patients' symptom presentations quickly became highly unpredictable. Their personalities sometimes became bizarre, with obvious departures from their previous personalities. I named these symptom and personality changes "partial recovery." Years later, when I understood the importance of *first* getting rid of self-induced pause and only then working on any remaining injuries, these cases made a lot of sense.

The reason that most people with self-induced pause also have unhealed foot injuries was discussed earlier. You will recall that it has to do with inhibition of non-crucial healing when on pause...and many people hurt a foot or turn an ankle at some time or another.

For an example of what I mean by "bizarre" physical and emotional behaviors of people in partial recovery, I already shared the case study of the person who could merrily chase his wife on a good day and was immobilized by fear of the dentist on the very next day. Here is another example: I had been working with a patient whose foot injury had healed up over the last few weeks. Her Parkinson's symptoms had suddenly become greatly magnified in response to negative thoughts. Oppositely, they now might cease altogether for hours at a time when she felt safe or calm.

During a subsequent session with her, I asked her to try using positive affirmations, a type of medical qi gong, during the coming week. I offered a few examples: "I am safe enough to relax all the time, I am safe enough to be calm all the time." I repeated this several times. She repeated them with me. When she was leaving, with her hand on the doorknob, I asked, "You remember the affirmations?"

She replied, with a strange glaze over her eyes, "Yes. I cannot be safe enough to relax, ever. I cannot be safe enough to be calm, ever." And then her mouth smiled at me in a strange, mechanical manner...nothing like the genuine smiles that had already replaced her previously "masked" facial expression – when she felt safe.

Although the look in her eye gave me the creeps, I wasn't too surprised to see it or to hear her response. Just disheartened. I'd seen that look before, in other people in partial recovery. Partial recovery symptoms can include bouts of mental incomprehension, twisting of reality, and/or even short windows of amnesia. And these symptoms *only* appeared after the old foot injuries had healed.

I wasn't the only one noticing these weird changes. Spouses and friends also observed, in response to my patients' old injuries healing up, the new, drastic come-and-go changes in symptoms, as well as the appearance of glazed eyes, periods of severe illogic and evasiveness, and even amnesia lasting up to an hour. These drastic mental shifts often followed immediately on the heels of a suggestion for making psychological changes or of a gentle inquiry as to whether or not the person's symptoms might have a psychological component.

Darting eyes

Very often, rapid, left and right, back and forth darting motions of the eyes preceded the amnesiac or altered-personality behaviors.

I pointed out to a patient in my office who had recently started having these types of mental breaks that he had just done the eye shift again. He replied, as if he was battling with himself to tell me, "Just now, when you explained what I was doing this moment, when my eyes darted sideways and you pointed it out to everyone (his health practitioner and spouse who were in the office with us), I *was* able to realize I'd done it. And at that same exact moment, I stopped being able to understand what you were saying. I can still *see* you and *hear* you, and I can tell that my wife and Suzanne, they're sitting here beside me, they are understanding what you are saying. But just now my mind put up a wall. I honestly don't know what you are trying to say, but my mind is telling me that whatever you say, you are wrong, you don't know. My brain won't let me understand what you are saying and instead it's telling me that I shouldn't trust you."

I heard something like the above many times from people in partial recovery.

My first experience with the mental irregularities of partial recovery occurred in a patient who was showing improvement in his PD symptoms. He showed up at my office and announced, "I want you to know, I called all my friends on the east coast this morning and told them that the treatments we're doing aren't working. I told them I'm getting worse."

I was baffled. He was one of the first patients who had slid into partial recovery after responding well to the foot treatments.

I replied, "But you told me that you're doing much better, having more feeling in your legs, moving better, all kinds of improvements, even though the improvements do come and go. Why did you tell your friends you're getting worse?"

"Because Parkinson's is incurable. There is no way that what we're doing can possibly be helping, because it's incurable. I refuse to believe that changing the energy flow in my body will stop my Parkinson's disease. So I told everyone I'm getting worse because I know that's what's going to happen. Just recently, I found myself moving easily. I know this must be because I'm kidding myself. I *can't* actually recover!"

He was among the first to tell me something like this. I was stunned. Now I'm used to it. Over the years, after working with hundreds of people with Parkinson's, I became accustomed to this type of attitude showing up when a person slides into partial recovery. Nearly all of the people who ended up in partial recovery *never* fully recovered. Many became increasingly psychotic, and their symptoms became increasingly powerful. As mentioned earlier, this is why we disbanded the PD Treatment Team in 2013, determined to stop working with people with Parkinson's until we could figure out what caused partial recovery.

Denial

Another manifestation of partial recovery was the inability to remember anything having to do with recovery that had previously transpired. People who still had Type I PD after healing from their foot injuries and who had a few, preliminary recovery symptoms often forgot that they had *ever* experienced any recovery symptoms or that their injury had healed.

One patient kept working with me after the foot injury healed and recovery symptoms started to appear. We had both assumed, incorrectly, that she was going to fully recover. At this time, I still didn't know about Type I PD and that it could still be present even after the foot injury healed.

About six months after her foot injury was healed, she said to me, "I don't see why you're wanting to work on my mental posture (what at that time I was calling the wariness and negativity of the Parkinson's personality), because you've never gotten rid of my foot injury. I've never noticed any improvement in my feet."

I flipped back through her chart to her sixth week of treatment. "Do you remember saying, on June 4, "After the last treatment, my right foot hurt right across the top of the arch?"

"No."

"Hmm. Do you remember saying, on June 11, "I've had a sharp pain at the base of my third toe all week."

"No."

"Well, do you remember saying, on June 18, "My foot pain is gone and my feet feel warmer lately, it feels really good."

"No, but I believe you."

"Do you remember saying, on June 25, "This last week, I stepped on a small piece of kitty kibble with my bare foot. It *really* hurt! There's no way I would have been able to feel something like that in the past. It really *hurt*!"

"Well, OK. I'd forgotten about that. So if my foot is better, then why did I stiffen up a week ago when I found out that my grandson was going to prison? I've barely been able to walk since then, and my tremor's gotten much worse. You obviously haven't fixed my foot injury."

"I think your foot is fine. It seems to me that you might be stuck in partial recovery. Let's get back to work on addressing the mental aspects that seem to make up a large part of that pattern."

"No! You have to fix my *foot*! My *foot* must be the problem: I never even feel it! My mood and my thoughts have *nothing* to do with my Parkinson's. My foot has reverted back to being injured."

"It's the foot, not the head!"

Most Parkinson's patients *loved* the Yin Tui Na foot holding treatments, once they got used to the idea of a stranger touching their feet or ankles. Many people with both Type I and Type II PD, after the injury healed, experienced a slight reduction in symptoms and maybe even a few recovery symptoms such as sensations of pins and needles in the foot followed by improved somatic and proprioceptive awareness of the foot. Most patients assumed that their Parkinson's must be going away.

But when, sometime down the road, an emotional jolt brought their PD symptoms back to the previous level or higher, they were certain that they needed more Yin Tui Na foot holding treatment because *the injury had come back*. Again: when an emotional blow triggered a higher degree of self-induced pause and brought their PD symptoms back to a previous level or higher, they were *certain* that their foot bones had become *displaced* again.

In retrospect, I can see why they made this assumption. But at the time, I could tell that their feet were still behaving as if healed. So this assumption seemed illogical to me.

In most cases, there was *no way* patients were going to work on anything related to mental or emotional behaviors. The problem – they were *certain* – was the return of the foot injury. And the people who *did* agree to try working on the wariness and negativity quickly developed amnesia, selective memory, and in some cases, paranoia towards anyone who was trying to help them.

Forgetting to have Parkinson's

Many patients who got stuck in partial recovery noticed that their Parkinson's symptoms had gotten worse, *except* during those hours or days when, as they often put it, they "forgot" to have Parkinson's disease. Some laughingly reported things like: "I forgot to have Parkinson's on two different days this week – both times I forgot for the entire day! But don't worry, it came right back when I remembered I have it."

The strange thing was, their symptoms had never actually *disappeared*, according to the spouses. The symptoms had been greatly *minimized*, as PD symptoms tend to do when a person with Type I PD doesn't think about them or *worry* about them. What had happened was that they'd forgotten to be *worried* about their symptoms. They had maybe even dropped into some degree of parasyampthetic mode for a while because their foot injury had healed. The circuitry in the *foot* was able to flow in the path of parasympathetic mode. But most of the channel qi *outside of the injury area* was still flowing in the pause patterns *except* during periods when they "forgot" to have PD. I can only presume that, during these "forgetting" times, the channel qi was running predominantly in parasympathetic mode.

I heard this from *so* many patients: "I forgot to have Parkinson's!" together with the incongruous, "But don't worry! It's back,"

Why on earth would I be worried about the Parkinson's *not* coming back? Several patients helped clarify this for me: They actually *did* have Parkinson's. They were *never* going to recover. So when they forgot to have Parkinson's for a few hours or a few days, they were living a *lie*, which was *bad*. So it was *good* when they remembered to bring the Parkinson's back. I should be *happy* that they were being honest and manifesting their fullest compliment of Parkinson's symptoms.

At the time, I thought this was a manifestation of illogic. Now, I see in retrospect that they were right: they *did* still have Parkinson's and they had no way to make sense of their conflicting feelings of healing in some small part of the body while *still* being on pause in the rest of the body. Or maybe they were even slipping into body-wide parasympathetic mode for a short while.

Dormancy

A variation on "forgetting" to have Parkinson's was the decision that the Parkinson's was still there but the symptoms were reduced because the PD had gone "dormant." The patients' explanations for what was going on ranged from "I don't *deserve* to completely recover," to "It *can't* be this easy to recover." Therefore, the Parkinson's was still there even if the symptoms *appeared* to be decreasing. Again, this seemed like illogic at the time. In retrospect, these people were in partial recovery. Because of injury healing that was out of the natural sequence for healing, their bodies were sometimes predominantly on pause and sometimes predominantly enjoying the parasympathetic physical and mental behaviors that can accompany healing.

Just like with the people who "forgot" to have Parkinson's, these patients' *knew* they had PD but their more severe symptoms might be "dormant" for hours during the day, whole days, or even weeks But when some distressing life event occurred, they would manifest their symptoms at the highest level again, or even worse than before. The resurrection of these more severe symptoms was usually deemed proof of incurable loss of brain cells. They assured me that they were never going to recover – which turned out to be true for most of them. The emotional blow of this "proof" often resulted in super-rapid worsening of symptoms. I *now* suspect that, in response to some negative situation, they inadvertently increased the *degree* of self-induced pause compared to how much they had previously been using, thus worsening their symptoms and wiping out the parasympathetic-inducing benefits of having healed from the foot injury.

For years, this kind of thing is what happened to *most* of my patients. I had no idea what to make of all this.

Recovery spurned

In a few cases, I had patients who had been in partial recovery call me on the phone to say that their Parkinson's was now completely gone, and they were moving normally, even dancing wildly, and that they were going to enjoy it because in a few days or in a specific number of hours, the Parkinson's would return and would *never* leave again. This self-fulfilling prophesy would play out, just as predicted.

I would plead on the phone with these people saying, "If it's gone it doesn't *need* to come back!" They would tell me that they *couldn't* permanently recover for various reasons. The single *most* common reason was "I don't deserve to recover." They would often add something like, "I'm being given one last taste of freedom as a gift and then I'll have Parkinson's forever, so I won't be working with you anymore. I don't want to be wasting your time."

One patient in partial recovery, after a few weeks of playing excellent tennis again after years of not being able to play because of the muscle rigidity and immobility of *moderate* Parkinson's, stumbled while going for a ball and very slightly hurt her ankle. When this happened, she suddenly realized that she didn't "deserve" to recover. She *immediately* went into a condition of advanced Parkinson's. She very quickly became unable to walk, move her arms or torso or even feed herself. She was suddenly much worse off than she had been during her years with mild symptoms of Parkinson's, prior to her Yin Tui Na treatments. At the time, the Yin Tui Na had brought new awareness to her foot, and had seemed to be turning off her PD symptoms. But as soon as she injured her ankle, she was suddenly far, far worse than she'd ever been. And she was certain she *should not* be able to recover.

A few weeks later, she told me, "I shouldn't have been able to play tennis like that. I hurt my ankle as a punishment for being arrogant." She was never able to play tennis again. However, her husband thought I should know that, after he put her into bed each night, she could move *perfectly normally* while she adjusted her pillow and got herself comfortable.

She snapped at him, "I don't *have* to have Parkinson's once I've gotten into bed. I only need to have it as a punishment when I'm trying to show off by having mobility." She was adamant that her symptoms did *not* have a psychological component.

She was a highly respected child psychologist with a history of early childhood sexual abuse from her father who "was a very respected and good man…I shouldn't have such negative memories about him." I repeat, she had a doctoral degree in psychology and was a highly respected psychotherapist. In other people, she was quick to point out that everything they did had a psychological basis.

She insisted that her own symptoms had *no* psychological component.

Her situation was not unique. Many, maybe most, of my patients who slid into partial recovery eventually decided that they didn't deserve to recover and/or that there was no psychological component to their come-and-go, mood-related and/or situation-dependent symptoms, so they certainly were *not* going to do exercises to improve or alter their thought patterns.

Utter illogic

I was non-plussed the first time a patient said, "The tingling sensations in my face (a *temporary*, short-term recovery symptom) has stopped, so I can't recover."

I pointed out that she had regained full facial expression and a sense of smell and taste. I reminded her, yet again, that the tingling only lasts during the healing process. Once the nerve healing has finished, the tingling ceases.

My explanation was countered with, "Even so, I guess this means I won't be able to recover." Nothing I could say or do could influence this person who suddenly knew she could *never* recover *because* her recovery symptoms were following the *correct* trajectory. She was right, of course. She still had Type I PD, so she wasn't actually recovering.

Back in the early days of the project, when I wrongly thought all my patients were just dealing with a foot injury situation, I had to wonder what was going with these seemingly illogical convictions. In these cases where Parkinson's symptoms were reduced in severity after the injury healed but then came back stronger in response to some stress, I asked myself: was the short-term (hours, days, weeks) appearance of *recovery* merely psychosomatic, or was the *return* of the Parkinson's psychosomatic?

Something didn't make sense. If Parkinson's was based purely on physical problems, it shouldn't come and go for short or long periods *or* be triggered by mood or environment. But if it was purely mental or emotional, how could I explain the similarities in the physiological recovery symptoms that patients experienced after their foot injuries healed? As I figured out *much* later, most people with PD had both: a psychological problem (Type I) *and* a physical injury problem (Type II) PD.

Before I figured that out, it was still clear that *most* of my patients who recovered from their foot injuries did get stuck in what I had named partial recovery, and the symptoms during partial recovery seemed to have exaggerated responses to *psychological* triggers.

The name "partial recovery" didn't do justice to these inexplicable symptom changes and the eerie, even creepy mental changes that occurred in response to healing of the old injury, but I had to call it something. At the time, because the injury *had* finally healed and the channel qi was now able to flow correctly *some* of the time, I sincerely thought that these people had merely hit a bump in the road to recovery. The bump seemed psychological. I assumed that, with time, they would get over their psychological bumps and join the others in full recovery.

In a way, I was right: these people had come up against psychological bumps. In a way, I was very wrong: time alone would *not* get them past those bumps.

As it turned out, nothing was going to *lastingly* change for the better unless they made some very specific changes in their mental habits, changes that would stimulate their brains' long-dormant striata and thalami. And if they didn't make the changes, their symptoms on their "bad" days would quickly become much more severe than they'd had in the past, before the foot injury was healed.

It took more than fifteen years to figure out that these people had both Type I and Type II PD. If they *first* recovered from Type II PD and self-induced pause mode was still up and running, they started manifesting the kinds of thinking and behaviors described in this chapter. And the few cases in this chapter are just the tip of the iceberg. I saw it in *hundreds* of people with Parkinson's disease. The chapters on recovery symptoms provide examples of the tremendous difference in perception between people who were fully recovered and those in partial recovery as they experienced changes in their bodies in response to healing from injuries. Ongoing self-induced pause co-existing and conflicting with parasympathetic mode behaviors in the vicinity of the healed injury was, I suspect, the underlying culprit in partial recovery.

Ever since I started promoting the idea that Type I PD must be addressed first, *before* working on the injury or blockage in the Stomach or Du channel, I no longer see the weird partial recovery symptoms.

Chapter Ten

Worrisome Observations and Single Case Studies

Didn't want to go there

I *really* did not want to find a psychological component. I wanted a straightforward biological explanation for what causes Parkinson's and a logical, corresponding cure. I thought I'd found one, but it only seemed to apply to about five percent of my patients with Parkinson's.

I also knew that most of my PD patients did not *want* a mental component to be contributing to their symptoms. Not At All.

Nearly all of my Parkinson's patients had told me, so many times, in so much detail, how their symptoms increased or decreased in response to various stresses or relaxation methods, or even in *anticipation* of stress or relaxation, and yet most of them were *adamant* that their syndrome was *purely* physical: not in the least mental.

For an example of the mental component that was clearly dominant in most of my PD patients, one of them was astonished to learn from me that some people have PD symptoms even after they come home from work. Puzzled, he asked me, "Why would they have symptoms once they're done for the day?"

He wasn't even in partial recovery. From the *start*, he had *never* had symptoms after six in the evening. As soon as he sat down in his lounge chair at 6:00 p.m., he was symptom free until the next morning. He refused to consider that there might be a mental component to his Parkinson's symptoms.

As for my patients who were now in partial recovery, my team members, the patients' spouses and friends, and I were all seeing new, mood dependent extreme come-and-go Parkinson's symptoms and personality swings. As for the sideways-darting eyes, the selective amnesia and/or glazed facial expression in response to suggestions about positive affirmations or to casual remarks about the symptoms appearing to have psychological triggers, those symptoms looked a heck of a lot like the behaviors of a person using two personalities.

As a professor of psychology, I know that *most* psychologists consider multiple personality disorder (now known officially as dissociative identity disorder) to be incurable. The *others* say that it doesn't exist. Many big names in psychology feel that this is the realm of freaks and frauds. I did *not* want to consider the possibility of multiple personalities in my Parkinson's patients.

Then again, why not? Was I afraid of the "messiness" of a psychological component such as multiple personality disorder? Was I afraid of the "incurability" label? Parkinson's was considered incurable and yet it clearly was not – for some people. So why should another "incurable" label worry me? Was I concerned about the credibility aspect of my research?

When a syndrome has a psychological component, it is much harder to isolate any research variables. Double-blind studies often don't make sense for such syndromes. The big cohort studies with thousands of people who are all similar genetically or who all have a similar syndrome are much harder to put together if the problem is mind-based. If, for example, the problem is a highly individualized mental construct designed in secret to keep the person from feeling pain, it might be nearly impossible to design a meaningful cohort study.

The single-case study

In the field of psychology, the single-case study, meaning a case report with just one patient, is increasingly considered a valid and important type of research. Compiled psychological research that builds upon single-case studies is almost the opposite of a double-blind study: often, everyone involved knows who is doing what process. [1]

Ever since the 1970s, in the field of psychology, the recognition of and significance of single case studies has been growing. Because each person responds to psychological therapies in a somewhat unique way, journal write-ups of *individual* treatments and *individual* results have become a respectable source of data for researchers and for people trying to find their way out of pathologies with a mental component.

By building on single case studies and observing how the methods used with one person get results, or not, when used with another person, it is possible to build up enough data to show that, *in general*, a certain percentage of people with a given mental quirk or pathology *do* or do *not* tend to have a particular response to a given therapy.

Cognitive behavioral therapy: an example

Since being developed in the 1970s and '80s, the original type of cognitive behavioral therapy has been tested on hundreds of thousands of people with depression. It has been shown to be effective in a majority of cases, and to be more effective than drug-based therapies.

The researchers who developed cognitive behavioral therapy, a therapy now recognized as a powerful tool in abating depression, started with single-case studies. Over time, compilations of single-case studies showed that, while not perfect, cognitive behavioral therapy had a far higher success rate for treating depression than did the pharmaceutical approach or the talk therapy / analysis approaches.

As cognitive behavioral therapy became more widely accepted, further research studies were done to investigate whether people could use the methods effectively by working on their own, from a book. It turned out that the percent of people that recovered from depression via working from a book on cognitive behavioral therapy was even higher than the percent of people who recovered by doing cognitive behavioral therapy exercises with a trained therapist.[2]

Bibliotherapy

The book-based, self-applied approach, called "bibliotherapy," is now considered a valid therapy track. In its early years, bibliotherapy was scorned by many practitioners of old-style psychological talk therapies such as Freudian analysis – therapies now proven

---

[1] *Single Case Experimental Designs: Strategies for Studying Behavioral Change*; Herson, Michel, PhD, Barlow, David PhD; Pergamon Press; Elmsford, NY; 1976; ISBN 0-08-0019512-1.

[2] From the introduction to *Feeling Good: the new mood therapy*; David Burns, MD; HarperCollins Publishers; 1980; p. xxviii. ISBN 978-0-380-81033-8.

to *increase* negative thought patterns if their focus is probing deeper into problems instead of looking for ways out. Bibliotherapy is a *zero*-blind process. The patient *reads* about the therapy and then practices the suggestions in the books. He brings about changes in his own brain. No therapist can do the actual work of changing the thinking patterns of his patient. The patient must do the work. Because the focus is on what the patient needs to do rather than on the relationship with the therapist, people using bibliotherapy tend to make faster progress. The effectiveness of bibliotherapy, which means working on one's own, from a book, has now been proven by tens of thousands of *single*-case studies.

Based on my years of experience working very closely with people with Parkinson's, I have concluded that bibliotherapy, not talk therapy, is also the *most* effective way for turning off Type I PD.

Single-case studies are considered highly valuable when dealing with medical problems that are presently regarded as incurable. Even if only one person in fifty in a very small study recovers from an "incurable illness," the findings of that single case is considered to be highly significant...*especially* if those unexpected results, however skimpy, can be replicated now and again by others.

At the time cognitive behavioral therapy was being developed, severe, disabling depression was considered to be more or less incurable. Therefore, even single case studies in which people recovered were of value.

After many years and many successful single-case studies, when cognitive behavioral therapy was firmly accepted by a large number of researchers in the field, then larger, quantitative studies were done. These studies further verified that the therapy was, in fact, helpful for a large percentage of people with depression.

This slow approach to confirmation of a theory might take decades. Along the way, the founders of cognitive behavioral therapy were, of course, despised by people promoting more traditional therapies: psychoanalysts and prescribers of pharmaceutical drugs for what they were then calling "chemical depression." Some therapists even accused proponents of cognitive behavioral therapy of "blaming the victim," because cognitive behavioral therapy helps patients feel better by changing their own mental habits.

When I started on the Parkinson's Recovery Project, I did not know of the latest standards for research in the field of psychology. Fortunately, one of my earliest advisors for my research, Dr. Fred Jones, PhD, had a background in teaching both medical research and psychology research. He suggested that I focus on single case studies in the beginning. Readers of the first few editions of this book will remember that those early books featured primarily single case studies in which people had unexpectedly recovered from PD. Those editions reflected much less *technical* understanding of what was physiologically happening in the people who recovered from Parkinson's, but those case studies certainly were fascinating. My readers with PD could relate to their stories, their personalities, their stoic responses to injury, in a way they couldn't relate to what their doctors said about dead brain cells. People from around the world sent me emails saying they could see powerful similarities between those patients and themselves, even though they *weren't* usually able to relate emotionally to other people, for the most part. These reports, and other similar statements from people with PD helped keep me going during the long years of self-doubt.

My early-on single case studies of people with inexplicable recoveries were hugely important over the long run. They provoked in me and in others a curiosity and even a passion to find the electrical, physiological, and/or mental common denominators in people with Parkinson's, so as to make sense of those intriguing single case studies.

Didn't want a psychological component

Even so, I really didn't want to find a mental component in people with Parkinson's disease. But there clearly was. The weird behaviors that looked a lot like a second personality – one that didn't always know what the other personality was doing – was the strongest proof yet that something psychological was going on.

I needed a name for the mental process driving the briefly or intermittently glazed eyes and amnesiac personality. I settled on "the Blocker."

Then I described the Blocker-driven behaviors in *Stuck on Pause,* a book that I posted online even though it was not yet completely finished. Many people in partial recovery who were not my personal patients but who were following my work online sent me emails after reading *Stuck on Pause*. They described their own interactions with their very real and sometimes scary Blocker when they tried doing positive thinking or positive affirmations. Nobody disagreed with the name I had given to this strange force that seemed to be living in these people's brains and resisting their attempts to alter the established course.

Some people said the Blocker manifested as a voice. Many people with western religious leanings said the Blocker was a devil. A patient from southeast Asia said it was a green ghost, a traditional form of demon from that part of the world.

In some patients, the Blocker was silent, but manifested as threatening visuals or cue cards. For example, when one patient tried to therapeutically imagine feeling the sense of pericardial expansion characteristic of parasympathetic mode, he saw in his mind's eye that his heart had little signs all over it saying, "Stop!" "Don't do this!" and "No!"

Another, trying to imagine that her heart and head were filled with bright and happy light, saw that the inside of her mind was a cave with barbed wire and a big "Keep out" sign across the opening of the cave.

Although inhibition of *positive* visualizations is normal during pause, visualization of *negative* scenarios is usually effortless. This makes good biological sense: when a person is motionless following an almost deadly attack, that is not the time for him to start imagining rainbows and merry dance moves. Being preoccupied with dangerous outcomes and *scary* visualizations might even *help* a direly injured person remain curled up and wary.

Happily, when people recover from Parkinson's, they often find that they can once again see fanciful images in the clouds or see "faces" in the bark or the light-layered leaves of a tree. But while a person is on pause, he usually cannot access the part of the brain that does *positive* imaginative thinking and/or visualization.

Getting back to the Blocker, its presence was a common problem for many people in partial recovery who were trying to do conventional types of mind- and mood-changing self-help and/or cognitive behavioral therapies in order to turn off their come-and-go pathological degree of wariness, wariness that triggered or amplified their PD symptoms.

The people in the previous chapter who declared they couldn't actually recover in spite of seeing positive changes, or who declared they didn't deserve to recover, were obeying the instructions of a part of their minds that I now called their Blockers. The Blocker can be utterly illogical and yet completely convincing.

As a licensed acupuncturist, psychological counseling is not within my scope of practice. However, I am legally allowed to instruct a patient in self-change therapies so long as they fit under the description of medical Qi Gong.

Medical Qi Gong is the art of using visualization, affirmations, the sensations of energy and/or specific physical movements, in order to bring about changes in the way a person uses or perceives his physical and mental energy.

I encouraged my patients in partial recovery to try various self-help therapies, both common and fringe, including Qi Gong and cognitive behavioral therapy. Some of my patients also worked with therapists or hypnotherapists. None of these methods seemed to help. Worse, repeated attempts at positive mental changes, even short affirmations, seemed to embolden and strengthen the Blocker.

– A reminder: as noted before, Qi Gong, yoga, positive affirmations and other *body*-awareness therapies ***do*** help in cases of *only* Type II Parkinson's.

Many people have written asking if they should avoid doing Qi Gong or other therapies that help Type II PD *if* they have Type I PD or have both Types I and II. Don't worry: whatever type of PD you have, go ahead and do whatever yoga and Qi Gong you have been doing. Be aware that, *if* you have Type I PD, these therapies will probably not bring you joy, body awareness, or any of their other benefits, nor will they help move you towards recovery. So long as you are using Type I PD, you will not be able to *do* these techniques in a correct, meaningful, effective way.

I've had PD patients who were *very* skilled in these arts, even long-time *teachers* of yoga and of Qi Gong. They had gradually developed Parkinson's disease in spite of doing these techniques for decades because they were never actually doing them correctly: they never did them with full *somatic* awareness while holding themselves in parasympathetic mode. They were just going through the *physical* motions while keeping their bodies on pause. There is not much risk that a person will inadvertently heal any dissociated injuries as he keeps doing his exercises *while* staying in self-induced pause.

As one patient said, "I did Qi Gong exercises almost daily for more than twenty years while slowly developing Parkinson's disease. Only after I recovered did I learn what doing real Qi Gong actually *felt* like. I realized that I *hadn't* actually been doing Qi Gong at all during those years. I had merely been going through the physical motions."

That having been said, a person with both Type I and Type II PD should *not* do Yin Tui Na treatments to help re-associate with and heal from any injuries that might be *helping* keep pause mode circuitry in place. Unlike your ineffective and incorrectly performed yoga and Qi Gong, which isn't helping you, the assist from another person doing Yin Tui Na might actually encourage you to re-associate with your injury(s) *before* you turn off pause mode. That would be bad.

If you have Type I PD combined with any other type of PF, recover from Type I PD first. *Then* deal with the injury. If the injury(s) doesn't heal spontaneously within a few weeks of pause mode turning off, then you can try using Yin Tui Na, Qi Gong, or whatever helps you pay attention to and feel safe about your injury.

Chapter Eleven

Weirdest of all: the epiphanies

Moving even further into the realm of the unexpected, *several* people with Type I *or* Type I *plus* Type II Parkinson's recovered *permanently*, almost instantly, within minutes, in response to an utterly unexpected epiphany.[1]

For example, one person had been in partial recovery for several years. She was finally bedridden most of the time due to the rapid worsening of her symptoms following successful Yin Tui Na treatment of her foot injury and a very short-term, come-and-go improvement in symptoms. Despite the eventual extreme severity of her symptoms, keeping her bed-ridden, she recovered almost instantly, within minutes, after her epiphany, when she unexpectedly found herself yelling to God, 'I *do* want to live; I *do* want to live!"

When I first met her, a few years after her recovery, she told me, , "I never even knew that I was thinking that I didn't want to live, but I guess I had been."

In each of these recovery-by-epiphany cases, the person had finally given up after decades of something along the lines of trying to be loving to *others* while staying strong, even stoic with regard to himself or herself: maintaining an extremely high degree of "noble" self-control and emotional numbness towards self. In each epiphany case, the person had unexpectedly exploded in an unplanned conversation, either silent or aloud, either angry with or surrendering gratefully to God or to some higher authority or a deceased loved one – all of whom I might refer to in this book as an "invisible friend." The invisible friend might previously have been silently spoken to *dutifully*, but nevertheless kept at an emotional arm's length.

The *cause* of the change was different for each person but each person did *consciously* decide to change a core attitude or opinion.

During their epiphanies, there was a sudden flip in their previous convictions: maybe the idea that one must always be on guard; that life wasn't worth living; that "I never asked to be born" (oh, yes you did); that life had been unfair (no it wasn't, ultimately); or some other long-held excuse for living as if half-dead. It was as if they stopped listening to the pause- and Blocker-produced arguments and started listening to the loving support of a different voice.

The change might involve allowing an invisible friend *or* the Love represented by the friend to take over, to be in charge of the patient's life. Or it might be a decision to finally accept the love of or the truth being spoken by an invisible friend. The change might be a decision to stop listening to the relentless, negative, internal voice: a voice proclaiming that the battle of life must be fought *alone*.

---

[1] Epiphany definition: (1) a *sudden* perception of the essential nature or meaning of something. (2) an intuitive grasp of reality through something (such as an event) usually simple and striking. (3) an illuminating discovery, realization, or disclosure.

In spiritual writings, handing responsibility over to a comforter is often referred to as "surrender." Surrender can be accompanied by enormous relief and relaxation. But in my experience, most people with Parkinson's have an inflamed dread of the very idea of "surrender," and associate the word with imminent death or increased suffering. A person with this limited understanding of surrender might do well to consider a young child who is having a tantrum due to some frustration. He makes himself increasingly miserable until he finally breaks down. He *surrenders* and allows the parent to hold him and comfort him.

In the epiphany recoveries, at some point in each one's harangue, the person with Parkinson's suddenly was overwhelmed with an internal feeling of love and safety, burst into tears, took deep gulping breaths, felt shivers going down the spine, and the Parkinson's was gone. Permanently.

A person who trembles following a nasty shock gives a strong shiver or two to "shake it off" and then snaps out of it. In the same way, these people had an epiphany that they were safe. They were not existentially alone. They were loved. And then they shivered and "snapped out of it." Their Parkinson's was permanently gone.

As noted before, following that almost *instant* change to *not* having Parkinson's, a person will still have to heal from the decades of nerve inhibition, muscle rigidity and, in other areas, muscle atrophy. But the *driver* behind the Parkinson's will be clearly gone...in an instant. And it's glaringly obvious. But instant recovery via epiphany made this syndrome seem even more like a mental disorder. You can see why my conviction of a mental component was growing stronger. While I wasn't happy about introducing the idea of a mental component, let alone the drama of multiple personality disorder, I was flat out determined *not* to go down the path of faith healing or epiphanies.

This was hypocritical of me, as my own recovery from Parkinson's disease had been of the epiphany type.

One of my medical advisors for the Parkinson's Recovery Project told me early on that regardless of how *I* recovered, my own case should *not* be of particular importance in my overall research. I could use it for yet another set of data points, but I should be careful *not* to lean too heavily on the fact that I too had recovered. My own data, my single-case study, was only important for what it contributed to the larger picture.

Because the spontaneous-epiphany style of recovery was fairly uncommon, and because it did *not* seem – at the time – to contribute to a biological understanding of Parkinson's, I minimized my own recovery in my earliest writing and kept looking for what I thought should be biological answers.

What I failed to connect, for years, was what led up to each person's epiphany: a vigorous, even bitingly honest and/or profoundly intimate – even laughing and irreverent – communication with someone or something loving, invisible, and outside of and separate from oneself: behavior that can *stimulate the striatum*, a brain area that is *inhibited* when a person is on pause.

I didn't learn about the striatal activation/ word-based communication connection until I stumbled across some radically new brain research in 2015. This research showed how specific feelings and communicative thoughts could increase activity in the thalamus and striatum: A person *feeling* resonant with something loving outside of himself had increased activity in the thalamus. A person who was even *thinking* about mentally *communicating* with something loving outside of himself had increased activity in the striatum.

After reading about this new brain research, I went back over my notes and confirmed that every person with an epiphany-type recovery also had a very *long* history of regularly talking to someone outside of himself, either a spiritual figure, a departed loved one, a totem animal or a spirit guide: an "invisible friend." During the epiphany, the person had taken the relationship to a higher degree of trust: very often it was trust that the friend was more capable of being in charge of the patient's life than the patient was, or could comfort the patient, or was at least qualified to give advice or help. The patient didn't have to "be in charge" or "be alone" in the world anymore. The patient had finally let go of some long-term mental and emotional distancing between the self and the invisible friend, and was willing to trust the friend *more* than he trusted his own mind. The word used by many who recovered from Type I PD was "surrender." They explained to me that they had to give up on their brain's controlling method of dealing with life. They "surrendered." They allowed their own positive-attitude embracing, loving self, a self long-stifled, to silently *communicate* with someone else who was loving and protective. They allowed that other someone be their protector. Then, they could let their guard down.

As I mentioned earlier, I had taken copious notes about as many aspects of my patients' lives as possible. I was able to confirm by my notes that all the epiphany-recovery patients had long maintained a *habit* of mental communication with some type of invisible friend. The communication might have been a regular conversation with a departed mother or childhood friend, or even a beloved deceased pet. It might have been a spiritual practice of almost constantly, if only dutifully, talking to some aspect of the Divine.

In my own case, it was a spiritual discipline, a habit practiced dutifully, if mechanically or, at times, resentfully, but practiced nonetheless. The discipline was obeying these simple laws: never let yourself imagine that you are alone; always know that God or a representative is right there with you; always be silently talking to God; the company you keep is stronger than your own will power, so stay always in the company of the saints and share your every thought with them.

These are basic precepts in *every* major world religion. For example, a New Testament adherent would understand all of this to be contained in the admonition: "pray without ceasing." [1]

Parasocial relationships

In the field of psychology, since the 1950s, the term "parasocial relationship" has been used to describe what was originally thought of as a one-way relationship, often between an audience member and the performer. The audience member feels that a relationship exists. He might even have silent, meaningful, imagined conversations with the performer *outside* the context of the performance: the performer becomes a personal, invisible friend. In the Freud-dominated 1950s, this relationship was presumed to be somewhat infantile, possibly related to the so-called "imaginary friends" that children often have and which parents often cruelly discourage.

Today, psychologists recognize that many people have a healthy, supportive relationship with a benevolent, invisible friend – and the relationship is *not* necessarily

[1] Thessalonians, 5:16.

one-way. Very often, the friend offers loving support and advice, even humor and insight. The term parasocial relationship is still used to describe these relationships, but with the new recognition that these relationships can be two-way, beneficial, and are even fairly common. [1]

In spiritual circles, this type of relationship with one's preferred saint, savior, guru, or totem animal has many names across many religions. "Practicing the presence of God" is a phrase that is currently seeing renewed usage across several religions. This phrase was famously used by Brother Lawrence of the Resurrection (1614-1691) and described in his book *Spiritual Maxims*. His book succinctly explains his spiritual discipline of constantly talking with and feeling tangibly close to God.

The spirit quests undertaken by Native Americans and First Nations peoples of North America are often a search for an invisible friend and guide. In these coming-of-age rituals, an adolescent must go off on his own until he develops a relationship with some totem animal, ancestor, or spirit with whom he can intimately communicate, and who will advise and protect him for the rest of his life. This rite helps an adolescent make the move away from relying on his mother or aunties for comfort. By finding an omnipresent communicant, he can learn to constantly commune with a vaster source of energy. By doing so, he stays in touch with his heart: learns to think with his heart.

In many western and eastern religions, the practice of constantly talking to some aspect of the Divine is encouraged. Sadly, both eastern and western cultures seem to be moving away from teaching children the importance of developing a relationship with a loving, invisible communicant as we grow into adolescence and grow apart from the tangible but ultimately unreliable support of our family members and friends. Maybe someday we will better understand the deep need humans have for this kind of omnipresent, loving support and once again encourage communicating with it, from either a secular *or* a religious standpoint.

The loving and steady advice and support from an "outside source," if *not* associated with a particular friend, is sometimes referred to as the voice of conscience or the voice of God. It can be thought of as our innate wisdom, a loving wisdom associated with the heart, as opposed to the constant, ego-based thought stream generated by the brain. [2]

In cartoons, this relationship is often portrayed by an angel sitting on a person's shoulder. Very often, the other shoulder has an ego-driven imp or devil. Both might vie for the person's attention.

---

[1] Secret Friends: Tapping Into the Power of Imagination. This 51-minute audio file interviews people "who have trained themselves to experience the invisible as real."
www.NPR.org/2020/01/27/7999635099/secret-friends-tapping-into-the-power-of-imagination

[2] Karl Jung, the famous philospher/psychologist/ explorer once asked Ochwiay Biano, chief of the Pueblo Indians, for his opinion of the white man. The chief said white men must be crazy because they think with their heads, and it is well known that only crazy people do that. Jung asked how the Indians thought. The chief replied that, naturally, they thought with their hearts. (From *The Sun*; "Sunbeams (Letters to the editor);" Laurens van der Post; Sept 2007; p. 48.)

Animals don't need to develop this connection. They already have it, always. Unless they have been hideously tortured to the point that they have become deranged, animals do not have the mental capacity to delude themselves into thinking that they are apart from the one Unifying Love.

The heart, or more accurately the highly conductive connective tissue *around* the heart, the pericardium, acts like a radio receiver/ transmitter. When a person lets his thoughts be guided by his pericardium, he can "tune in" with the heart-type frequencies of loved ones, saints, or sages, whether they are living or have passed on. According to ancient Vedic physics, this heart communication uses gravitational waves, which are faster and less disrupt-able than the mere electromagnetic waves of brain-based thoughts.[1]

Most of us have had the experience of unexpectedly thinking fondly of a dear friend and then the phone rings or a letter arrives in the mailbox: it's the friend! This process uses the "radio" of the pericardium, not the habit-controlled thought-ruts of the conscious mind. Great saints have often developed the power of this connection to the point that they testify to conversing directly with some aspect of the Divine, an aspect with which they can tune in via their hearts.

A strong habit of mentally conversing with someone who loves you and with whom you can laugh and comfortably be yourself, whether it's your late cousin Larry or some aspect of God, helps keep your attention on the waves generated or received by the heart. Conversing with a trusted, irreverent friend *also* stimulates the currents that run through the *midbrain*, keeping the striatum and thalamus activated and keeping the body circuits running predominantly in parasympathetic mode patterns.

Oppositely, staying wedged in a chronic distrustful, negative monologue keeps one blindly repeating the ego-driven, negative thought habits collected and accumulated on the *sides* of the brain. This keeps one oriented towards sympathetic and/or pause modes and actively *inhibits* parasympathetic mode. You cannot be neutral with your thoughts. You are always doing one or the other: either you are encouraging positive thoughts or reinforcing negative ones.

---

[1] Vedic (ancient Indian) physics holds that matter comes into existence through the condensation of subtle waves: the foundational, "original" waves of creation are generated by the consciousness of God (The Word, in Judeo Christian scripture, or The Sound or The Voice, in the Vedic). These pure waves of consciousness, also known as "Sound" or "Divine Sound" waves, can condense into the denser waves of "Movement," modernly referred to as gravitational waves and also referred to in the Vedic as waves in the Air phase. From there, gravitational waves can condense down into light waves. Light waves can condense into subtle types of electromagnetic waves, and these can condense into the most dense waves of all, the electromagnetic waves associated with the electron behaviors in tangible matter.

The five phases of waves used in the creation of the illusion of matter are, translated from the Vedic, Ether (Sound, or God's Consciousness waves), Air (movement or gravitational waves), Fire (light waves), Water (subtle electromagnetic waves) and Earth (densest, easiest to perceive electromagnetic waves such as those generated by tangibles). These five phases are sometimes referred to poetically as the five "elements" or, in Sanskrit, the *pancha tattva*.

We are made "in God's image" in the sense that we too have the capacity to generate, transmit, and receive all of these types of waves – but only if we use our *heart*-based ability to generate ideas and receive and transmit wave information – *not* our very limited, *brain*-based, ego-based minds.

Epiphanies in the presence of the friend

My patients' epiphanies occurred – and the Parkinson's turned off – when the conversation was, for some reason (usually desperation from pain or fear or just giving up), taken to a deeper, more passionate, intimate, and trusting level than before so that the *feeling* of being mutually connected was enhanced *or* the un-self-conscious *quality* of the communication was enhanced. Or both.

Based on the new brain research, this surge of feeling connected would have stimulated the thalamus and striatum, and thus allowed the person with PD to mentally let go of his ferocious, pause-amplified sense of isolation and need for self-control. This change occurred as my patients mentally allowed themselves *finally* to be consoled, comforted and/or lovingly laughed at by the invisible friend.

Following this, the self-induced pause immediately turned off – as pause is *supposed* to do when a person begins to 1) feel stable inside and 2) confirms that he is now safe enough to come back to life.

In 2015, given the new striatum and thalamus research, those epiphany-type recoveries no longer seemed as random and unrelated to my research as I had first supposed.

An epiphany case study.

In the late 1990s, a couple of years after starting my PD research, I was diagnosed by a close friend and colleague while describing to him the symptoms of Parkinson's disease à propos the Stomach channel.

"What are you trying to tell me?" he asked.

"I'm just telling you about how all the symptoms of Parkinson's fit with backwards-flowing channel qi on the Stomach and Large Intestine channel," I replied.

"What are you trying to tell me?" He asked again, more slowly.

"What do you mean?"

"You've just described every symptom with reference to yourself and symptoms that you say you've had increasingly for some years now. Even your tapping with your index finger when it's idle is getting more frequent."

"Oh…" followed by a long silence. "Well, I don't have Parkinson's. Don't be ridiculous." I abruptly walked away.

I was dismayed by his diagnosis, with which I eventually had to concur.

I hadn't been able to explain to myself a recent episode with festinating gait. I had fallen, spread-eagled, on nasty gravel when my legs suddenly moved in slow motion and couldn't keep up with my torso during a six-mile run when I had temporarily dropped my mental focus on my legs in order to look at a passing cement truck. For the last few years, it had been getting harder and harder to turn over in bed.

I was only in my late forties, but I often needed a hand up from family members to get up off the sofa if I sat down for "too long," even though I was an avid runner.

Lately, when strolling around town, I often caught myself mirrored in the shop windows. My body was increasingly hunched over, elbows bent at a ninety-degree angle. My posture was positively distorted. I would straighten up my spine and relax my arms. Continuing my stroll, I would see in the next shop window that I was hunched and bent again.

I could no longer coordinate my hands enough to play classical piano. I fell back on playing only ragtime – where the timing didn't matter so much.

For about the past two years, my face in the morning mirror was expressionless. I would pull my mouth up into a smile to start my day. Increasingly, people on the street said to me in passing, "Hey, it can't be that bad…smile!" or something similar. In decades previous, total strangers had been wont to say, "You've got a beautiful smile!"

People were starting to have trouble reading my handwriting. In the evenings, while reading before bed, my right index finger tremored steadily.

I made a list of my Parkinson's symptoms. I had, though to a modest degree, *all* of the classic symptoms of Parkinson's, and more than two *dozen* of the more obscure ones such as the inability to separate the second and third toes (the terminus of the Stomach channel) on the more affected side and an oppressive feeling of pressure against the upper chest while raising the arms above the head. This pressure is due to the rigidity of the pectoral muscles – which lie on the path of the Stomach channel.

Another example of an "obscure" symptom is the very specific way in which most people with Parkinson's turn over in bed at night – while they are still able to. While laying on the back or side, one brings the knees up as far as possible towards the chest. Next, the head and shoulders are pulled forward, bringing the body as close as possible to a tight fetal position. Then, using a powerful sideways jerk, the whole body is hoicked over as a unit toward the desired side.

In comparison, a healthy person rolls over languorously, leading with the head, the shoulders, or the hip and leg and then letting the rest of the body smoothly follow.

For a few years prior to my friend's diagnosis of me having PD, I had been rolling over using the fetal-position jerk.

I had also trained myself, over decades, to produce a very slight, constant exhalation whenever food was in my mouth, in order to prevent aspiration of food particles and the choking and throat spasms that accompany the aspiration. I had even seen a doctor, nearly fifteen years earlier, because of frequent, spontaneous "choking on my own saliva." The MD had assured me, "You can't choke on your own saliva. It's physically impossible. There's nothing wrong with you. It's all in your head."

But since starting the Parkinson's project, I had already learned from my patients that many of them had trained themselves to practice this cautionary, faint but steady exhalation while chewing. And even with this precaution, they often had spontaneous choking, "choking on their own saliva." A person who is on pause has a very poor swallow reflex, and can easily choke on his own saliva whenever saliva slips down into the windpipe instead of into the stomach tube.

Most of the more obscure symptoms are not known to neurologists, but a thorough intake of even just a few dozen people with Parkinson's will create a long list of symptoms that are not common in the general population and very common in people with Parkinson's disease. I had nearly all of these "obscure" symptoms.

More significantly, at the time my friend offered his diagnosis, I had already seen people recover from Parkinson's. I had *seen* people recover. And yet, almost my first thought upon being diagnosed was, "I won't be like them…I won't be one of the lucky ones who can recover."

This thought startled me, and them made me furious at myself. This attitude that "I won't be one of the lucky ones" had already been stated by *most* of my new recruits from the PD support group…and had never been stated to me earlier, by what turned out to have been Type II or Type IV patients.

Then again, a *few* people who were stuck in self-induced pause did have a powerful conviction, based on their self-perceived ability for "mind over matter," that they *would* be one of the "lucky ones"…but they weren't able to turn off pause despite their determination. As it turns out, an ability to emotionally surrender or enjoy self-deprecating humor or laughter at one's own expense is a better predictor of recovery than an ultra strong will power and a ferocious determination to succeed. The latter are both characteristics of the pause personality. The pause personality cannot turn itself off. Only the person/personality who set pause *in motion* can turn it off.

People with Type I either *knew* they couldn't recover or they *knew*, incorrectly, that they could recover through the use of their rare and powerful will power.

Oppositely, the Type IV patient discussed in chapter 2 had laughed merrily about the possibility of recovery shortly before it occurred: "Ha ha! Wouldn't it be funny if *I* recovered?!"

Prior to my own diagnosis, this breezy denial of hope in most of the new recruits had filled me with resentment. After all, I had seen people recover from this syndrome. Why were so many of the new patients so negative about the possibility of their *own* recovery? And now, here I was displaying the exact same, uncharacteristic (for me) negativity with regard to my own possibility of recovering.

Many of the new recruits from the PD support group had wanted to meet and talk with someone who had recovered in order to combat their cynicism. In the very early days of the Parkinson's project I set up meetings so that people with PD could meet one or two of the people who had recovered.

Instead of being inspirational or instructional, these meetings *always* had the opposite effect. *Everyone* with PD said, after meeting with a recovered person, "*I'm* not like that person. *I'm* different. So *I* won't be able to recover even if *everyone else* does."

I also heard a lot of, "That person [who recovered] looks perfectly normal. Their Parkinson's couldn't have been very bad. Mine is more advanced, so *I* won't be able to recover."

I really resented their negative attitudes and yet, for several days after being diagnosed, I couldn't help having it myself. I sulked around, certain that I was doomed. I was different from those people who had recovered. Recovery couldn't happen to me. Rats. And just when the arc of my life had finally started looking higher and brighter than it ever had.

Then again, my new diagnosis helped me understand why I had always felt as if I could finish the sentences of my patients when they were trying to describe what their symptoms felt like from the inside.

And maybe my immediate conclusion that I could not be one of the lucky ones wasn't *me*. Maybe it was part of the Parkinson's personality!

After a few days, I abruptly decided that I didn't have Parkinson's after all. All I had was doctor's disease: the sudden, psychologically induced manifestation of symptoms in a person who is *studying* a syndrome. So I sat myself down and wrote a more thorough list of all the somewhat idiosyncratic physical and *behavioral* traits I'd noticed in myself that might *possibly* be related to Parkinson's *and* their approximate date of onset.

Some of my symptoms went back fifteen years or more. The highly memorable pre-PD brain-spin event, probably triggered when the Stomach channel first short-circuits from ST-8 into GB-14 and GB-7 (see page 4 and chapter twenty-eight), had occurred when I was seventeen years old. Some people remember this event. Others do not. I hypothesize that, if the event occurs while sleeping, one will not remember it.

One symptom went back to around age seven or eight. I secretly, now and then, pulled off the entire toenail on my right-side smallest toe, pulling it off the nail bed all the way down to the cuticle because for the next few days the faint throbbing sensation gave me a rare awareness of my increasingly numb foot, an awareness that I found strangely reassuring.

I hadn't yet shared with my patients the alarming news of my diagnosis. The day after making my new, longer list, I casually asked some of my Parkinson's volunteer patients if they had ever experienced some of the symptoms on my new list.

I asked my first patient of the day, "Did you ever pull off your little toenail all the way to the root because the consequent throbbing sensation felt sort of good, was sort of a relief?"

His wife exclaimed, "No! That's gross!"

The patient gaped. He was speechless. I waited. Finally, he whispered fearfully, "*How* did you know that?"

The commonality of that symptom turned out to be *very* low. Most of my patients with PD had *not* done this. It was only a happy chance that my first patient of the day had done the same thing as me, for the same reason. Still, by the end of the week, I had learned that many of my idiosyncratic behaviors were *not* so unusual in people with Parkinson's. Many of my PD-related behaviors and nascent PD symptoms went back at least ten years, if not all the way back into childhood.

I had only been doing the Parkinson's project for less than two years. So my symptoms weren't doctor's disease.

I had Parkinson's.

I then decided that I might be able to take advantage of having Parkinson's to better help my patients. After all, the way the western medical theories described this syndrome did *not* fit with how we all *felt* inside. I had to say "we" now.

But I was still feeling depressed, uncharacteristically bitter towards God, and certain that I would not recover. I was ashamed of all three.

As a medical professional, I had always seen that the patients who do the best are the ones who find some way to look on the bright side, some way to be grateful in spite of the way things are playing out. I wanted to be like those people.

And so, early one afternoon, more than a week after my colleague diagnosed me with Parkinson's, I forced myself to go into my meditation room for a long talk with God. I told myself I couldn't leave the room until I was genuinely grateful. I didn't know or care what I would be grateful for, specifically, but I did know that when inexplicable difficulties arise, I should always seek the kindest possible explanation, in order to be closest to the truth.

I started mentally talking to Paramahansa Yogananda (1893-1952), a saint from India to whom I'd long felt close. I refer to this generically as "talking to God." For me, God is too vast to imagine, so when I "talk to God" I'm actually focused on some human who, to me, represents sweetness, love, wisdom, protection and, most importantly, a sense of humor and the ability to gently tease me, mocking my frequent foolishness.

A few hours later, joy radiating from my tear-swollen face, I staggered from the room. I was indescribably tired. I was also spilling over with gratitude for the many, many positive things in my life and especially for the utterly unexpected foreign-feeling waves of joy that had surged within me, swamping me and repeatedly overwhelming me during my hours-long, alternating bitter and grateful knock-down, drag-out confrontation with my saint.

In our silent conversation, I'd detailed all the terrible, unfair, negative experiences of my life. He'd responded by telling me he'd always been there, protecting me. But I'd never really wanted his advice or help. I'd wanted things to go the way I wanted. I'd been sulking. He assured me that every seemingly negative event had transpired for a reason and for my own good.

Eventually, grudgingly, I "surrendered" to his steady insistence that he was there for me, he'd always been there for me, and that everything God had "allowed" to happen had been part of a Divine plan. He assured me that I had done my best. More importantly, he had always loved me whether I had done my best or not. I decided to let go of my life-long, bitter version of the "unfair universe." I could admit that, in the big picture, I didn't really know what I was doing. In a metaphysical sense, I didn't know what was best for me or what I karmically deserved. I didn't know what prayers I might have uttered in a past life – possibly on behalf of others – that were being incomprehensibly fulfilled in this one. And my saint *did* seem to know. I decided I would trust his version of this loving but mysterious universe, a universe in which everything is ultimately fair and comes out beautifully okay in the end. The epiphany in my case was that I abide in a universe in which I never am, and never have been, alone. And everything happens for my highest good. And then I found myself overwhelmed with love...and I allowed myself to accept that love. This was followed by sobs of joy and waves of relief as the weight of forty-plus years of hidden resentment and stifled self-pity fell off my shoulders.

It was mid-afternoon when I left my meditation room. I went to bed and slept deeply.

When I woke up from my atypical mid-afternoon nap, I realized that something inside me was gone. The profound stillness (lack of internal tremor) made me think that I must have died in my sleep.

Then I inhaled. So I wasn't dead. But I was still just as motionless inside as before I'd taken the breath. I breathed again, just to test the waters.

Since I was breathing, I concluded that I wasn't dead, even though the internal stillness felt utterly unfamiliar, as if I was in an altered mental state.

The passing idea that "I must be dead" is fairly common in people with PD when the *internal* tremor ceases. Others have far less dramatic thoughts, such as, "The washing machine inside me just turned off."

I could sense energy moving just under the skin of my right foot, from ST-42 over to the Spleen channel near the ball of the foot – a healthy, sympathetic mode pathway and one that had probably been numb and non-functional in me since my right foot was smashed in a car door when I was around five years old. After my initial scream of shock when the car door shut, I had not cried from the pain, knowing that if I made a fuss, my sister who'd closed the door and maybe I, too, would be beaten by my mother: very likely whipped with a leather strap until my deeply troubled mother collapsed into tired satisfaction.

Due to regrettable family dynamics, I had taught myself to dissociate from and not react to painful events long before that foot injury.

Now, after the epiphany, while I was still lying in bed and *not* feeling agitation inside (!), I felt physically lighter, as if my body was less dense and heavy. I was filled with inexplicable joy. I suspected that the thing that was gone was the thing that had driven the Parkinson's symptoms. I was filled with new energy and radiance and my muscles were strangely soft. I *knew* I no longer had Parkinson's disease.

But what was going to happen to my research? I had already decided that one of the many reasons to be grateful for having Parkinson's was because it could help others via my research project.

I marched back into the meditation room. I told God, via Yogananda, that I didn't want to recover from idiopathic Parkinson's unless everyone else could.

I sensed silent words that seemed to come from all around me. "Everyone can. Most people do not want to."

Suddenly much less confident, I told the voice that I didn't believe him.

I set out to prove him wrong.

Years later, when the Blockers showed up, and second personalities, and I saw just how many people were determined that they didn't *deserve* to recover or couldn't recover even if everyone else did, I had to wonder, "Is this what that Voice was talking about when it said that most people do not want to recover?"

I now understand that, while most people in my experience *do* want to recover from the *symptoms* of Parkinson's disease, most people do *not* especially want to change the personality traits that they think are keeping themselves free from harm. They do *not* want to get rid of the personality they created that is stronger, faster, and somewhat impervious to pain: an effect created by pause mode combined with the intensity of a powerful norepinephrine override.

It is a medical truism that most people would rather die than change. Consider the many seemingly simple changes that a person might make to improve his quality of life or even save his life: stop smoking; exercise more; eat minimally and eat foods that aren't highly processed to help prevent high blood pressure, weight gain, or diabetes; and so on. Most people know perfectly well that making changes in their life-style might bring enormous health benefits. And yet, as we learn in medical school, most people would rather die than change. When I started this project, I assumed that this medical law would *not* apply to people with Parkinson's disease. I was wrong.

When it comes to changing core aspects of ourselves, we each have the right to make up our own minds on whether or not we want to do this. Most of us do not want to.

Oppositely, people who do recover often say something like, "Before recovering, I wanted to go back to the way I used to be before Parkinson's. Now that I've recovered, I *never* want to be that person again! That person was miserable and didn't even know it."

Returning to my own cases study, because I've been asked what type of PD I had, I would have to say both Type I and Type II. I remember commanding myself to be numb. I was in high school. I was staring hard into a mirror at the time (Type I PD). I also had a significant injury to my foot when it got slammed in a car door at age five or so. It had never healed: that foot was always a full size shorter than the other (Type II PD). A few weeks after my epiphany and the turning off of self-induced pause (turning off Type I PD), my long-injured and somewhat numb foot suddenly collapsed and wouldn't support my weight. It felt as if all the bones spread out, making my foot go utterly flat. And then, the bones slid painlessly into their proper places. My right foot was suddenly the same length as my left foot and had a new springiness. Within half an hour, the bones were stable. I was able to walk almost normally. This spontaneous self-healing of an old injury when pause turns off is not unusual. When Type I turns off first, old injury(s), if any, including any that might be contributing to Type II PD, often re-associate on their own over the next few weeks or months, as they should when one gets to a safe place. After that, the injury is able to quickly heal.

So. I'd had an epiphany and recovered from PD, and then my old foot injury spontaneously healed with no treatments from anyone. At this time, when people asked me who had done holding (Yin Tui Na) therapy on my foot, I was too shy about my spiritual inclinations to tell the full truth. So I merely said in a vague sort of way that I'd been helped by "a friend." In truth, it was the *invisible* friend's tangible presence during the *epiphany* that was my "help." That, in turn, led to all the other aspects of healing.

But the epiphany model didn't really help further my research...right away. After my own epiphany, I did try, for a few years, to encourage people to talk vigorously to God or some invisible friend in hopes of triggering an epiphany, but no one was able to have a healing epiphany by mentally reciting rote words to the silent walls.

As it turns out, there's a specific way of talking (friendly and laughing) and a specific type of relationship (trusting, *mutual* friendship) that leads to an epiphany. Completely and forcefully tuning out the constant, negative monologue of Type I Parkinson's and replacing it with constant, silent talking to the right kind of invisible friend in a loving, laughing, usually irreverent way *does* help lead to recovery because it stimulates the striatum. As you will read in chapter twelve, this is *one* of the two techniques I came up with that, used together, can turn off self-induced pause.

How long does it take to induce an epiphany?

And here is that question again: how long does this take?

Once in a while, self-induced pause turns off in a matter of moments after the person with Parkinson's starts to talk silently to a loved one. But most of my patients had no history of cultivating a parasocial relationship. They needed to spend months, sometimes years, before these techniques become habitual and strong enough to be effective.

But whether the response is quick or takes a few years, these techniques that involve working with an invisible, trusted loved one – one with whom the patient can laugh – *can* eventually turn off self-induced pause. Oppositely, talking respectfully to a distant God who is emotionally aloof or who has rigid and unforgiving rules for right and wrong behavior will *not* do the trick. Thinking about *this* type of God stimulates the amygdala, the fear and rage center, *not* the striatum.

That finding was years in the future. Until I understood the brain biology at work when silently talking to a trusted and invisible friend, one with whom the patient could *laugh* and be utterly honest, I didn't understand how to *teach* people how to have a healing epiphany. I couldn't explain how to have what should be a most natural, effortless type of silent or spoken conversation with someone or something that's invisible, loving, and located outside of oneself.

Immediate personality changes

The *immediate* behaviors following recovery were similar in nearly all patients, and in a most unexpected way. People who had been using self-induced pause, when they suddenly, fully recovered, often laughingly, light-heartedly, said something like, "Ha ha! I was doing this to myself!"

To appreciate this, you need to know how hard it is for most of the people I've known with Parkinson's to un-self-consciously laugh at themselves for having made a mistake. For example, many of my patients, when asked, admitted that, if they were walking down the street and suddenly remembered that they had to turn around and go back the other way, would not pivot, but would continue walking straight, turn at the corner, and go all the way around the block so that none of the strangers around them would perceive them as having made a mistake or as "behaving strangely" by turning around in mid-stride.

During the week that followed a person's complete recovery event, in response to some situation that previously would have been a *really* big deal, even a mortifyingly *shameful* really big deal, such as arriving one minute late to an appointment with me, the person very often said to me laughingly, and I quote, "So what. It's not like someone's going to die, after all."

A post-recovery statement about "not going to die" was so common that, in one week, I heard it *twice*. Two people who, a week earlier, would never have made that statement because *everything* was crucial and everything should be done *right*, said laughingly, about an error or screw-up on their part, "So what. It's not as if anyone's going to *die*."

This type of statement was *so* common after a person turned off pause that, for a short while, I asked people who were stuck in partial recovery to say this phrase or one like it as often as possible, in case it might trigger turning off the Parkinson's. It didn't, of course.

As an example of how utterly uncharacteristic this phrase was for these people, one of them laughingly told me that she'd talked to an old friend on the phone the evening before. She hadn't seen her friend in a very long time and the friend had no idea about her Parkinson's diagnosis or her very recent recovery. Her friend had asked what her plans were for the upcoming season, and my newly recovered patient had replied, "Oh, I don't know, I'll see what I want to do when the time comes."

A long pause had followed, and then her friend had asked carefully, "Are you OK?"

My patient laughed again and told me, "I've always been the Great Planner. I always know exactly what I'm going to do and when I'm going to do it. When I told her I didn't know just what I'd be doing next season, she was shocked. She must have thought I was sick or dying. Ha, ha, ha!"

I'm trying to get across just how freaky it was to have this type of person suddenly *not* worrying about the future or *not* dreading the reveal of some dire character flaw such as being the sort of person who might arrive at an appointment one minute late, and instead casually telling me, “Ah, I really blew it. Ha ha! So what. It’s not like anyone’s going to *die,* after all.”

I eventually began to wonder if maybe these people had been using a personality that was constantly reminding them that they were on the cusp of death, and only vigilance was protecting them from dying. As I was to learn more than a decade later, keeping alive while on the cusp of death is the whole point of pause mode.

When people recovered, when pause turned off, it was as if that pre-death personality disappeared. They cheerfully *laughed* at themselves and their shortcomings and said, “It’s not like someone’s going to die…”

Those patients who, in retrospect, had probably been using self-induced pause, instantly underwent a glorious personality shift when they recovered. They were able to laugh at themselves, to be spontaneous in speech and action, and *feel* the expansion of their chest in response to things beautiful or poignant: they could *feel* joy again.

But sadly, most of the people who were now in partial recovery, both my patients and my email correspondents, stayed there. By most measures, because of the increased severity of symptoms when wary – a problem that spiraled in intensity as they learned to be wary of wariness itself – they were far worse off than they had been prior to receiving the Yin Tui Na therapy and healing from their injuries.

I eventually decided that, in order to help them, I would need to find a consistent method for turning *off* their weird, often paranoid, second personalities if that’s what they were – thus preventing the descent into partial recovery. Relying on spontaneous epiphanies wasn’t going to cut it.

But neither Chinese theory nor western research in medicine *or* psychology told me how a person could go about turning *off* what seemed to be a deeply imbedded instruction to feel no pain. And in case you’re wondering, hypnosis didn’t help, nor did any of the many, *many* modern techniques that my patients worked at, including currently popular techniques for changing brain behavior. Neither did the purchased gimmicks and gizmos that promised to increase energy or provide inner calm. Nor did their various dietary changes make any difference. I have *never* seen a person recover due to a dietary change; not from Co-Q10, thiamine, diets with no fat, or with no meat, or with no alcohol, or “magic water” and other formulas that promised recovery via some external change. Very often, these programs did cause a period of improved symptoms – the placebo effect. But at the first sign of danger, wariness, or negativity, the PD was back, working away even harder than before.

The helpful Blocker

In the end, accepting the fact that *some* people had a Blocker personality was helpful. It *forced* me to venture past the overly simplistic ideas that 1) everyone with Parkinson’s had the same underlying cause and 2) the problem was purely a physical one with no psychological component. The idea that a person in partial recovery might have two personalities, an idea backed up by symptoms observed not just by me but by so many spouses and friends, and even some circumspect patients themselves, was alarming but enormously helpful in the long run.

Ordinarily, a person who is using normal pause mode *cannot* access parasympathetic mode at *all*. It’s a biological *law*.

The possibility of two personalities, one of whom could clearly be in parasympathetic mode when conditions were "safe," provided an explanation, at least an hypothesis, for why most patients were sometimes, *temporarily*, able to feel joy, or able to have greatly diminished symptoms, or no *visible* symptoms at all.

At some point it occurred to me that possibly, when *originally* commanding himself to be numb, the person had *not* actually put himself into pause mode. Instead, maybe the instruction had inadvertently created a *personality* that was on pause mode by using techniques of self-command that resemble self-hypnosis. That somewhat numb but physically powerful and intensely focused personality might have been so helpful, especially considering some of the childhood settings that I learned about from many of my patients, that it became the *dominant* personality.

But in partial recovery, these patients' new, post-Yin Tui Na capacity for sensory awareness and the joy, yes the joy of having a foot that they could *feel*, that joy and feeling could only manifest in the personality that could do parasympathetic mode: the non-pause personality.

This might explain why so many people in *partial* recovery behaved as if they had two distinct personalities. The dominant, default personality was the one stuck on pause. This is the one that developed a Blocker - especially if and when other people suspected or asked if there might be a *psychological* component involved.

Maybe the healthy (non-paused) personality was still *able* to use parasympathetic mode but, I hypothesized, this personality had increasingly been snoozing in the background as the pause personality had steadily gained in strength through the years. In response to the supportive Yin Tui Na treatments, this healthy self had been awakened in the part of the body that had recently re-associated with and recovered from an old injury.

It might be worth mentioning that, of all my patients who *had* always remembered commanding themselves to not feel pain, including myself, not one had ever told *anyone* what they had done. The action had always been a very private event. For some it was even a shameful secret…until I came along with my nosy intake questions.

As for why people in partial recovery were now so much worse off when they needed to use their protective personality, the one that the Blocker worked for, I hypothesized it was due to the re-association with the *foot* injury while the rest of the body remained numb, according to the old, secret instruction to "feel no pain." That healed foot, complete with restored sensory perception and linked to a trusting aspect of the patient's personality, might have served as a threat to the numbing protection system that had long ago been put in place.

Biological laws, for good reason, prevent a person or animal on pause from going into parasympathetic mode until the brain signals the all-clear.

By re-associating with their unhealed injuries and letting them heal, a parasympathetic mode behavior, I had to wonder, had people who'd also been using *self-induced* pause cracked open the door to their healthy personality that had been waiting in a back room? Had this then threatened their body-wide game plans for staying impervious to pain? Or created some kind of brain confusion?

In response to Yin Tui Na, usually on the foot or ankle injury, the patient had re-associated with the injured area – a behavior that is *not supposed to happen* so long as a person is on pause. Maybe the foot or ankle part of their consciousness had opened a door to their healthy, normal, real personality, a personality that could use parasympathetic mode, and thus move normally. Which *isn't* supposed to happen if you are on pause and at risk of imminent death.

Whatever the reason, when there was any hint of risk, the people now in partial recovery certainly fell back on the pause-using personality to a much stronger degree than they had before. And in some cases, it was now re-enforced by the recent creation of a Blocker.

I also hypothesized that the re-association with and healing of the old injury was, for some reason, disabling the use of the emergency override with norepinephrine, which had previously been used for motor function instead of using dopamine.

You'll recall that norepinephrine, or something like it, enables a person to override the motor inhibition of pause mode. Maybe, with the foot or ankle injury now re-associated and healed, with the brain dipping now and then into parasympathetic mode, the pause-related emergency norepinephrine override was no longer as readily available, if at all. But the motor *inhibition* from pause mode was still available, and could be activated when deemed necessary.

Or maybe summoning up the emergency norepinephrine override was no longer possible because being in partial recovery meant there was no more *actual* sense of emergency any more…only the *habit* of using pause.

In writing the above, I'm just pondering and proposing possible explanations for why some, only some, people in partial recovery become unable to activate their norepinephrine override as well as they did *prior* to recovering from the old injury.

But *if* a person could no longer access the norepinephrine override, he might, when using the paused personality, suddenly be *horribly* immobilized, far more than before. Which is what I was seeing in some people who were in partial recovery.

And at the same time, when these people were using the healthy and at-peace personality, the one that was only allowed to manifest when everything seemed completely safe, they might move almost normally. And every patient had a different idea of what constituted "safe."

Meanwhile

During these years, still more people, a small percentage, completely recovered from Type II Parkinson's in response to receiving Yin Tui Na treatments from spouses or friends or even by doing the treatments on themselves.

In people with *only* Type II Parkinson's, this type of treatment helps the patient re-associate with and heal from a long-dissociated injury, and this turns off the electrical behaviors that mimic those of pause. I often learned of their recoveries via emails.

But most people with Parkinson's who tried to recover did not. They slid into partial recovery. I heard from many of them, too, via email.

By 2013, I was semi-retired from my acupuncture practice. I was working steadily on finishing a set of textbooks for acupuncture students. When I had been a student in acupuncture college, all we had were poorly translated, confusing books in English translations that had been approved by the Chinese government. I was writing what I hoped might become replacements for, or at least additions to, these terrible texts. I was still teaching one class per semester and following closely the new research and trends in neurology and psychology. I was still working with patients two days a week and seeing a few people with Parkinson's, but no longer taking new patients.

Nearly all of the patients who'd gone into partial recovery had drifted away or lost touch. Which makes sense: I had nothing more to offer them. Some started taking antiparkinson's medications and suffered horrible, horrible adverse effects very quickly. If a person is in *partial* recovery and is able to go in and out of PD symptoms, the medications seem to be much more powerful and addictive than if a person still has full-time idiopathic Parkinson's. This altered reaction to the medication also suggested that their brains were now using more attributes of parasympathetic mode than a person with classic idiopathic PD does.

In May of 2013, the Parkinson's Treatment Team agreed that we should disband because there was clearly something that we didn't understand, and partial recovery was usually, or eventually, far, far worse than no recovery at all. Partial recovery also seemed to create the Blocker. By this time, I no longer was willing to work with new patients until I understood what was happening in partial recovery.

Considering that, in many ways, partial recovery was worse than Parkinson's, I did NOT want to provide injury-healing treatments that made people slide into partial recovery, or make them more susceptible to the dangers of the medications *if* they decided to start taking the medications sometime down the road.

I kept the website up and running, so that the small percentage of people who were able to recover in response to Yin Tui Na might work at doing so at their own risk. But until I understood who was a good candidate for that and who would instead end up in the nightmare world of partial recovery, I was no longer willing to work with new patients.

I made my new position clear to the patients I was still working with. A few of them wanted to keep working with me anyway, or to stay in touch via email. Since, at this point, these people had recovered from their injuries, if any, and the remaining problem seemed to be psychological, there was no need for me to meet with these people in person: emails would suffice.

Why was there no need to meet in person? The epiphanies, the psychological changes that had led to recovery in people with Type I PD, had *never* been brought about by working with a therapist or someone on the PD Team. In almost every case, the breakthrough came when the person felt that we had nothing more to offer. Then, when the person with Type I was desperate enough and finally willing to surrender, able to let go of some deeply personal reason for being angry with or grieving because of God, or because of the universe, or the world, or his mother, or some fateful event in his past, *then* he could move forward. He could turn to an invisible someone or something outside of himself. *Then*, his talk with his invisible friend could lead to a healing epiphany.

The epiphany was nearly always the result of a *decision* – not information, instruction, or encouragement from a paid professional. The people who'd had epiphanies were people who had, for the most part, given up on working with us and were stewing in misery until they decided to change their mind about some core belief. A very few who had only *recently* been diagnosed and/or who had very mild symptoms did *not* need to get rock-bottom desperate to have the epiphany, but most patients did.

The PD Team had already seen that people who regularly worked with us were *never* able to make, maybe weren't desperate enough to make, this type of decision. In every case, they were determined that we, the health practitioners, should be able to heal them, guide them, instruct them. So long as we were willing to meet with them and work with them week after week, they were apparently not interested in or desperate enough to make the drastic decision to change their mental alignment. Our "work" usually consisted of just talking, because their injuries had already long-since healed.

The people who had the epiphanies were, for the most part, people who had *given up* on the possibility of a cure coming from a doctor or therapist. The only thing they had left was the possibility of changing their own outlook – a deeply challenging mental shift: a shift that one must make on one's own. Of course, there are always exceptions and variations, as there will be with any self-created, primarily mental, syndrome.

For an example of an exception, in 2017, two years after I'd come up with the "talk to an invisible friend" therapy, a PD patient with very mild PD symptoms, who wasn't particularly desperate, had the epiphany within minutes. During his first visit to my office, I suggested he start talking to an invisible friend. He asked if he could talk to his late grandmother. When I said "Sure," he immediately stopped talking to me. He closed his eyes and I could see that he was silently engaged with someone. He began to smile gently. A shudder ran over his body. His Parkinson's symptoms ceased, never to return. Right there in my office.

It was his first visit. He was a friend of a friend who I agreed to see even though I was officially no longer taking new patients. He had never read my books. He had no idea about this type of therapy until I described it to him that day and warned him about some of the recovery symptoms. He didn't think he actually had PD, which is not uncommon in the early stages of this syndrome. Patients in the early stages of PD often think their doctor's diagnosis is wrong. Based on his dozens of symptoms, his unhealed foot injury, his personality profile, and his channel qi flow, he PD. And he had Type I and Type II.

He was also my first and only PD patient who immediately stopped talking to me and started talking with an invisible friend when I suggested that he should do this very thing.

I have asked *so* many patients to start talking to an invisible friend and all they have wanted to do is talk to *me* about what that might be like, or who they should talk to, or how often, and so on. This man was my only PD patient who ever understood immediately what I was saying: your invisible friend is more important than your doctor, your therapist, or me. Be always talking to your invisible friend who loves you *so* much.

I've never seen a person with Type I PD recover so quickly. Right before my eyes. I hadn't even finished telling him about what he was going to need to do, *how* to talk to his friend and so on. His case was an exception – a very rapid recovery from Type I PD: he started to have the facial spasms typical of recovery before he left my office. But for *most* people with this type, the epiphany came from a place of utter desperation, and in some cases, took years of work.

Epiphanies great and small

Not everyone who recovered from Type I PD had the huge, all-or-nothing, life-changing epiphany. More people who recovered from Type I Parkinson's had slow, *gradual* changes in mind-set: small breakthroughs in mental focus spread out over weeks, months, or years.

After 2015, as patients worked on the exercises that increase activity in the striatum and thalamus but most still wavered between a habitual fear-based monologue and their new ability to *feel* safe once in awhile, many had *small* moments of insight:

mini-epiphanies. The most important mini-epiphanies for many were the repeated realizations that their PD symptoms at any given moment *were* in fact directly related to their mindsets at that moment. They had repeated proof that they *could* influence and even retrain their own mindset by doing the exercises that stimulate the striatum and thalamus. After that, their observations that their mind was, in fact, causing their symptoms sometimes helped them to throw themselves more vigorously into their silent conversations with their invisible friends and turn their metaphorical backs on their negative, bitter, or wary mental habits. They often increased their intermittent efforts to change their mental habits when they made this connection. As the mind *slowly* changed its habits and they were able to feel safe more and more of the time, they observed their symptoms slowly decreasing in frequency and/or intensity, and recovery symptoms starting to appear.

Many patients have said to me, "I can't really be recovering. My symptoms are decreasing in intensity, and I'm starting to have recovery symptoms. But I can't be recovering because I haven't had the *Big* Epiphany yet!"

Please remember: not everyone has One Big Epiphany. No two people put themselves into self-induced pause for the same exact reasons or in the same exact manner. No two people turn off pause in the same exact way. If you feel safer, if your symptoms are less frequent or sometimes less intense, and/or if you are having recovery symptoms, then you are recovering. Whether the Parkinson's turns off in a flash or subsides over several years, you are going in the right direction.

Those people who had the dramatic, sudden epiphanies, after which they knew that the Parkinson's was gone, were hugely important to my research. Like the people with the Blockers, the people who recovered in a few moments following an epiphany forced me to confront the uncomfortable fact that mental behaviors play a role in self-induced pause and in Type I Parkinson's. However, the dramatic epiphany with its sudden and utter change is *not* the only way to recover. Small and gentle mental changes can also serve. Their effect can accumulate over time and lead to a gradual, more measured recovery.

Either way, full recovery is delightful and worth working towards.

2013

Getting back to the 2013 decision to stop working with *new* patients, I was still working with some people with Parkinson's, most of them via email. I had much less confidence that a cure for *everyone* with Parkinson's might come about in my lifetime.

Meanwhile, though now semi-retired, I was still extremely busy, especially with my writing. I hoped to record for posterity what I had learned so far about Parkinson's, pause mode, Yin Tui Na, and Chinese medicine in general. I had boxes of patients' file folders filled with notes written in my scrawling, near-incomprehensible shorthand. This was back in the days before electronic recordkeeping became the norm for doctors. Plus my head was packed with hypotheses and general observations that I had not yet written up about my patients with Parkinson's.

I wanted to get as much information into shareable form as possible. Even if I hadn't figured out how to help *most* people with Parkinson's, I hoped my observations might give the *next* researcher a leg up.

By 2013, I strongly suspected that there were four ways to induce pause-type flow of channel qi but until I could come up with a way to systematically, predictably turn *off* what I had recently named self-induced pause, I couldn't even be sure that there were *only* four ways to trigger Parkinson's. Until I could figure out effective treatments for curing all the types of PD, I couldn't even be *sure* how many types of PD there were.

Chapter Twelve

2015

The last part of the puzzle – how to turn off self-induced pause – was solved with information based on brain scan findings in the very new field of neurotheology. Neurotheology is a multidisciplinary field linking neuroscience with religious and spiritual phenomena. The puzzle's answers were found in the types of mental behavior that can activate the brain's striatum and thalamus: brain areas involved with the release of dopamine for movement and with somatic awareness, respectively. Activating these areas can lead to turning off self-induced pause.

In 2015, I found myself agog at the implications of the work of Andrew Newberg, MD, a leading neuroscientist. [1] Using brain scans, his research showed which areas of the brain manifested an increase in activity when people of various ages and religions were asked to "think about God." *Different* areas of the brain were activated in different people. The increased-activity area depended on what type of God one had.

For example, if a person's God was a critical or vengeful God, then thinking about God would bring about increased activity in the brain's amygdala (fear and rage centers). If a person's God was presumed to be knowable through word-based study such as memorizing of scriptures, then thinking about God increased activity in certain word-driven zones, in parietal (sides of the brain) areas.

Here's what jumped out at me: if one's God was feel-able and/or something one could physically resonate with, then thinking about God increased activity in the *thalamus*. If one's God was someone or something with whom one could *communicate*, then thinking of God increased activity in the *striatum*.

In pause mode, sleep mode, and in Parkinson's disease, electrical flow through the striatum and thalamus is significantly inhibited. As you'll recall from chapter 4, the striatum regulates dopamine release for motor function, positive imagination, and anticipation of joy. The thalamus processes somatic feelings and regulates how and where we sense that we exist.

I'd noticed since the beginning of my research that nearly all of my PD patients not only couldn't somatically feel themselves, they also didn't think it was *right* for them to talk intimately with God, saints, sages, saviors, or even loved ones who had passed on. Most were certain that it was good for *others* to talk to God or to saints, but for my patients with Parkinson's, this type of communication wasn't "morally right" for *them*. This bizarre idea – held by my patients who were devoutly religious but also by my many patients who were religious *professionals* – will be discussed in depth in chapter sixteen.

---

[1] *How God Changes Your Brain*, Andrew Newberg, M.D., Ballantine Books, 2010, chapter 3. Some of his other books are *Why We Believe What We Believe*, *Words Can Change Your Brain*, *Why God Won't Go Away*, and *The Metaphysical Mind: Probing the Biology of Philosophical Thought*.

So here's what I was looking at: new research showing that 1) thinking about a God with whom *conversational* communication is possible increases activity in the striatum. Again, activity in the striatum is *inhibited* in people on pause and in people with Parkinson's and 2) thinking about a God with whom a sensation of internal resonance, of resonant somatic feeling is *possible* increases activity in the thalamus. Again, activity in the thalamus is inhibited in people on pause and in people with Parkinson's. This new research started a revolution in my brain. Based on these findings and on the experiences of the epiphany recoveres, and working with my remaining patients, I developed two simple mental exercises that I hoped could re-awaken healthy activation in these two brain areas *despite* the pause-induced tendency for those areas to be inhibited.

My goal was for patients to self-stimulate their striata and thalami by doing these exercises. My thinking was, this could cause them to feel feel safe, which would then turn off pause – just as it had done in the epiphany recoveries. [1]

The new exercises

In the first of the two exercises, the person should treat all thoughts throughout the day as a two-way conversation with an invisible friend. Even during spoken conversation with some tangible human, with someone *other* than the friend, the person should assume that the invisible friend is in on the conversation. The invisible friend might be a deceased friend or relative, some saint or sage, a fictitious character or a person admired from a distance but never met, or even a beloved, deceased pet. And when I say "two-way" I mean *potentially* two-way. Grandma or Yoda might be silent, but the assumption has to be that she or he is listening and *could* reply either via the patient's intuition or even audibly, if and when she or he feels like it.

The friend has to be someone you can *laugh* with, someone who loves you in an easy-going, honest manner. It *cannot* be a stern or spiritually "superior" critic. Talking to a judgmental or "superior" god will stimulate the amygdala: the fear and rage center. An

---

[1] Further confirmation of the relationship between loving, word-based communication and the striatum comes from research done in 2019 using brain scans to show which brain areas are activated in children when being read to, as opposed to when children use computers or other "screen" devices for self-amusement. While books are read out loud to children, the children's brains' striatums become highly activated.

This finding is from a study done by the Reading and Literacy Discovery Center of Cincinnati's Children's Hospital. "This is your child's brain on books: Scans show benefit of reading vs. screen time"; CNN Health, Sandee LaMotte; Jan 16, 2020; www.cnn.com;2020/01016/health/child-brain-readubg-book-wellness/index.html .

In this study, looking down from the top of the skull, the children's scans show increased activity in a diamond-shaped zone centered at the striatum. Most of the activity is centered at the mid-striatum, and tapers off in the areas just anterior to and posterior to the striatum *and* off to the left and right sides of the striatum. The four tapers create a pattern of a four-pointed diamond shape with slightly inwardly- curving sides. The diamond shape exactly resembles the diamond shape of the fontanel, the "soft" area at the top of a newborn's skull that hardens as the skull matures. The fontanel is at the surface, but the activity in the diamond shape from being read to is deep within the brain at the striatum, directly *below* the area where a newborn's fontanel is found.

individual might or might not want to talk directly to God. Many patients assumed they *should* choose God, Jesus, Mohammad, or the Buddha as their invisible friend. As one patient put it, "You know, go straight to the top."

Whether or not talking to God is a good idea depends on whether or not the person's God, if any, is non-judgmental and if the person can share a good, even irreverent laugh with God. Most of my patients with Type I Parkinson's have come to realize that their idea of God was *not* intimate and fun enough to help in turning off pause. They were better off talking mentally with someone a little more down to earth and more irreverent.

I've had patients who only wanted to talk to God and no one else. But many of them also told me things such as, "God doesn't laugh." Or even "God doesn't like it if we have fun." For these people, God could *never* be a good invisible friend for this exercise. Thinking about *this* type of God, as the researchers had seen, stimulates the fear and rage centers in the brain – not the striatum. This *increases* the tendency to feel fear or anxiety, which in turn, moves one further into sympathetic and/or pause mode.

The person's thoughts needed to become *conversation* and not the usual, non-stop, even obsessive, silent monologue that is characteristic of most people with Type I Parkinson's. This new, chatty duologue, I hypothesized, would stimulate the striatum, the brain area that manifests increased activity when a person talks with a loving and understanding friend, a laughing, gently *teasing*, personable, even *irreverent* friend.

While this exercise might seem to have spiritual overtones, treating your conversations with your friend as a sacred, emotionally distant rite won't help you, and might make you worse. On the other hand, having a laugh with your late cousin Larry, the only one who knew the truth behind the infamous spaghetti incident, or giggling with your auntie Cassie, the one who always humored your penchant for mismatched plaids, has a much better chance of helping you turn off pause because they share love with you. This is more helpful in turning off pause than cowering before some amygdala-stimulating, perfectionist God.

The second exercise

The second exercise could begin when, in response to the first exercise, the invisible friend begins to seem *real* and trustworthy enough. Developing this sense of a real relationship took some people a few minutes to attain. Others needed *years*. Most were somewhere in between.

Once attained, a person could work on the second exercise: regularly ask the friend to manifest as more *physically* present: "Let me *feel* your presence near to me!" or "Hold my hand!" A patient might ask the invisible friend to palpably hold him or her, or manifest as some sort of feeling or sensation either on the periphery or even inside of the patient's body. The expectation is to feel as if the friend is giving physical comfort or gentle stimulation to some part of the body that wants support or stimulation, or maybe feel as if the same loving energy that is present in the friend could manifest inside the patient: a *feeling* of self-awareness inside of the patient's previously numb body.

If a person had some part of the body that was particularly vulnerable or injured, or a place on his body that he really didn't like to have touched, he might ask his constant friend to "help me feel your presence" or "your loving energy" in that body part. I hoped that this might stimulate the thalamus, the brain area that exhibits increased activation if your idea of God is something subtly energetic that you can *feel* or resonate with.

This type of therapy is exercises, not counseling. It is referred to in Chinese medicine as Medical Qi Gong (mental energy and thought regulation).

I hoped these techniques *might* not activate or stimulate the Blocker, if any. Unlike every previous attempt at imposing a psychological change upon the mind, this type of therapy did *not* seem like it would significantly challenge or try to change the self-protection behaviors of a person with self-induced pause.

I had reason to think this technique might actually work to jump-start the process that turns off pause. My thinking was this: if a person could *directly* stimulate his own thalamus and striatum, this should eventually create electrical midbrain behaviors that mimic those that occur following sensory confirmation of external safety: step two for coming out of pause.

As it turned out, I was sort of wrong about the Blocker. The Blocker *might* try to prevent a person from doing these exercises. Even so, the Blocker's influence was *much less* powerful against these techniques than it was with other cognitive behavioral therapies we'd tried: with these new exercises, the Blocker's voice *competed* with that of the friend. The patient now had voices that could help him ignore the Blocker: the patient's *own* voice while talking to the friend *or* the voice of the invisible friend. *If* the patient chose to keep up a constant conversation with his invisible friend, he could even *tune out* the voice of the Blocker. The Blocker was no longer The Boss. The Blocker was reduced to being a choice, an option. Sometimes the Blocker was pushy, or even scary, creating terrifying short-term scenarios and negative moods when given the chance, but thanks to the new friend, the person was usually able to stay aware that there was always a *choice*. As it also turned out, I *was* correct about the benefits of brain stimulation from these exercises.

I asked the Parkinson's patients I was still working with to try these techniques. I also send out descriptions of these techniques to the people with PD with whom I was still exchanging emails. Over the next few months, I was completely gratified by the slow but definite changes that some people started to experience. I was also not too surprised that some of my patients were completely baffled by my extremely simple suggestions. Some did not even want to risk doing something that seemed crazy to them and/or their Blockers.

Many needed to ask me a seemingly infinite number of questions that had to be answered before they dared to attempt something as simple as, "Imagine your thoughts are a silent conversation with someone who you trust, who can make you laugh, and who is not in a physical body. It might be a beloved, late grandparent or a deceased childhood friend. It might be Fido or Fluffy. It might be a "good person" or buddy of your own mental creation. All day long, direct your thoughts towards him or her, *not* towards your own mind." But the ones who trusted me enough to do this "risky" exercise eventually noticed a difference.

A third exercise

I should also mention that a *third* exercise is necessary for some people, though not for all. This exercise increases the *amount* of energy flowing in the long-repressed Du channel. People who simply cannot force themselves to do the above two exercises might need to practice imagining large amounts of energy surging into the body at the back of the neck and powering into the head along the path of the Du channel. (See Fig. 13.2 on p. 141.) This is explained at length in the book *Stuck on Pause*.

At the same time, they must practice mental attitudes of power and strength. If/when the menacing Blocker shows up, a person is going to need to feel like a warrior, not like a North American opossum, an animal that "plays dead" at the least startle. Practicing living as though powerful and strong, while imagining energy streaming into the back of the neck and up into the head, can help a person do the above two exercises and prepare him to turn his adrenal glands back on after years of them running at a fraction of their normal strength.

I've had patients whose Blockers only appeared when they started working on feeling more energy flowing into the body. The Blocker threatened one of them in an *audible* voice. This patient had turned off self-induced pause but felt himself repeatedly tempted to turn it back on.

Using pause instead of sympathetic mode

If a person who has successfully turned off pause mode finds himself in a situation that is scary, angering, or even merely unpleasant, he might find himself automatically reverting back into self-induced pause mode.

A mentally healthy person in the same situation will slide into a higher degree of *sympathetic mode* to deal with the unpleasantness, *not* pause. Pause is a drastic mode, to be used in case of imminent *death*. But in many people who have been on pause for a long time, their whole sympathetic system has gone somewhat dormant. They might not have used adrenaline for a very long time. When they first start to use adrenaline it can feel unfamiliar, unsafe, even dangerous.

One patient, when he started feeling adrenaline after turning off pause *most* of the time, wrote to me that it felt like constant, mild stage fright: a mild sense of always being ready for something. He'd never felt anything like it before. He wrote that it wasn't a negative thing or a problem: he didn't mind it at all. It showed up when he stopped feeling numb inside.

Patients have come up with many ways to re-activate sympathetic mode. They might imagine themselves pulling more energy into their bodies at the neck, in the vicinity of Du-15 and the medulla oblongata, thus increasing the energy in their overall systems. Then they can use this energy to practice feeling strong and fighting back. They might beat their chests like a gorilla, or yell out loud, or throw punches at the air – perform the physically assertive behaviors that a person on pause usually will *not* want to overtly perform. But do them he must if he needs to reawaken his ability to fully access sympathetic mode – if sympathetic mode *doesn't* turn back on automatically. This subject is addressed in *Stuck on Pause*.

Getting back to the patient whose Blocker audibly threatened him, when he realized that he was re-activating pause mode over and over in response to any negative situation, he started doing exercises that can re-awaken sympathetic mode. He practiced pretending to be a *physically* powerful animal, as opposed to coldly, *mentally* summoning up norepinephrine-driven power in his mind. Going into pause at the drop of a hat is something an animal (other than an opossum) will *not* do in response to a *frisson* of fear. But a person who is accustomed to using self-induced pause *might* do this, over and over.

The above patient successfully got sympathetic mode running again. He felt the strange sensations of having his body flooded with adrenaline, and at the same time, he heard the Blocker. That's when the patient emailed me: "I actually *heard* it [the Blocker] *tell* me, out loud, he was going to get me with a vengeance while I was doing exercises to stimulate my adrenal glands!"

When some people successfully turn off pause, they automatically experience full access to sympathetic (fight or flight), mode. After turning off pause, subsequent events that are scary, angering, or stressful will *automatically* increase the use of *sympathetic* mode: the channel qi circuitry in the body will be re-routed into the sympathetic mode patterns in order to conserve energy, provide more energy for the increased heart rate and deeper breathing, and more life force energy will automatically be pulled into the body at the medulla oblongata, at the back of the upper neck. This is the *healthy* response to fear, rage, and stress.

For others, accessing adrenaline does not automatically resume when pause is turned off. Instead, even after turning off pause for good, they might, from habit, automatically want to *re*-induce pause mode to deal with negativity or stress. In these people, it can feel as if pause mode is trying to reassert itself, with the help of the Blocker, any time stress appears. Until they increase the *amount* of energy that flows into the body *and* practice physical moves that *use* that power, thus increasing sympathetic mode behaviors, they might find themselves sliding back into pause mode from sheer habit: behaving and thinking in a manner similar to people in partial recovery.

Cognitive behavioral therapy

In addition to the above exercises for stimulating the midbrain (and for turning on the adrenal glands, if needed) many people had to first learn how to be circumspectly *aware* of, let alone in charge of, their own thoughts. Simple cognitive behavioral therapy teaches a person how to 1) recognize the types of thoughts that are associated with negativity, depression, and hopelessness; 2) come up with specific positive *replacement* thoughts that a person can use when he finds himself, from habit, looping back into his negative thought patterns. [1]

Between the cognitive behavioral therapy retraining for replacing negative thoughts with positive ones *and* learning to turn off the inherently-negative, pause-driven internal monologue by mentally talking with a supportive invisible friend with whom one could laugh, patients were able to either quickly or slowly turn around the mental processes that were keeping the striatum and thalamus dormant.

---

[1] *Feeling Good*, by Dr. David Burns, is the original self-help book of cognitive behavioral therapy. If a person has no idea how to go about changing a habit of negative self-talk, the suggestions and instructions in this book can be a huge help. Some of his examples are now extremely dated, but his ideas are very clearly explained. Many of my patients *really* didn't like this book even as they found themselves saying, "Oh my God! He's describing *me*!" And even though many patients agreed with everything explained in the book, they still couldn't "find the time" to do the exercises. They did, however, find the time to continue their self-harming habits of *negative* thoughts. These exercises are extremely effective in learning to be circumspect about your own mental habits and changing them by substituting more positive and more honest ones, but they only work if you do them.

The epiphany people already had a habit

Prior to coming across the striatum-activating research, I hadn't realized that all my patients who recovered during a quick epiphany had already spent decades or even most of a lifetime regularly talking to a higher power or a deceased loved one. It might have been a habit developed as part of a spiritual discipline or a habit that started upon the loss of a loved one. When they spontaneously, maybe from desperation, took this long-established habit and made it either deeper or more surrendering, they had an epiphany that turned off pause.

But none of the people I was working with now had *any* experience doing this normal, human behavior of frequently talking to an invisible friend. Many thought it would be *abnormal* to do this. Some thought it bordered on insanity.

Talking by rote or requirement

Then again, merely having a *habit* of talking to a spiritual authority figure was *not* necessarily a guarantee of good results. For example, one of my patients was a long-time monk, a lama. He had constantly practiced talking perfunctorily, by rote, to his departed guru. He spent hours every day reciting memorized prayers. He never actually *felt* there was anyone listening or, *if* someone was listening, that someone was listening in a critical and superior way. In this monk's mind, the guru was *not* a personal friend with whom an irreverent or forgiving laugh could be shared. Maybe the guru was a laughing, loving friend to *other* people, but not to him. However, my patient was determined to use his guru and only his guru for his invisible friend. After more than four years of being unable to change his rigid ideas about his relationship with his guru, he still couldn't laugh or even feel relaxed in the presence of his deceased guru, his "invisible friend." Though he was constantly talking to his guru, his Parkinson's symptoms steadily worsened.

When it came to recovering from Parkinson's disease, it turned out that just having a decades-long *mechanical* habit of talking or praying wasn't enough. And it also wasn't helpful to have a critical or stern, no-nonsense God or friend. These constructs actually *increase* activity in the amygdala and can worsen the symptoms of Parkinson's. A loving, trusting, *fun* relationship with the invisible friend was needed.

Risky behavior

Most of my patients with Parkinson's had, as long as they could remember, spoken silently to *themselves* in a non-stop, fairly circular monologue, a judgmental, constantly-assessing monologue that ran on even while outwardly conversing with other people, while listening to music, and while going through all the motions of life. The moments of their lives weren't *experienced* so much as *analyzed* and critically *judged.*

When I came up with the idea of talking to someone *outside* of the self – having a duologue instead of a monologue – most of my patients and correspondents with Parkinson's who ran a constant, pathological monologue with themselves told me that it's not *normal* to talk to an invisible someone who is *outside* of oneself.

To many, the idea of directing their silent, secret thoughts to someone else seemed unsafe, even alarming: the behavior of a crazy person. I was even told by some patients that only religious people could talk to an invisible friend. These patients were clearly forgetting that lots of young children even talk out *loud* to what we call "imaginary friends." Some of my patients, completely missing the point, asked why atheists don't all have Parkinson's, as if *failure* to religiously talk to God *causes* Parkinson's.

Some assumed that *only* religious people could talk to an invisible friend or feel connected to a listening, loving universe. This isn't the case, of course. The above ideas and questions are packed with fallacies. So I purchased the rights to use two cartoons from Bill Watterson's famous comic strip, "Calvin and Hobbes," for this book. I thought the cartoons would serve to show that, in healthy people, this type of conversation is, in fact, the norm. I hoped that my patients would see these two cartoons and say, "Oh! I see what you mean. Talk sincerely to something outside yourself. How simple!"

A couple of cartoons

In the first strip, Calvin is relying on his mom to save a dying baby raccoon that was hit by a car. The mom seeks comfort in talking to Hobbes. Hobbes, a stuffed tiger toy, is Calvin's best friend. Calvin and Hobbes are usually in constant conversation.

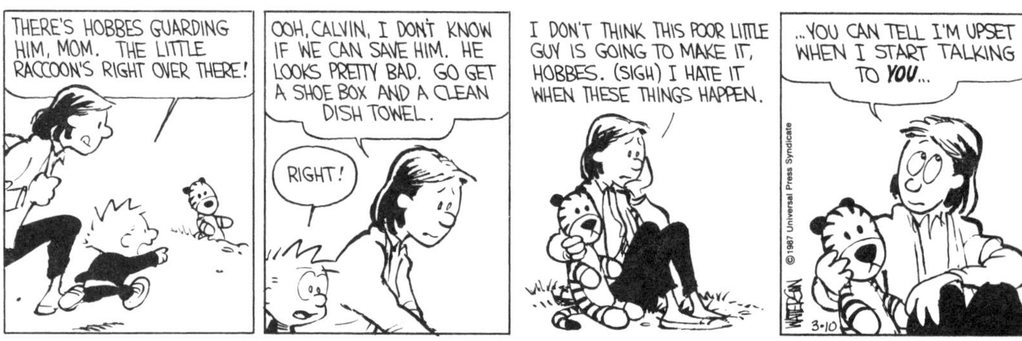
THERE'S HOBBES GUARDING HIM, MOM. THE LITTLE RACCOON'S RIGHT OVER THERE!
OOH, CALVIN, I DON'T KNOW IF WE CAN SAVE HIM. HE LOOKS PRETTY BAD. GO GET A SHOE BOX AND A CLEAN DISH TOWEL.
RIGHT!
I DON'T THINK THIS POOR LITTLE GUY IS GOING TO MAKE IT, HOBBES. (SIGH) I HATE IT WHEN THESE THINGS HAPPEN.
...YOU CAN TELL I'M UPSET WHEN I START TALKING TO *YOU*...
© 1987 Universal Press Syndicate
WATTERSON
3-10

1

In the second strip, Calvin is desperate. Hobbes has been missing for a week after being carried off by a stray dog. So Calvin talks to the universe at large.

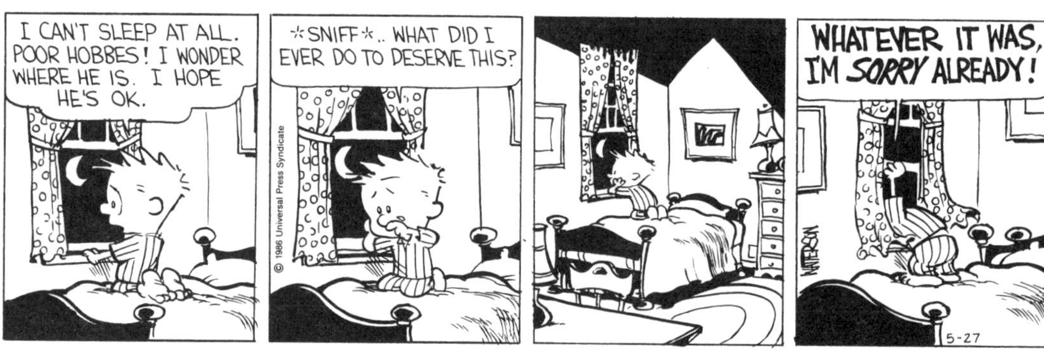
I CAN'T SLEEP AT ALL. POOR HOBBES! I WONDER WHERE HE IS. I HOPE HE'S OK.
SNIFF.. WHAT DID I EVER DO TO DESERVE THIS?
© 1986 Universal Press Syndicate
WHATEVER IT WAS, I'M *SORRY* ALREADY!
WATTERSON
5-27

2

[1] CALVIN AND HOBBES © 1987 Watterson. Reprinted with permission of ANDREWS MCMEEL SYNDICATION.

[2] CALVIN AND HOBBES © 1986 Watterson. Reprinted with permission of ANDREWS MCMEEL SYNDICATION.

For decades, this beloved comic strip resonated deeply with millions of readers because the strip almost always drew on core human behaviors, behaviors that nearly all of us can relate to – including Calvin's constant, two-way conversing with Hobbes, his stuffed tiger and very best friend, in nearly every strip. The two strips shared here derive their poignant humor from the inherent human need to call out to or talk intimately, even if *seemingly* illogically, to something or someone other than the self, when seeking comfort.

When most people see these strips, they chuckle because they have found themselves in a similar position – distraught and therefore un-self-consciously talking to an unknown, despite the seeming illogic of it. But so many of my *Parkinson's* patients had no idea what was going on in these strips. Most of my PD patients *didn't* read the cartoons and say, "Oh, I understand." Instead, most of them said things like, "Why is Calvin's mother talking to the stuffed tiger?" and "So who is Calvin talking to out the window…the reader?"

So many of my highly intelligent Parkinson's patients couldn't even understand what these characters in a comic strip were doing, or why! One of my patients even asked me, "Are you trying to imply that the boy in the second cartoon is religious"?

No. Calvin is a bratty, self-centered six-year old whose primary invisible friend is a stuffed tiger doll named Hobbes. I don't think most of this comic strip's readers would assume that Calvin was a particularly religious or spiritual child. However, when he is desperate and he doesn't have Hobbes to talk to, he instinctively screams out the window to someone or something that he knows is listening.

Calvin constantly seeks and receives comfort and answers from Hobbes. Hobbes' replies are often teasing, funny, and irreverent. Oppositely, most of my Type I Parkinson's patients are very hesitant to seek comfort from others. Some have told me they would rather die than be "reduced" to asking for help.

As an aside, collections of the Calvin and Hobbes strips are available. I recommend that people with Type I PD study these strips.

The Parkinson's support group

Here's an illustrative vignette: When I attended the local Parkinson's support group to recruit my first dozen volunteers, before I knew *I* had Parkinson's disease, I took a chair while people seated in a circle took turns telling how they were doing.

One of the women with PD said, "This week, I was at the grocery store and I needed something from a top shelf. I just couldn't reach it. Though I didn't want to, I asked a young man if he could reach it for me. He did. He was so nice. But what I want to share is that he seemed to actually be happy *because* he could help me. It never occurred to me that asking for help might make another person feel happy. So maybe it's OK to ask for help sometimes."

I was puzzled that this most human of interactions had been eye-opening for her. I'm quite short, and asking total strangers for items on high shelves is just part of my life. Then again, I too had long been a member of the I'd Rather Do It Myself club, so I understood her humiliation and chagrin. The other members of the group nodded in silent accord when she said "so maybe it's OK to ask for help." But I could just tell, somehow, that every one of them was thinking, "Yeah, but I hope I never have to…"

While I'm on the subject of the support group, I want to share another observation from that meeting. The first time I walked into the church's community room where the Parkinson's support group met, I was instantly overwhelmed with a strange, pleasant feeling of what I now think of as electromagnetic resonance.

Usually, I was uncomfortable in large meetings of people, especially if they were strangers. But I felt physically OK, safe, even. I felt as if, for the first time in my life, I was in a roomful of people many of whom felt I could relate to as fellow humans. Although I hadn't ever before used what I thought of then as a "corny" expression, I found myself thinking, "I have found my tribe." However, I still felt that about *half* of the people sitting in the circle weren't especially resonant and safe. They were just regular people.

This isn't to say that I was usually paranoid, but I'd always felt a *physical* discomfort, almost an internal agitation, in the presence of large groups of people, and in this group of people with PD, that discomfort was far less than I'd anticipated.

Shortly after the meeting started, the head honcho said, "So now, the caregivers will go to room C, down the hall. The people with Parkinson's will stay here." And all of the "ordinary" people, the people with whom I did *not* feel this new resonance, got up and left the room! I was now in a room full of people that felt *real*, that felt normal and safe. For the first time in my life, I *physically* felt like I fit in. At the time, I just wondered if I had some sort of morally superior compassion that made me feel good about willingly being in a room full of people fighting a powerful illness.

Much later, after I was diagnosed and then recovered from PD, I found myself losing my chronic defensiveness and my internal physical agitation when around large groups of people. I conclude that the weird electrical configurations of pause in my body had long made me feel what I now refer to as an electrical dissonance with nearly everyone else in the world…everyone *except* for people who had the same, pause-type electrical configurations that I had. My internal feelings of agitation and electrical dissonance with most others ceased as soon as pause turned off.

Prior to my recovering, in large groups of people or when given a friendly hug by others, including loved ones, the feeling of dissonance would sometimes be physically painful. But the first time I was in a room full of people who, unknown to me, were all running the exact same electrical currents that I was, I felt myself relax. After the non-Parkinson's people left for room C, another silent platitude popped up: "I've come home."

Which takes me further afield, to a class I taught in Reading, England, in which about thirty people with Parkinson's were sitting in a circle going around introducing ourselves and each saying a few words about their battles with Parkinson's. Two-thirds of the way around the circle, a woman in her thirties introduced herself and then said, "I don't belong here. I'm not like any of you. You're all so clever and, well, you're all *different* from me. I'm just a *regular* person."

She then told us how, after injuring her shoulder at work, the next day she couldn't move her right arm. She saw an MD and was immediately diagnosed with Parkinson's. She had no other symptoms of Parkinson's other than "lack of automatic arm swing." I popped her humerus bone back into the shoulder socket and she was immediately able to swing her arm for the first time in three years. She had been *inexcusably* misdiagnosed. Her mother, who had come with her, burst into tears.

But the point is, this woman was absolutely correct. Electrically, she was *not* like the other people in the room. She knew it intellectually and I suspect she physically *felt* it.

I wonder if, by being in a room filled with people with Parkinson's, she was feeling the same discomfort that I had always felt in a room full of people who *didn't* have the electric circuitry of pause. Whether or not our bodies are resonant with those around us is an extremely important factor in how connected and how safe we feel.

Waxing philosophical for a moment, a good life goal might even be to learn to be resonant with something far larger than the mere individuals around us. For example, if we are resonant with all the love in the universe, we are less likely to be thrown off course when in the vicinity of some individual whose currents are running a bit differently from our own. But I digress.

Getting back to the previous point, which was the idea of conversing with an invisible friend, people with Type I PD are very often reluctant to do this, let alone ask for help, cry out for help, or physically reach out for a comforting hand, even an *invisible* comforting hand: the normal, healthy human behavior of a person who has been highly traumatized.

Many of my patients with Type I Parkinson's, by secretly commanding themselves to feel no pain – often for *very* good reason – had inadvertently shut the door on this type of *instinctive* behavior of talking to an invisible friend or reaching out: healthy behavior that should be *automatic* during times of stress or emotional suffering. The secret command that triggers self-induced pause serves to deaden a person's innate ability to somatically *feel* and to have a sense of being connected with something outside of oneself. It also inhibits the ability to have a sense of communication with someone/something outside of oneself. Pause mode puts your brain in a twilight zone between life and death.

Getting back to 2015, when I shared with my patients my new ideas for self-stimulation of the thalamus and striatum by developing a parasocial relationship, most of them were eventually willing to give it a try. Even though it made no sense to them, or seemed a bit dangerous, or bordered on the insane, they all agreed to give it a run. Within a few months, some of them noticed their social and mental behaviors were slowly changing…and their symptoms of Parkinson's were a bit less constant, and/or a bit less powerful. Most importantly, many started recognizing an immediate relationship between their thoughts and their physical symptoms at any given moment. Others worked at it for two or three years before they noticed the correlation. But once they noticed it, they were on their way.

Auxiliary exercises to hasten recovery

With the realization of the role the striatum plays in pause and in Parkinson's came additional techniques and exercises that can be done together with the primary exercises of talking to and feeling close to a friend. The ultimate goal of *all* the therapies for Type I PD is increasing the amount of energy moving through the midline of the brain. To this end, the following therapies can also help.

1) Mentally imagine as much energy as possible in the vicinity of Yin Tang, the point between the eyebrows. This creates a pull on the Du channel, drawing more channel qi through the midline. When meditating with the eyes closed, the eyes can be gently lifted as if looking at this location. When the eyes are open, one can still imagine that this area is glowing with light or that this site has a powerful amount of energy in it, as if there is a magnet or a glowing ball of light in the center of the forehead. This can be done as

constantly as possible. Do *not* do this when trying to fall asleep, as it might keep you awake.

2) Mentally imagine energy moving along the Du channel path through the middle of the head. This energy moves from the base of the neck to Yin Tang. Many people with Parkinson's cannot imagine anything positive, let alone energy moving through the head. However, even *trying* to imagine energy moving along this line can be helpful. How often? As often as possible. Even if it seems that you *cannot* do this, or that you feel nothing, do it anyway. You are working at overcoming a deeply entrenched habit, and being on pause makes your brain want to resist having this current activated. You might need to do this unsuccessfully many thousands of times before your brain even starts to think about changing.

3) Mentally say thank you. It doesn't matter for what. Whatever happens, especially if something untoward happens and you would just love to go down a rabbit hole of self-pity or bitterness, say thank you. Say it over and over, until your immediate impulse to think something negative or stare in the mirror to self-console or self-instruct has been redirected to gratitude or something positive that will stimulate the striatum. Remember: negative thoughts *inhibit* flow through the midbrain.

If you like, your invisible friend can be the one to whom you offer the thanks. Much more on this subject is shared in *Stuck on Pause*. When you get good at this, you will be able to feel a subtle shift in how you *feel* when you mentally say thank you – if you mean it. This shift in how you feel inside suggests that your thalamus is being stimulated.

Say thank you for your meals, for your ability to breathe, for your Parkinson's symptoms. Say thank you for everything. You *don't* need to be a spiritual convert to the School of Gratitude, but you *do* need to change the way currents flow through your brain. Saying thank you to an invisible someone does two things: it temporarily replaces the flow of negative thoughts with a positive one *and* it strengthens your relationship with your invisible friend. Thus in *two* ways, it encourages flow through the striatum.

4) Meditate. If you know no particular technique of meditation, just sit quietly and mentally say a positive, simple phrase, over and over. Or watch your breathing. Or do some gentle meditation technique you learn from a friend or from a website. Websites with instructions on meditation abound. Sitting in silent meditation can be extremely difficult if you are running an internal tremor and/or if you are stiff and uncomfortable. But please don't be discouraged. Forcing yourself to do something good for yourself for a few minutes even if your PD-brain doesn't want to is still do-able. You might find that the battle for regaining authority over your own mind is very hard, especially if the mind has long been long caught up in an unnatural level of wariness and negativity due to being on pause. Even if it's hard, it's do-able. You created your brain's behavior; you can un-create it or replace it with something different.

My favorite meditation website offers lessons in meditation techniques that are suitable for followers of any of the major world religions: www.yogananda-srf.org .

More about the time frames for recovery

As mentioned earlier, one new patient with very early Parkinson's symptoms unexpectedly, permanently, turned off pause within less than a *minute* of starting to talk silently with his lately deceased grandmother. He also sped through the recovery symptoms faster than most.

Most people, after turning off pause, don't have the recovery symptoms of uncontrolled, infantile movement in previously numb tissues for a few weeks or even a few months. But this patient started having recovery symptoms almost immediately. He exhibited a bout of the infant-like facial spasms of recovery within twenty minutes of turning off pause, while he was still there in my office. He was alarmed. He exclaimed, "Those things you warned me about [recovery symptoms] are actually going to happen? I didn't believe you!"

Within just a few days he found himself grabbing his previously atrophied, now burning, aching biceps, in a fruitless effort to prevent the new, automatic arm swings that were now occurring thousands of times a day, one healthy arm swing with every footfall.

I should note that this person was very young: in his late twenties. He also had long forced himself to keep a positive, trusting outlook even as he found himself increasingly *inclined* to be wary and non-trusting. He had constantly, actively, fought with and rejected the wary and increasingly dominant voice in his mind.

For all my other patients, physical and/or internal changes after starting to talk to an invisible friend took longer. Often, much, much longer: years, in some cases. But those who stuck with it, teaching themselves to constantly direct their thoughts and questions to loving, invisible friends, slowly found themselves feeling safer. They were gradually learning to keep themselves constantly – and I mean constantly – as if in the presence of someone or something that loved them and with whom they could laugh and be themselves, warts and all. This felt drastically new to all of them. For many, it felt ridiculous, at first. They were embarrassed to be "talking to nothing." And yet, if they stuck with it until their friend seemed real and then eventually added the thalamus-stimulating request of "let me *feel* your presence" or "let me *feel* your joy and love inside of me," their long-running use of pause mode eventually turned itself off.

When these people with Type I Parkinson's disease finally felt internally stable and *safe* enough to come back to life, pause turned off. Instantly or gradually, Parkinson's symptoms ebbed, then ceased. The weird recovery symptoms, symptoms that are the opposite of Parkinson's disease, began.

Many people never recover

I want to be clear: many of the people I worked with who were on self-induced pause did *not* recover. The reasons tended to fit into four categories.

1) They couldn't "remember" to pay attention to a positive duologue with an invisible friend: they felt their habit of dwelling on the negative was too strong and compelling. They eventually became convinced that they could never change, and stopped working at it.

2) They didn't *want* to change their thinking or "surrender" to universal forces of goodness and felt they shouldn't have to. They preferred to focus on dietary changes, "energy machines," ozone therapies: you name it. In my limited experience, *none* of these gambits have ever worked for the long term, though many provide a temporary placebo period of reduced symptoms.

3) They decided to go the medication route because they needed to "not have Parkinson's" right away. They felt that recovery wouldn't be fast enough.

4) Most tragically, many people felt they didn't deserve to recover, wouldn't be able to recover even if everyone else did, or that they "deserved" to have Parkinson's as some sort of punishment or a manifestation of "the will of God."

A *majority* of my patients fit into the above four categories.

The voice I'd heard in my meditation room had been right. A majority of my patients didn't *want* to recover from the underlying cause of Parkinson's disease. They *did* want to get rid of the symptoms. But they didn't want to, didn't think they could, or didn't think they *deserved* to get rid of the underlying cause: a decision to stop feeling the physical and/or emotional pain of this world.

Chapter Thirteen

The Biology of Pause

Setting aside, for now, the unfinished discussion of recovery-related questions and the chronicle of my research project, the next six chapters will cover the more "technical" aspects of Parkinson's disease: the biomechanics of pause mode, the specific locations of the various types of Parkinson's symptoms, how to diagnose Parkinson's, and then how to diagnose which *type* of PD a person has.

This chapter presents a more complete discussion of the electrical behaviors of pause mode than you were offered in chapter one. This lengthy chapter is quite technical. It is oriented towards a person with a background in medicine who wants to know the details of the circuitry and physiological mechanisms at work during pause. This information is also included as support for my statements that the electrical schematics of Parkinson's disease are a perfect match for the electrical schematics of pause. The level of detail in this chapter might feel like Too Much Information for a person with Parkinson's who just wants to know how to recover. If you get bogged down in this chapter, please, just skip ahead to chapter fourteen. If you have Parkinson's, chapter fourteen is definitely going to hold your interest.

Most of this chapter was lifted from chapter fourteen in my book *Tracking the Dragon*. That chapter explains how normal, life-saving pause – a hopefully *short*-term mode – behaves in a healthy person. Most of the information about pause in that chapter is not *specifically* about Parkinson's disease. Still, a person with PD will be able to see the similarities between healthy, short-term pause and the chronic pause of Parkinson's. For this book, I've added some introductory material and a few Parkinson's-specific modifications to the material from *Tracking the Dragon*. There are also a few bits that are somewhat redundant, discussing aspects of pause presented in previous chapters.

Tracking the Dragon has instructions on how to feel channel qi, describes the general channel schematics for each of the four neurological modes and explains, in everyday English, how the bio-electric circuitries that underlie the channel theories of Chinese medicine might go wrong, causing physical and emotional problems. If you *do* enjoy this chapter, there's more where this comes from: the full text of *Tracking the Dragon* is available at JaniceHadlock.com.

Not all or nothing

Pause is not usually an all-or-nothing mode. Like the other three neurological modes, 1) parasympathetic (content, curious), 2) sympathetic (fight or flight), and 3) sleep, pause mode (coma or near-death) can manifest its particular neurotransmitter, organ, and thought behaviors on an amplitude continuum from mild to strong *and* on a behavioral continuum with sleep mode, sympathetic mode, or both being at the opposite end of the continuum from pause mode.

At the mild end of the amplitude continuum, pause symptoms might manifest as slight paired-muscle tension in certain muscles and slight limpness in the opposing muscles, as well as slight wooziness and/or the release of pain-reducing endorphins. At the extreme end, symptoms can include immobility and/or coma.

Although a doctor might say that a person is "in sympathetic mode," what the doctor actually means is that the person is sympathetic-mode *dominant* at that moment: using a somewhat *higher* degree of sympathetic mode and a somewhat *lower* degree of parasympathetic than is average. At any given moment, a person is almost always using a blend of two or more modes. Even a very healthy, happy person uses a blend of sympathetic and parasympathetic modes. As the person's mood fluctuates, his subdermal electrical currents shift accordingly: negative thoughts shift the channels more towards the sympathetic circuitry; positive thoughts towards more parasympathetic. Neurological and physiological behaviors and body chemistry shift in a way that reflects the electromagnetic waves given off by a person's thoughts – thoughts that influence channel qi behaviors, which then influence everything else.

A person on pause who is walking around – meaning he is not in a coma – is in a *partial* degree of pause mode. Some of his body circuits might be running in pause patterns, and other circuits might be running in the circuitry or amperage variations characteristic of sympathetic mode. Some portions of his channels might be flowing in more of a sleep-mode or a pre-sleep mode pattern. A person using pause might even be running a *small* amount of parasympathetic mode circuitry. But *if* he is using *any* amount of pause mode, it's likely that the overall *amount* of channel qi in his entire body is correspondingly decreased to *below* normal levels.

For example, a person with early-stage, Type I Parkinson's who is *eating* has *some* pause circuits running *but* his digestive tract might be moving in the right direction (running some circuits of parasympathetic mode in the digestive organs). Digestion might not be *optimal*. He might be subject to constipation because his gut might be *somewhat* inhibited, reflecting his use of some degree of pause mode. At the same time, his chewing muscles and swallow reflex might be working, reflecting that he is also running *some* parasympathetic channel patterns, albeit at a far lower amplitude than is ideal. The net effect is that some currents might be running in pause circuits, at low amperage, even while some other parts of the body have currents running in parasympathetic *or* sympathetic mode directions, also at a lower amperage than the ideal. The point is, different parts of the body might be using the circuitry patterns of different modes, and *all at the same time*.

A person using a blend of low amounts of pause circuitry and low amounts of parasympathetic circuitry might still swallow and digest *moderately* well. Then again, some of my Parkinson's patients have had chronic, almost life-long digestive problems – lack of appetite, constipation, or a "cast-iron" (numb) stomach. Some have compulsive eating problems. Others never feel hunger and must force themselves to eat. The swallow reflex might be working, but still might be less than ideal: for example, my own use of constant exhalation while eating to try to prevent food going down the wrong way – into my windpipe – was a long-term problem due to the impaired swallow reflex typical of pause mode.

The point is, a body might be running some pause circuitry and some circuitry from sympathetic or sleep modes, and even a little bit, enough to power digestion *somewhat*, of parasympathetic mode.

Blended modes

To better understand blended modes, consider *mechanical* systems that use a blend of changeable electrical currents: a computer can run two or more programs at the same time. A split screen can show two files at the same time. Or the computer can be on, but "sleeping." The screen might be bright or putting out a low glow: seemingly endless possibilities and variations.

Now consider the parasympathetic / sympathetic continuum. In humans, all the Primary channels flow to or from the tips of the fingers and toes when in *parasympathetic* mode. If alive, energy is *always* flowing into the body at the back of the neck at the medulla oblongata, known in ancient times in the Mideast as "the mouth of God." The amount flowing in at any given moment is variable and depends to a large extent on how much power the person *wants* to be feeling in his body. This energy enters the body in wave form. It converts in the inside of the spine into the electrical charges of channel qi. The channel qi then flows from inside the spine out through the coccyx and out into the Du channel.

Excess channel qi is always being discharged from the fingers and toes. During an emergency, one that requires expending extra energy, the channel qi flow diverts away from the fingers and toes, to prevent loss of energy at these discharge locales.

As a person glides into a higher degree of sympathetic mode, a corresponding amount of channel qi is diverted *away* from the fingers and toes and shunted directly into the subsequent channel from a location that *precedes* the digits.

For example, in a high degree of *parasympathetic* mode, most of the Stomach channel qi flows all the way to the tips of the second and third toes. The channel qi then discharges into the ground or travels across the tops of the toes to the tip of the big toe, as needed. At the tip of the big toe, the current changes names and is referred to as the Spleen channel. The Spleen channel flows from the big toe, up the inner side of the foot, up the leg, and into the torso.

But as a person moves towards a higher degree of sympathetic mode, less Stomach channel qi flows to the tips of the toes. More of the Stomach channel qi flows sideways from the top of the foot and into SP-3, near the ball of the foot, thus bypassing the tips of the toes.

The incredibly complex schematics of the body allow for different *amounts* of current to be shunted into the most appropriate pathway at any given time, depending on the thoughts and needs of the moment. The electrical possibilities of a human are *infinitely* more complex than a computer's. Our bodies can manifest an almost infinite number of variations on the combinations of pause, sympathetic, parasympathetic, and sleep modes. Yes, even sleep mode has variations, such as REM cycles. Some of the channel qi variations that occur during sleep influence the nature of our dreams.

As an aside, the paths of the Primary channels, presented in basic books about Chinese medicine and displayed on posters on many an acupuncturist's wall, only show how the channel qi flows in a person who is in *pure* parasympathetic mode, is conscious, is in perfect health, and is not moving. The channel flow patterns for the *other* modes are *never* shown in these basic diagrams, nor are they taught in most acupuncture schools. "Primary" channel means "pure, ideal, parasympathetic route."

The ancient texts say that there are "ten thousand" possible routes of channel qi. In both ancient Chinese and Sanskrit, the phrase "ten thousand" was used poetically to convey the concept of "infinite" or "beyond comprehension." Sadly, the phrase is usually translated into English quite literally, making people wonder why the body has exactly ten thousand channels, or ten thousand distinct bits of currents. It doesn't. It has a potentially *infinite* number of possible flow patterns or, as they said in olden times, "ten thousand."

No two people will have currents that run exactly the same. For example, in response to an alarming stress, a person might do a mini, localized version of sympathetic mode, or maybe even pause. For one person, that might manifest as tightness (a "lump") in the throat. Another might feel a "knot" or maybe nausea in the stomach in response to the exact same stress. Yet another might experience the same stress as causing a "kick" in the gut. Or wooziness. Or a wave of confusion. No two people will respond to a stress in the *exact* same way. No two people will do a modified pause response in the exact same manner. No two people with Parkinson's have the exact same symptoms.

When I write about pause in this chapter, I am describing the generalities that present in a relatively high degree of pause-related circuitry and symptoms, *as if* pause mode is all or nothing, and *as if* pause mode manifests the same way in all people. But at any given moment, in response to the *same* external events or emotions, people activate *different* modes, to *different* degrees, and even in *different* parts of the body. The activators behind an individual's specific channel qi behaviors are primarily his thoughts, memories, and genetics, but they can also be influenced by the person's history of injuries, illness, diet, scar tissue, allergies, and so on.

The following is copied from chapter fourteen of *Tracking the Dragon*

Pause mode is the correct, healthy neurological response to severe blood loss or other near-death traumas such as concussion or potentially mortal injuries. Pause might also be triggered by excessive perforation of the skin, which can include self-cutting and, to a mild degree, excessive acupuncture needling.

During pause one might experience, to varying degrees, a *decrease* in heart rate, shallower or slowed breathing, and a *drop* in blood pressure. Blood might leave the skin and muscles and shunt deeply interiorly to the spine and brain – *not* to the heart and lungs. The skin might be clammy. Temperature regulation might be poor, especially in the extremities. Release of endorphins and a concomitant decrease in awareness of some types of pain might occur.

These alterations in physiology might be life saving. For example, the pause-driven inhibition of heart-force *greatly* slows the rate and strength at which blood is pumped. If blood vessels have been broken to a dangerous extent during an injury, this inhibition of heart rate and strength might help reduce blood loss.

The body might either become limp or curl into a fetal position. This fetal positioning occurs because, in the parts of the body where channel qi suddenly flows *backwards*, the muscles become rigid. Oppositely, where channel qi is *cut off*, muscles become weak. The backwards and the turned-off channel qi flow occurring over paired, oppositional-muscle sets can cause pulling up of the legs and maybe a curling in of the torso and arms, and the pulling forward of the neck: the fetal-esque position observed in some people who are on pause.

The voice, if any, might be faint. The senses of taste and smell might diminish greatly or become altered. The senses of hearing and vision might be *heightened* while on pause. The *type* of hearing and vision is more analytical and behaves more as it does in sympathetic mode.

For example, in sympathetic or pause mode, a person is *less* able to see fanciful images in the clouds or in tree bark. The ability to visualize positive images or playfully imagine shapes and faces while gazing at something is a feature of *parasympathetic* mode. The ability to do this type of playful imagining diminishes as a person slides into a higher degree of sympathetic mode or lurches into pause.

Sound perception is altered during sympathetic mode and pause. Hearing becomes attuned to sounds of possible danger. Background sounds become a source of agitation instead of pleasure. For example, if a healthy person gets lost while driving and becomes concerned, one of the *first* things he usually does is turn off the music or radio in the car. As the driver transitions from parasympathetic-dominant to sympathetic-dominant, the sounds from the music or radio transition from pleasant to distracting, even annoying.

In a high degree of parasympathetic mode, a sudden burst of bird song might evoke laughter, or at least a smile. Oppositely, in a high degree of sympathetic or pause mode, the same sudden song might elicit a startle response or a sharp intake of the breath.

As a Parkinson's-related aside, many of my PD patients have told me they used to enjoy listening to music, but that now it distracts them. "Distracts you from what?" I ask. "From the things I need to be thinking [or worrying] about," is the most common response. More accurately, they no longer enjoy music because they can no longer, or only rarely, access parasympathetic mode.

Other pause-specific behaviors also occur, but this should be enough get you started – giving you a mental picture of a person who is on pause and letting you recognize that this is *not* a variant of adrenaline-releasing sympathetic mode. It also is *not* the pre-sympathetic hesitation that we refer to as "deer in the headlights." A deer in the headlights is surprised. He has not yet activated the appropriate dash for safety – but he isn't almost dead. A person on pause, in preparation for possible death, is switching over into suspended animation, feeling no pain, and most likely perceiving himself from outside his body. Observing oneself as if outside the body is referred to in western medicine as dissociation.

Dissociation

Unfortunately, the term "dissociation" has been adopted by several fields of scientific inquiry, each with a very different meaning of the word. In the field of medicine, *biological* dissociation refers to perceiving oneself from outside the physical body, a change in perception that often occurs during pause. In the field of *psychology*, the term refers to a separation or compartmentalization of some mental data away from normal consciousness. *Psychological* dissociation involves mentally blocking awareness of some event or body part to the point where the person has no memory or a distorted memory of the event or body part. This is the most common meaning of the word dissociation for today's general public.

While on pause, a person might experience *biological* dissociation. He might *observe* his own body from outside of it, while having a diminished level, or even none, of the usual physical sensations of being inside his own body. He might lose both somatic awareness (*how* the body feels inside) *and* proprioception (awareness of *where* his body parts are if he can't see them). While the idea of a person perceiving himself as if outside his body might strain credulity for some readers, *many* people who've had a concussion or severe, life-threatening injury or anesthesia during surgery describe the strange experience of a shift in self-awareness, so that they are somewhat numbly *looking* at themselves from outside of their body instead of *feeling* as if they are inside their body. The *skin* isn't necessarily numb. The internal, *somatic* self-awareness feelings might be missing. [1]

Pause-driven shifts in channel qi

Changes in the Stomach channel schematics

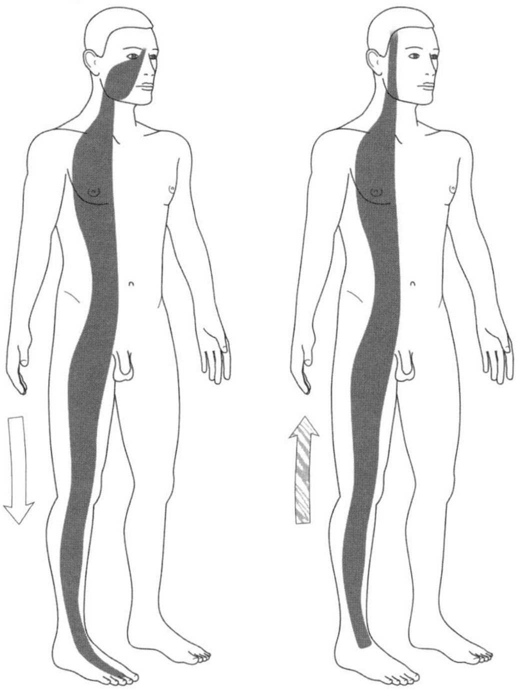

In pause mode, the channel qi in the Stomach channels runs backwards from ST-42, on the foot, to, depending on severity, the leg, torso, or even the head. This backwards flow of the channel qi can be felt by hand.

When you feel the Stomach channel qi of a person on pause, you might detect a sensation of it flowing *up* the leg, rapidly vibrating back and forth, or even seeming to disappear. All of these behaviors are referred to as "backwards."

If the backwards-flowing Stomach channel qi makes it all the way up to the jaw, it is shunted from ST-6 on the jaw to ST-8, on the forehead. From ST-8, it can flow into the Gallbladder channel at adjacent GB-14, on the forehead, and from there join into the flow of Gallbladder channel qi. (See Fig. 13.6, p. 150.)

Fig. 13.1 Normal Stomach channel flow / Stomach channel while on pause

[1] In my earliest writing on this subject, I decided to refer to some strange aspects of the Parkinson's personality, aspects that I now know to be characteristics of pause mode, as "dissociation" because so many of my patients with Parkinson's perceived themselves as if outside of their bodies. Using the word dissociation was a bad choice. The multiple meanings for the word dissociation led to lots of confusion. I have since changed the name of this mode to pause, but some of those early editions that refer to a "dissociated mode" are still out there on copyright-violating web pages, keeping the confusion alive.

I am constantly writing up-dates. Please, do not try to be helpful by posting my quickly out-dated writings on your own website. Instead, if you want to share this material, please consider making a link to the Parkinson's Recovery Project website so that your readers can always get the most up-to-date information. Even though all my Parkinson's-related writing is provided for free download at the PDrecovery.org website, it is copyrighted and legally cannot be copied, excerpted, or otherwise shared or used without permission. Thank you.

In a high degree of pause, Stomach channel qi does *not* flow from ST-42, on the top of the mid-foot, down to the tips of the toes (the parasympathetic pattern) *nor* does it flow from ST-42 over to SP-3 on the side of the foot (the sympathetic pattern).

In healthy people, when awake, the channel qi always forks in two directions at ST-42. Some channel qi goes to the tips of the toes, some goes over to Sp-3: a blend of parasympathetic and sympathetic schematics. How much goes in each direction at any given moment depends on the person's mood and thoughts at that moment.

On pause, in addition to flowing backwards from ST-42 towards the ankle and on up the leg or higher, some channel qi in this area might seem to vibrate back and forth between the top of the foot at ST-42 and the center of the sole of the foot at KI-1, or from ST-42 to KI-3, on the medial ankle between the ankle bone and the Achilles tendon.

As an aside, Stomach channel qi can flow backwards in response to situations other than pause. *Any* channel will flow backwards when doing so is the path of least resistance. A severe blockage at *any* point along the path of *any* channel might cause that channel's qi to run backwards or sideways from that point.

The path of least resistance and a water analogy

Electricity and water both always flow in the path of least resistance. If a non-conductive bit of the body such as scar tissue inhibits the flow of subdermal electrons, or if a dam blocks the flow of water, the electrons or the water will either back up or get deflected in some other direction.

In clinic, I have seen the backwards Stomach channel pattern set in motion by appendectomies, C-section scars, and by childhood foot injuries from which the bones were still displaced, to name just a few *non*-pause examples.

The Du channel

The healthy Du channel begins at the anus. Du channel qi flows up the back, directly over the spine, just under the skin. At the neck, it flows into the head and through the midbrain. After emerging at the forehead, it flows down to the upper lip. It then flows into the mouth, down through the gut, and out the anus.

From the anus, it again flows up the back, keeping a continuous loop going. The high level of energy in the Du channel as it travels through the striatum, thalamus, and frontal lobe helps drive automatic movement, joy, mental alertness, and consciousness.

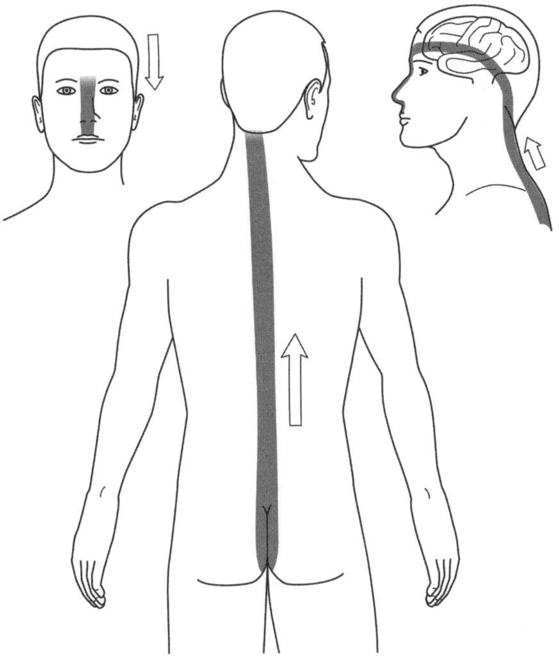

Fig. 13.2 The Du channel in parasympathetic mode

During sleep, the amount of energy flowing in the Du channel is greatly diminished. A reduced level of current flowing in the Du channel activates a shunt at the top of the neck: the reduced-energy current is shunted into a path that runs over the *top* of the head, just under the scalp, instead of running through the center of the head and frontal lobe. This sleep-time shunt *greatly* diminishes activity in the midbrain regions and the frontal lobe. This diminished activity allows for the drop-off in consciousness that accompanies sleep, as well as inhibiting release of dopamine in the striatum, thus inhibiting most motor function while snoozing.

The Du channel on pause

When on pause, the torso portion of the Du channel qi becomes a standing wave. It stays between the sacrum and the base of the neck.

During pause, the Du channel does *not* noticeably flow up the neck and into the head in the parasympathetic pattern *nor* does it flow over the top of the head in the sleep pattern. When detecting the Du channel qi of a person on pause, the Du channel might feel as if it stops at the base of the neck, stops somewhere lower down the spine, or is missing altogether. Or the Du channel qi might feel to an observer as if it is making tiny up-and-down movements, rather than flowing steadily in an upward direction. On pause, the *amount* of channel qi in the Du, and therefore in the whole body, might be greatly reduced.

As a gross generalization, the *midbrain* areas (the brain parts located *between* the left and right hemispheres) regulate the brain functions that are dominant during parasympathetic mode. The bilateral brain areas (left and right sides) regulate brain functions that are fear- and/or ego-driven (sympathetic and pause modes) or sleep-based. While a person is in a higher degree of sympathetic mode or in pause mode, the currents that direct fear- and ego-based behaviors carry more current, and the Du carries less.

The brain can be active during sleep, but not along the Du channel, except during certain sleep pathologies such as sleepwalking. For example, consolidation of memories, a side-of-the-brain process, occurs during sleep, in brain areas that are regulated by the Gallbladder channel

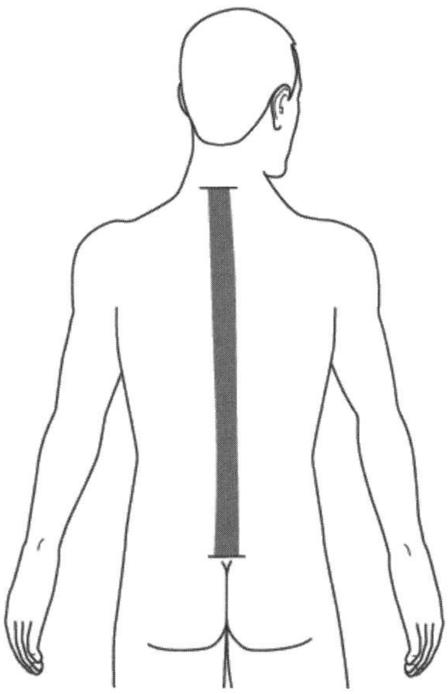

Fig. 13.3 The path of the Du channel while on pause. Note: there is no directional arrow.

When a person is in a high degree of parasympathetic mode, he is highly aware of being *conscious*. He is predominantly oriented towards enjoying his sense of resonance with others, with nature, or with joy itself. His Du channel runs at full strength through the midline of the brain – the area of the brain that regulates dopamine release for playful imagination and effortless, "automatic" motor function. Again, a high amount of energy flows in his Du channel when predominantly in parasympathetic mode or sympathetic mode. The amount of energy is reduced when sleep or pause modes are in use.

In pause mode, when most of the Du channel qi stops at the base of the neck, brain functions are driven primarily by channels on the sides of the head, especially the Urinary Bladder (UB) and Gallbladder (GB) channels. These side-of-the-head channels influence activities in the brain areas that regulate speech, risk assessment, fear, rage, and *command*-based (emergency) motor function, to name just a few.

On pause, the amount of energy flowing in the *entire* Du channel is reduced. In the *head* portion of the Du channel, it is even *more* reduced. Depending on the degree of fear or trauma, it might be moderately reduced or almost not flowing at all. When on pause, with the brain portion of the Du channel significantly inhibited, the energy level in the midbrain – where the striatum and thalamus are located – is correspondingly inhibited. Therefore, dopamine release from these areas is inhibited. Instead, when a person is on pause, his brain functions are predominantly oriented towards self-preservation: side-of-the-brain behaviors.

The Urinary Bladder (UB) channel on pause

The UB channels normally run from the eyebrows, up over the upper sides of the head (directly over the brain's amygdala), down the *sides* of the neck, down the *sides* of the spine (directly over the connections where the spinal nerves meet the spinal column), and all the way down to the littlest toes.

During pause, the same electrical obstruction that causes the Du channel qi to stop at the base of the neck might cause the UB channel qi to stop at the neck. When the current in the UB channel is stopped at the back of the neck it might convert to wave form and shunt off into space at the base of the neck, just above UB-11. On pause, the UB channel qi *often* flows from the neck out into the air instead of staying under the skin and flowing down the torso. After a moderate amount of training, one can easily detect the waves of this electromagnetic divergence.

The UB channel streaming outside of the body during pause mode might cause two shifts: 1) an *increase* in the "speed" (voltage differential) of the UB channel qi that flows over the head and over the amygdala – the fear and rage center of the brain. This can amplify the degree of wariness, anxiety, fear, and/or rage that a person feels.
2) a *decrease* in the amount of channel qi past Du-11. This decreases the amount of stimulation of the spinal nerves. The spinal nerves ordinarily stimulate the *sympathetic* nerve responses in all the torso organs and the torso and leg muscles.

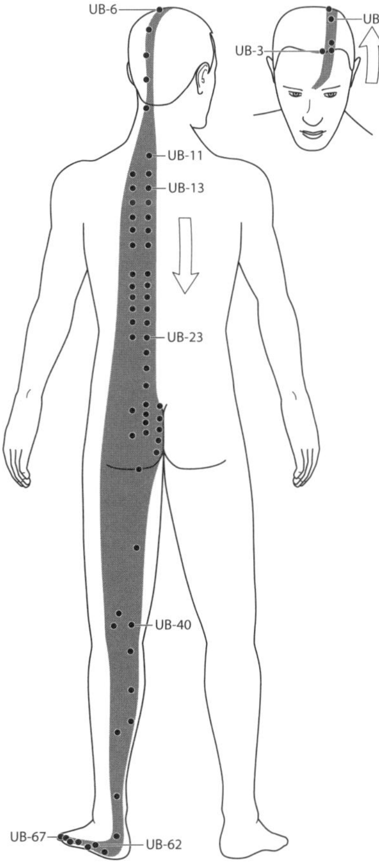

Fig. 13.4 The path of the UB channel in parasympathetic mode

On pause, the blockage of the UB channel at the neck diminishes or blocks activation of the spinal nerves. This decreases or inhibits the sympathetic nerve impulses that go to the organs in the torso and to the muscles. The decrease also diminishes or inhibits pain signals that are heading *towards* the brain *from* the torso and limbs.

An absence of UB channel qi flowing over the roots of the spinal nerves where they meet the spinal column also turns *on* the release of endorphins at these locations. Endorphins are neurotransmitters that inhibit transmission of pain signals. An absence of UB channel qi below the neck prevents the release of adrenaline from the adrenal glands. The adrenal glands are located right next to the kidneys.

This means that, on pause, with both the UB channels and the Du channel running in pause-type schematics, the release of adrenaline from the adrenal glands is inhibited *and* the release of midbrain dopamine is inhibited. This combination of neurotransmitter inhibitions allows the extreme stillness and lowered metabolic functions, such as coma, that can manifest when a person is on pause. Even so, in an emergency in which physical movement is required in *spite* of being in the throes of a potentially fatal trauma, the brain can release norepinephrine. This allows for intense, command-driven physical movement even while the release of adrenaline from the adrenal glands and dopamine release from the midbrain are both inhibited.

As an aside, the *parasympathetic* nerve instructions for organs are regulated by the vagus nerves, cranial nerves that are regulated by the brain portion of the Du channel, and which emerge from the base of the skull, slightly to the left and right sides of the neck bones. Like the spinal nerves, the vagus nerves are inhibited while on pause. The greater degree of pause, the greater the degree of inhibition.

Going back to the previous discussion of the UB channel flowing out of the neck and into space from just above UB-11 when on pause – instead of staying just under the skin where it usually flows – this phenomenon might be related to the feeling of "being outside of the body" that is a common feature of being on pause.

This might also be the reason that ancient Chinese tradition holds that the UB channel is the "closest channel to the exterior," meaning "most likely to flow into the air." Most of the other channels are equally close to the under-surface of the skin in terms of physical distance, but the UB channel is the most likely to *exit* the body, converting its currents into electromagnetic waves that flow *outward* from the skin. [1]

---

[1] Full medical anesthesia puts a person into a high degree of pause mode. It does *not* put a person to *sleep*, despite the popular euphemism. The phenomenon of "watching my surgery from the ceiling" is *not* unusual during lengthy surgeries, and is even somewhat common in heart-related surgeries. While *western* medicine has no explanation for the normal biological dissociation that is a common feature of being on pause, it is simply the re-centering of one's Source waves, one's Yuan Qi, to a location outside the body.

Normally, electromagnetic waves created by this energy, a type of lightwave associated in ancient Asian scriptures with the immortal part of one's soul, are centered in the pericardium, the conductive tissue around the heart, but they can actually be centered anywhere. This aspect of a person's overall energy departs the body after death. During pause, these waves may relocate to outside the body but usually stay nearby. The association of waves of energy with the ancient Chinese concept of "soul" is one reason that the *atheist* Chinese government has outlawed the medical study of channel qi. Another reason channels are illegal in China is that the existence of channels has long been mocked by western doctors, causing Chinese doctors to "lose face."

In recovering from Parkinson's, this UB channel "escape" pattern usually corrects itself automatically when pause turns off. However, if the UB channel stays stuck in this pattern due to inertia, a person might need to spend ten minutes or so visualizing this current of Bladder channel qi returning to its correct location – staying *under* the skin and flowing down the torso. This will help turn off a chronically elevated amygdala response. A chronically elevated amygdala increases negative emotions which, in turn, can make a person with a strong habit of inducing pause feel that he needs to return to pause mode.

Until this UB channel returns to *under* the skin, it can be very hard, if not impossible, for the person to perform the "shimmy" that travels down the spine in Step 5 of turning off biological pause. It is possible that the shimmy, the *frisson*, that healthy people experience when coming out of pause is a physical response to the return of the UB channel qi coming back into the body and resuming its flow along the sides of the spine, turning the spinal nerves back on. That's certainly what it *feels* like.

In many cases, if a person *cannot* bring himself to let a shudder or shimmy travel down his spine after doing the first four steps for turning off biological pause, it may well be because the UB channel is still flowing out into space. If the UB channel fails to automatically return to inside the neck even after pause has been *nearly* turned off, simple visualization of the channel flowing correctly can usually retrain this channel back into its correct path, provided there is no unhealed injury in the neck or spinal vertebrae. Then again, if a person feels a strong reluctance to or simply *cannot* mechanically force himself to shake the shoulders or shimmy the spine, it might be that either there is still an unaddressed injury in the head or spine *or* that the pause mindset has not yet been turned off. Whether pause is being sustained physically from an injury or mentally from a self-command, a hard and fast biological rule prohibits the bobbling of the neck and head and the shaking of the spine so long as pause is in place.

This biological prohibition is a life-saving rule. You do *not* want to recklessly move the neck or spine while on pause. This shiver down the spine can turn the sympathetic nerves systems back on and get you physically moving, which you do *not* want to do if there is a potentially life-threatening injury in the neck or spine *or* if a predator is still in the vicinity, staring at you and looking for signs of life.

As an aside, if a person regularly experiences the UB channel spinal shiver when urinating, this means that there is no *physical* neck or spine blockage, no unhealed injury in these areas. It means that the person *can* physically experience the spinal shimmy. In these cases, a blockage at the base of the neck most likely has a mental origin such as self-induced pause, not a physical origin: physical blockages such as scar tissue and tissue displacements do *not* come and go in response to urination. However, the opposite does *not* hold. Just because a person is having a hard time getting his UB channel to stop flowing out into the air and instead flow down into his torso does *not* mean he necessarily has an unhealed injury in his neck. He might have a pause-type mindset that hasn't turned off.

The Ren channel on pause

When a person is calm and contented, the Ren channel qi flows from the anus to the front of the torso, up the midline of the torso, and up to the lower lip. From the lower lip, the Ren channel qi flows into the mouth, down through the gut, and out the anus. At the anus, it flows up the front of the torso again.

Both the Du and Ren channels begin at the anus, flow up the back and front of the body, respectively, flow into the mouth, down through the gut, and out the anus. These huge, powerful currents are present on the outer surface of the early embryo when in "blastula" phase: when the cells are a ball-shaped cell cluster with a hollow tube running down the center. The *internal* portions of the Du and Ren channels, the currents flowing down the tube of the blastula, pave the way for the digestive tract. The embryonic Du and Ren channels are flowing before the twelve primary channels even begin to take shape. The Du channel also provides the energy for the area that will become the embryo's brain.

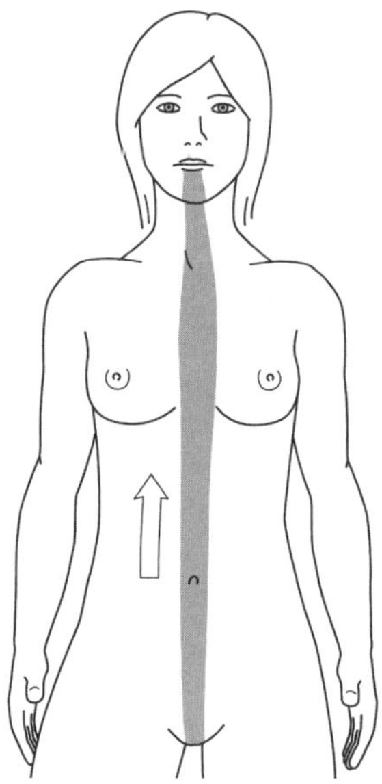

Fig. 13.5 The Ren channel in parasympathetic mode

The Du and Ren channels provide the energy for all the other channels, as well as providing much of the energy that moves the digestive system. The Du and Ren channels are the strongest (largest amperage) channels on the body.

The word "Du" means governor, and refers to the subordinate relationship that the brain and sympathetic mode should have with the heart / pericardium and parasympathetic mode. The heart / pericardium is considered the "King" of the body. The King is the soul, considered to be knowable through the heart, and manifesting in the heart and in the heart's resonance with the *mid*brain. The "Governor," the brain, is considered to be, at best, a servant to the heart. At worst, the brain is constantly trying to usurp power from the heart. The sides-of-the-brain, ego-based intellect, unless well regulated, is always trying to overthrow the King soul.

"Ren" means person, people, and/or humanity. The Ren channel provides back-up channel qi support for any organ or channel that needs a boost. For example, during sympathetic mode, some amount of Ren channel qi in the vicinity of the chest is diverted deep inside to the heart, to help with the need for increased heart rate.

During pause, when blood is diverted deep inside to prevent further loss of blood from the possibly-injured perimeter, the Ren channel qi also diverts deeply inside the body, towards the spine, becoming undetectable by hand. The location from which it dives deep is variable, ranging from just below the pubic bone to the bottom of the sternum. The sternum is the "chest" bone that connects to the front ends of the upper ribs. On pause, the Ren channel qi only rarely gets as far up the torso as the mid-sternum.

When on pause, the *amount* of channel qi in both the Du and the Ren is greatly diminished. When a person is on pause, his appetite and digestive tract function can be diminished or even severely inhibited. If pause lasts quite a while or becomes chronic, constipation can become a problem. On pause, sometimes, in the absence of adequate energy flowing down through the digestive tract and in combination with the *backwards* flow of Stomach channel qi, the digestive tract might even move backwards now and then, causing chronic low level nausea or even a tendency to vomit. During surgical anesthesia or following a concussion, pause-mode channel qi patterns predominate. This is why, during anesthesia or after a concussion, the possibility of vomiting while unconscious or asleep is always a significant concern.

The other channels

The alterations in the Stomach, Du, Ren, and UB channels when on pause *might* lead to further changes in channel qi flow in other channels. The possibilities include backwards or inhibited flow in the Large Intestine channel and/or rerouting, diminished power or other altered behaviors in the Heart, Pericardium, Gallbladder, Liver and Triple Burner channels.

Confused qi

In English translations from the classic Chinese medicine, the pause-related shifts in channel qi are customarily referred to in English translations as "Confused [channel] Qi." There is *nothing* "confused" about these shifts. The axiom we are taught, "Terror Confuses the Qi," is a poorly translated reference to the *logical* and even *life-saving* channel qi changes that occur during pause. Pause does *not* trigger an incorrect or *random* flow of channel qi, as the word Confused implies. The changes of pause are *healthy* and *correct* responses to severe, imminently life-threatening damage. Pause can be a life-saving mechanism. However, channel qi remaining *stuck* in some pause-related electrical circuitry after the crisis has ended might sooner or later lead to serious health problems.

The joy of inner stillness is not the same as pause

Many people have asked me if pause mode is the same as the deep stillness and joy of meditation. No. The stillness and joy attained by regular practice of single-focus meditation during which breathing and heart function might become slower or even greatly diminished is *not* pause. Just the opposite: this type of joy is a manifestation of a very high degree of parasympathetic mode: a state approaching resonance with Universal Love; what the Chinese gospel of *Nei Jing* calls "In tune with the Divine."

Allowing the body to become gently, lovingly motionless during intense focus on some aspect of love or the Divine while practicing single-focus types of meditation allows much more of the channel qi to recede from the skin and muscles into the spine and from there to specific locations such as the pericardium, the point between the eyebrows, the midbrain, or the inner-spinal chakras (locations *inside* the spine where lightwave energy and electromagnetic energy convert back and forth: your spinal "solar panels"). In deep meditation, in response to diminished energy in the Primary channels and the sides of the brain, *physiological* movements and sensory functions such as hearing and awareness of somatic sensations might diminish or even cease. Then, in the physical stillness and mental focus of deep meditation, one finds that superconsciousness, and awareness of the heart's attunement with joy (increased pericardial amperage), and the presence of subtle, light-based energy throughout the body are all easier to perceive.

The Du channel's route through the brain

According to the Chinese texts, in people with poor mental focus, the energy in the brain portion of the Du channel "meanders" through the left and right sides of the brain. Highly focused thought and/or single-focus meditation makes the Du channel run in a much straighter line through the center of the head.

In certain types of single-focus meditation, a person might learn to greatly straighten his Du channel: keep the Du channel energy in a thin line right up the center of the spine and through the center of the brain, as opposed to having the Du channel energy constantly zigzagging distractedly to the left and right – especially in the sacrum and head.

If the Du channel flows in a straight and narrow path up the back and through the midbrain to the forehead at the location of the "third eye," sometimes called the single eye, this unwavering current goes straight up the spine and curves gently as it travels through the brain. It forms the shape of a shepherds's crook.[1] When highly centered, not veering randomly left or right as it does in most people who have not learned to focus it, this current can function as an antenna. Via this narrow, straight "antenna" of channel qi, one can literally tune in with the various frequencies, the waves of energy, that carry the joy of one's own soul as well as the frequencies of Cosmic Joy. As Jesus is quoted in the gospels, "Straight is the gate, and narrow is the way." [2]

The delusion of being *defined* by the body, a delusion sustained by activities in the right and left sides of the brain, is thus destroyed. Tuning in, radio-like, with the soul and/or the frequencies (various wave-rates) of Universal love via this Du-channel antenna is then possible. This is *very* different, almost the opposite, from the *ego-identified* sense of self that *usually* perceives itself as being primarily defined by the physical body and imagines itself to be distinctly *apart* from everything else in the universe. In a high degree of parasympathetic mode, a person realizes that his real nature is vibratory energy, energy that is connected to endless waves of loving, consciousness-bearing vibrations throughout the universe. A person realizes that he is not, primarily, a physical, ever-changing body. In this joyful state, distracting neuronal activity on the *sides* of the brain is deeply stilled.

Oppositely, during pause, a person might feel as if his consciousness has been expelled from his physical body and that he is outside of his body: not just apart from everything else, but also teetering on the verge of dreaded and permanent annihilation. While on pause, it is *extremely* difficult to sense the electromagnetic wave variations and amplifications in the pericardium, sometimes called "heart-feeling," that are associated with joy. On pause, awareness of heart-feeling sensations is *greatly* inhibited. Fear and anxiety dominate: the *opposite* of joy. On pause, a person or animal is struggling to stay alive so that he can get back inside his precious, unique body. If he is conscious, the *side* structures of his brain and especially the risk-assessment area – *not* the midline – are *extremely* active. Assessment of the situation's risk is elevated until the risk level comes down, physical stability is attained, and pause is turned off – or the person or animal dies.

Research using brain scans of highly experienced meditators, including some Hindu and Buddhist monks, shows them having narrowed, highly focused *midline* brain

---

[1] Ps 23:4. "Thy rod and thy staff, they comfort me."

[2] Matthew 7:14. Another related scriptural quotation states, "When thine eye is single [all the attention is focused at the third eye and the Du current is running in the "Middle Way," [neither to left or to right], thy whole body will be full of light": your consciousness will be attuned to the uplifting frequencies of specific types of lightwaves. These waves are just behind the illusion of the solid body. The body illusion is created via rivers and glaciers of electrons and protons: condensed light waves. When your Du channel runs in the straightest possible line through the spine and head, your consciousness can resonate with the creative forces *behind* the illusion of solid matter.

activity during meditation. A person in this nearly pure parasympathetic condition can know his body as a temporary residence in which and from which he might lovingly experience various sensory events without having ego-based attachment to his observations.

Oppositely, a person on pause, with his Du channel stopped at the base of his neck, has a greatly diminished amount of current flowing through his brain's midline and a greatly diminished ability to resonate with joy. Instead, he will have increased energy-flow through the sides of his brain. He might have an elevated level of ego-driven desire to protect and preserve his precious body. (The word "ego" is used here to mean "sense of identity that imagines oneself to be apart from, separate from, the rest of the universe.")

The almost dead mouse

Many of us have seen an animal in pause mode. A very common example of pause occurs when a cat catches a mouse. As the claws of the cat sink into the mouse (excessive perforation of the skin), the mouse immediately goes into pause. The mouse becomes rigid. Its body might curl up into a fetal position. Its skin becomes cold. Its breathing is minimal and nearly silent. It might appear to be dead.

If the cat was hunting merely to amuse himself, and not to satisfy hunger, the cat might biff the rigid mouse around a few times, seeking a response. If the mouse remains cold and rigid, the cat will soon lose interest and go off in search of livelier sport.

After a few minutes, when the mouse is no longer bleeding at the clawed sites, so that blood pressure has stabilized, the mouse's sacrum and brain will begin producing a small "starter" electrical signal that causes a sense of internal tremor. This tremor, in turn, stimulates the risk assessment area of the mouse's brain to shift into a higher gear.

When the mouse no longer sees the cat, hears the cat, smells the cat, or feels the cat, allowing its risk assessment area to determine that the vicinity is now safe, it will take a deep breath, wobble its head slightly to turn back on its vagus nerves at the base of the skull, allow a visible shiver to run down its spine activating the spinal nerves, and then it will scamper off to safety. Many people have seen this "dead mouse" behavior. Sometimes, people imagine the mouse is just "playing 'possum," meaning "*pretending* to be dead." [1]

The mouse was not "playing dead." A mouse does not have the intellectual capacity or self-control to *pretend* to be dead. The mouse entered into an involuntary condition of pause brought about by perforation of its skin by the cat's claws or teeth. This collapse into the inert immobility of a high degree of pause renders the mouse cold, rigid and corpse-like, and may well save the life of the mouse.

---

[1] A North American opossum's pause response to being startled is not a trick. An opossum has a hair-trigger, *involuntary*, full-body pause response when startled. The opossum isn't making a decision: he is hard-wired to go into pause in response to just about any startle event.

"Penguins," the 2019 Disney full-length nature movie, has footage in which an Adèlie penguin goes into pause after being attacked by a seal. The penguin survives because the seal loses interest in the seemingly lifeless bird. Again, this is very different from the frozen "deer in the headlights" phenomenon, which is a *pre*-action assessment phase of the sympathetic mode response. As with pause mode, this is a neurological phase in which a person *might* become stuck.

Of course, this type of *full-blown* pause mode, a condition in which a person or animal is cold and motionless, is not usually seen in an acupuncture clinic. However, patients with a modified degree of pause or a situation in which some *portion* of channel qi has become stuck in the channel qi circuitry of pause might very well come to your office. Long-term use of even a portion of the pause-type channel qi circuits can cause significant health problems, including chronic syndromes of "no known cause," or "incurable" syndromes and health problems. The word incurable in these cases only means that MDs don't know how to fix the problem. The actual syndrome might be perfectly curable, if a treatment is administered that restores the correct flow of channel qi.

Getting back to the pause-mode changes in the Stomach channel

Perhaps the most important Stomach channel shift during pause is the shunt to ST-8, on the forehead. As mentioned earlier, when Stomach channel qi runs backwards, this shunt prevents the Stomach channel qi from going backwards all the way up to Yin Tang (the point between the eyebrows) and then *backwards* into the mid-brain – a routing that might induce coma and autonomic irregularity.

ST-8 is *not* on the Primary route of the Stomach channel. Stomach channel qi is only routed through ST-8 when the Stomach channel is running *backwards* up to the jaw.

When Stomach channel qi is flowing backwards, *if* it backs up to ST-6, at the back of the jaw, it is shunted up to ST-8, on the forehead. There, it either builds up, causing a headache, or it short circuits into the nearby GB channel. If the backwards flow is mild, qi might merely accumulate at ST-6 or ST-8. Tooth or jaw pain at ST-6 or a pressure-type headache at ST-8 might develop, brought on by the localized channel qi build-up. If *enough* channel qi builds up at ST-8, the channel qi might surge out of ST-8 and short circuit into the nearby GB channel, causing an increase in amperage of GB channel qi.

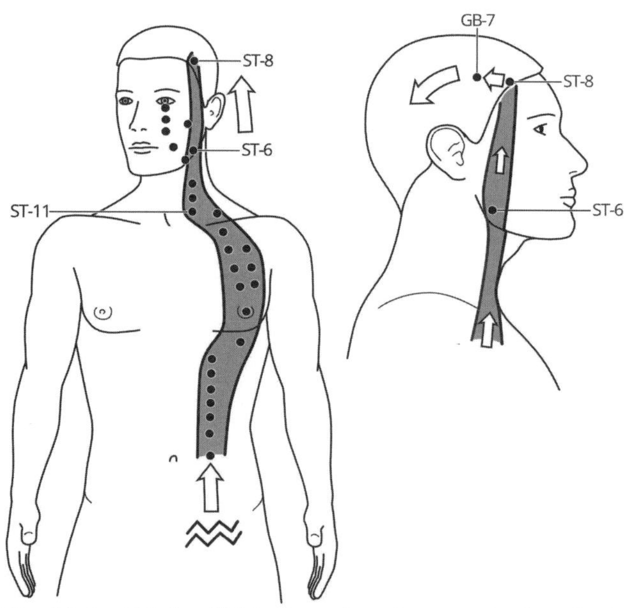

In this diagram Stomach channel qi is flowing backwards due to a blockage represented by zigzag lines on the lower torso. This blockage location was selected at random. The blockage might just as easily have been drawn on the neck part of the Stomach channel or on the foot part of the Stomach channel.

Although the GB channel is not shown, a large arrow on the side of the head demonstrates the direction of flow in the head portion of the GB channel qi. The addition of Stomach channel qi (the short arrow) to the channel qi already flowing in the GB channel increases the overall amount of channel qi in the Gallbladder channel path.

Fig. 13.6 ST-6 to ST-8, the safety shunt on the jaw for backwards-flowing Stomach channel qi.

This drawing is just a reminder of the head portion of the Stomach channel's *parasympathetic* and *sympathetic* paths: In these two modes, Stomach channel qi flows down from the forehead, flows over the cheeks, down the neck and down the torso to the feet.

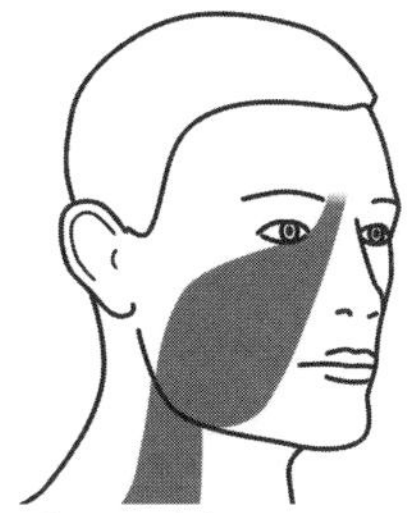

Fig. 13.7 Stomach channel in parasympathetic mode

As an aside, sleep mode is usually activated by a night-time circadian surge of energy in the GB channel. When a nightly surge of increased current runs through the head portion of the GB channel, which runs from the front of the head to the back, there will be a corresponding *decrease* in the amount of channel qi running in the opposite direction: from the back of the head to the front...the direction of the Du channel.

Again: an *increase* in amperage in the head portion of the GB channel will cause a *decrease* in amperage in the head part of the Du channel, including in the energy flow to the striatum, thalamus, and the center of the frontal lobe – the primary brain locations for maintaining alert consciousness and will. This decrease in consciousness allows a person to drop off to sleep.

(To learn more about the electrical schematics of sleep mode, please read chapter 13 in *Tracking the Dragon.*)

When, due to backwards flow, a person's Stomach channel qi surges into the GB channel from ST-8, the person, if awake, might experience a sensation as if the inside of his head is spinning, or as if he has temporarily experienced an altered consciousness or even a momentary loss of consciousness.

If the backwards flow becomes *chronic*, a new, *constantly open* path into the GB channel might develop. This situation, if chronic, might make a permanent increase of energy in the Gallbladder channel This, in turn, can make it easy for a person to fall asleep quickly, every time the person feels safe enough to do so.

Again, during pause, backwards flow building up at ST-8 might flow into the nearby GB channel, thus *increasing* the power in the GB channel. As the power in the GB channel *increases*, the power in the Du channel *decreases*. If the Du decreases in power enough, sleep or even coma might ensue: the person or animal might pass out and stay passed out until the body stabilizes and pause turns off.

It is easy for the backwards-flowing Stomach channel qi to flow into the GB channel: the GB channel is very wide across the forehead and offers little resistance.

Sometimes, the amount of backwards Stomach channel qi flowing into the GB channel is so small that the traumatized person might merely feel woozy or go in and out of alertness. This wooziness can be temporarily overridden by norepinephrine, released by emergency-type thinking. If/when the emergency-type thinking is turned off, a person running a pause-type pattern in the brain might be able to drop off to sleep *very* easily due to the excessive level of channel qi in the GB channel.

As soon as pause mode turns off *or* the Stomach channel blockage heals and then opens up, the Stomach channel qi will *usually* resume flowing in the correct direction automatically: any previous build-up of charge at ST-8 will disperse by flowing back down to ST-6 and then down the torso and leg to the foot.

As mentioned earlier, almost any significant blockage along the Stomach channel might eventually cause the Stomach channel to flow backwards. Although most of my Type II Parkinson's patients have had backwards-flowing Stomach channel qi due to a *foot* or *ankle* injury, other damage along the Stomach channel can also set the pause-type channel patterns in motion.

For example, some of my patients have had Stomach channel qi blocked and flowing backwards due to an appendectomy scar. Others have had the Stomach channel blocked and flowing backwards due to a side-to-side C-section cut.[1]

[1] "Having your appendix removed trebles the risk of getting Parkinson's disease, suggests largest study"; *The Telegraph News/Science*; Bodkin, Henry, science correspondant; May 9, 2019.

This study led by Dr. Mohammed Sheriff, a physician at Case Western Reserve University and University Hospitals Cleveland Medical Center, was looking for a better understanding of the relationship between gut proteins and Parkinson's disease.

What they found was, among 488,190 who had appendectomies, .92 % went on to eventually (more than six months later) develop Parkinson's disease. Of the 61.7 million patients *without* appendectomies, only .29 percent went on to eventually develop Parkinson's disease.

Although they posit that this might mean something in the gut causes Parkinson's, I would propose that pause mode causes gut inhibition, thus altering the gut's microbiome *and slowing* the peristalsis in the gut – one of the main causes of appendicitis. Pre-Parkinson's pause mode might make a person more likely to have appendicitis in the first place. In this bit of research, doctors might be confusing cause and effect: pre-Parkinson's might lead to appendicitis. Then, the appendectomy's surgical scarring across the Stomach channel adds to the other blockages in the person's body. This hastens the severity of the backwards flow of the Stomach channel due to blockage at the appendectomy-scar site, on top of whatever else was causing the pre-Parkinson's pause mode behaviors.

Oppositely, a case of appendicitis *not* related to any pre-Parkinson's slowing of the gut might start a person down the path towards Type II PD *because* of the surgical scarring blocking the Stomach channel.

Scar tissue, like rubber, is non-conductive. It presents a high level of resistance to electrical currents in the fascia. Deep scars, such as those created by abdominal surgery – including internal laparoscopic scarring which is *much* harder for the body to heal from than clean surgical incisions, especially those *really* damaging, hard to heal scars inside the umbilicus area – almost always make a fairly complete blockade against the flow of channel qi in the vicinity of the scarring.

Also, there is a powerful relationship between the gut microbiome and the mind. Thought waves are the single largest factor in determining what types of gut microbes are thriving at any particular moment. Being on pause affects the microbiome.

At the same time, the electromagnetic signals generated by the microbiome can affect one's thoughts. For example, if a pathogenic "bug" gets into the microbiome, or if the microbiome gets grossly out of balance, the signals from the microbiome can overwhelm the mind's capability for self-determined thoughts. Researchers recognize that the microbiome of people with Parkinson's has a different composition from most people who *don't* have Parkinson's. When the brain is using pause mode, the digestion is significantly inhibited. The brain's signals to the microbiome correspondingly somewhat suppress or even inhibit those biota involved in healthy digestion. Hence the altered microbiome in people with PD.

Turning off biological *pause*

Turning off *biological* pause requires going through a very specific set of feelings and movements. These are not *attitudinal* thought processes, but very specific sensory feelings and observations that *start* with the resonance that occurs when physiological trauma ceases and the body's crucial life systems such as blood pressure regulation and heart rate are stabilized. This resumption of internal resonance allows a subtle, "*almost* back to life" electrical agitation to start up in the sacrum and thalamus. This small "starter motor" agitation is a *call* for assessment. If large enough, this internal electrical agitation can also cause *physically obvious* tremor or shaking in the body. This type of tremor might temporarily activate when a person is coming out of pause *or* coming out of anesthesia.

As an aside regarding pause mode, Parkinson's disease, and the thalamus: researchers have long recognized that, in people with Parkinson's-related tremor, the thalamus gives off "static" in rhythmic time with the tremor. During the 1980s and '90s, many people with PD were horribly paralyzed when surgeons removed portions of their thalami in hopes that this would stop their tremoring. It didn't work, of course, and the patients were usually much worse off after the removal of a crucial brain part, one that helps sustain consciousness and somatic awareness.

I had one patient who'd had a thaladotomy. He and his wife never got over their bitterness at how this procedure drastically and immediately reduced his quality of life, changing him from a person who could get around by himself, although tremoring, to a person who was completely wheel-chair bound, barely able to talk, and unable to care for himself at all. He lived another twenty years in this condition. His tremor continued unabated.[1]

Feeling biologically stabilized is a reflection of the person's *internal*, physiological environment. The next step for coming out of pause is assessment of the *external* environment. Sensory assessment using eyes, ears, nose, and/or touch, *or* the caress or gentle verbal reassurances of a fellow animal or helping human can confirm that the immediate danger and risk of imminent death has now passed.

After sensory confirmation that the *external* situation is now safe, the animal or person automatically takes a deep, audible inhalation, an audible "sigh of relief." Next, the vagus and spinal nerves that have been turned down or off are physically turned back on with specific, automatic neck and spinal movements. These physical movements allow a surge of healthy energy to pour through the sacrum, brain, and vagus and spinal nerves. Specifically, a quick left-right head bobble stimulates the vagus nerve and allows resumption of flow in the Du channel. The surge of flow in the Du channel turns off the sensation of electrical agitation or "static" that was due to *minimal* energy flow in the sacrum and brain. This ends the internal tremor sensation and the physical tremor, if any. A shimmy or *frisson* down the spine allows the spinal nerves to resume normal function, including re-activation of the adrenal glands.

---

[1] In 2020, a greatly modified thalamus-altering procedure, one using ultrasound waves to selectively destroy a small number of thalamus cells over an area the size of a sesame seed, has been promoted as helpful for essential tremor – but *not* for tremor from Parkinson's. I have not found any information yet about the risks and/or side affects of this procedure. As of this writing, this procedure has *not* been used successfully for Parkinson's tremor that I know of. It does, of course, cause permanent brain damage.

However, as with any channel qi variation, it's possible for the channel qi flow to get *stuck* in some or all of the circuits related to pause, and in the pattern of insufficient energy flowing in the sacrum and thalamus. Being *stuck* in some aspects of biological pause that occurred in response to a physical or emotional trauma might quickly *or* slowly, eventually, over decades, lead to Type IV Parkinson's disease.

Self-induced pause

The channel circuitry of pause mode can also be set in motion in response to a person's forceful command to himself to "Feel no pain." Very often, this command refers to emotional pain as well as physical pain.

The body does have a mode in which many types of pain are minimized: pause mode. Many of my Parkinson's patients who've been stuck in pause mode's electrical patterns got that way by telling themselves "don't show pain," "be numb," or something along the lines of "I don't want to be a part of this world."

The usual biological steps for turning off pause will *not* work for self-induced pause. Instead, the numbness to somatic feeling that was triggered by the mental instruction must be ended. A person doesn't need to remember the specifics of the pause-inducing instruction that he used. However, he must learn how to create the midbrain electrical behaviors of biological stability and safety that sets in motion the other steps for turning off pause. Only then will his brain be able to go through the steps that turn off the pause-type neurological and channel qi shifts that he unwittingly set in motion with his self-instruction.

Self-induced pause can lead to Type I Parkinson's disease.

Pseudo pause: pause-like channel qi flow from unhealed injury or channel qi blockage

In response to an unhealed injury, pause-type electrical circuits might develop quickly, within hours, or slowly, over decades. Pause might develop slowly if an injury only *partially* blocks a channel. In my limited experience, pseudo pause circuitry usually starts with an injury along the Stomach channel or on the neck or spine portions of the Du channel. Again, this is *not* true pause: the patient hasn't necessarily lapsed into a state of neurotransmitter inhibition, decreased mobility, and lowered blood pressure – at least not at first.

Rather, the unhealed injury creates a condition in which channel qi behaviors might eventually *resemble* those of pause. In the case of displaced bones or soft tissue in the ankle or foot, the pause-like channel qi behaviors might come on gradually. With a *significant* leg injury or a significant neck injury, the pause-like symptoms might appear almost immediately. For example, in the case of a broken femur (upper leg bone), the Stomach channel might become immediately blocked: pause-type channel qi flow might begin almost immediately and the patient might pass out.

If an injury or blockage on the Stomach or Du channel fails to completely heal, psuedo pause can lead to Type II Parkinson's disease.

For an example of *gradual* onset of pseudo pause, in the early years of a dissociated and therefore somewhat painless unhealed foot injury featuring slightly displaced soft tissue and/or bones of the foot or ankle, the Stomach channel qi might be only partially blocked on the foot. Due to increased resistance in the channel qi on the foot, *some* amount of the channel qi might back up or diverge on the side of the leg, upstream from the blockage, maybe going sideways into the medial ankle at Ki-3 or Ki-6 or maybe flowing sideways from the middle of the lower leg over into the nearby Gallbladder channel at GB-35.

These not unusual divergences might cause weird, unsettled feelings or maybe tension on the side of the leg, or even restless leg syndrome, but there will be no backwards-flowing Stomach channel qi getting up to the forehead, and no significant symptoms of pause...yet.

If the electrical confusion at the site of the blockage expands in size over time, the backwards Stomach channel qi might back up a little higher up the leg or even into the torso, where it might then flow sideways into any nearby channel. If the Stomach channel qi flows backwards as high up as the neck, it might intersect with the Large Intestine channel qi and cause the Large Intestine channel qi to flow backwards.

After a few hours, days or most often, after several decades, as the channel qi in the vicinity of the injury /blockage continues to spread out sideways or back up, at some point almost *no* Stomach channel qi can get past the injury site.

Meanwhile, the force of the backwards-flowing channel qi might gradually become severe enough that Stomach channel qi flows backward all the way to ST-6 on the back corner of the jaw and thence to ST-8, on the forehead.

When the build-up at ST-8 is large enough, the channel qi might shunt into and augment the Gallbladder channel, which flows from the front of the head to the back. This can cause, to varying degrees, inhibition of the Du channel, which flows from the back of the head to the front. This diminishing of the Du channel leads to diminishing of or inhibition of certain midbrain behaviors such as dopamine release for motor function.

When this occurs, the *mental* changes associated with pause, including heightened wariness and emotional numbness *might* be set in motion – even though the origin of the pause-like currents was *not* an imminently life-threatening injury. Then again, *some* people with pseudo pause from a dissociated injury do *not* develop the pause-related mental components. The mental components contribute to what is called the Parkinson's personality. A person with pseudo pause might not develop the mental components and the personality, or at least not develop them to the same degree, as a person with pause or self-induced pause.

Pseudo pause can lead to Type II or Type III Parkinson's disease.

Channel variations caused by pause

When pause-type routings of channel qi remain uncorrected for years, all bets are off with regard to how the channel qi flow in channels *other* than the Stomach, Du, Ren, UB, and Large Intestine might change, and over what time frame, and what symptoms might then arise.

Pause-type currents in the Du, Ren, UB, Stomach and LI channels can be set in motion by pause and by self-induced pause. They can be set in motion by pseudo-pause from non-life-threatening, incompletely healed injury, surgery, or physical or emotional scarring that has slowly expanded into a channel obstruction. They can be set in motion from pseudo pause from a dissociating self-command to never feel a specific injury, so that the injury remains unhealed and leads to a pause pattern (Type III PD). No matter how the pause-type currents were set in motion, if the electrical system becomes *stuck* in the electrical patterns of pause in the Stomach, Du, Ren, and/or UB channels, pause-related channel qi behavior in all the *other* channels might eventually manifest.

Once electrical currents start flowing in the pause directions for the long term and are, for whatever reason, unable to perform healthy self-correction, the only certainty when it comes to the other channels is that the channel qi will *always* flow in the path of least resistance.[1]

Pause-based alterations in the brain supply of channel qi

On pause, when the Du channel is blocked at the base of the neck, the other currents flowing over and through the head (primarily the UB and GB channels) can still provide support and direction to the currents inside the brain.

As noted earlier, when the head portion of the Du channel is greatly inhibited or blocked, as it is in pause, the energy level, the *amount* of channel qi flowing through the midline of the brain is severely diminished. This causes inhibition of some of the functions of the brain structures that straddle the midline such as the striatum and thalamus.

At the same time, the brain experiences *increased* activity in the sides of the brain: the locations for fear-based risk assessment, hyper-analysis (anxiety), and increased amygdala (fear-and-rage center) activity – areas located directly under and influenced by the UB and GB channels. Analytical thinking, word-based thinking, and word-based self-expression is also increased.

Dopamine is used in both the midbrain *and* on the sides of the brain. For example, the risk-assessment area in the right lobe of the brain, in the right anterior caudate, uses dopamine as its main neurotransmitter. As mentioned earlier, in people with Parkinson's disease, dopamine levels are *elevated* in the right-side anterior caudate area even though dopamine release is *inhibited* in the midbrain areas. [2]

---

[1] Here's a plumbing analogy: blocked plumbing in a house causes the wastewater to flow *seemingly* unpredictably as it follows the path of least resistance through the pipes that are hidden in the walls. Sometimes a mild blockage will cause bubbling noises in the toilet while water moves transversely into other lines until it slowly drains, but a severe blockage beneath the house might result in raw sewage from upstairs spewing up from the downstairs shower drains.

When plumbing flows backwards, it can *seem* unpredictable or even illogical as to direction because you can't see what's happening inside the walls. But rest assured, the sewage *always* flows in the path of least resistance.

Water movement is impelled primarily by gravity and influenced by route availability. Channel Qi flow is impelled primarily by voltage differentials (analogous to water's relationship with gravity) and conductivity. With channel qi, these impelling factors can be influenced by physical damage and scar tissue, as well as the distinct brain signals associated with each of the four neurological modes. Other influences on channel qi flow include wave signals that come from thought waves, including subconscious thought waves and thought habits, *and* the electromagnetic signals generated by one's cellular and mitochondrial DNA. Channel qi flow might *seem* random, but there's always a logic behind it based on the simple laws of physics.

[2] "Personality traits and brain dopaminergic function in Parkinson's disease"; *Proceedings of the National Academy of Sciences USA* 98:13272-7*;* Valtteri Kaasinen, MD, PhD et al; 2001.

When people refer to dopamine as the "feel good" neurotransmitter, they are only talking about dopamine that's used by the midbrain, not the dopamine that's stimulating anxiety and other negative or ego-based processes on the sides of the brain.

In summary

Pause mode is a short-term, potentially life saving mode.

During pause, many specific channel behaviors are set in motion and possibly some side effect behaviors in other channels. While on pause, aside from the backwards flow in the Stomach channel, stoppage in the Du at the base of the neck, deep internalization of the Ren, the "escape from the body" at the neck of the UB channel, and very likely backwards flow in the arm part of the Large Intestine channel, all other channel bets are off.

These various channel qi behaviors work to reduce bleeding, reduce the need for oxygen, hold the body as motionless as possible, and make the body less noticeable and attractive to a nearby predator.

Pause is designed to turn off automatically as soon as the near-death situation has been resolved and the metaphorical coast has been confirmed as being clear.

This 2001 study describes the utterly unexpected discovery that people with Parkinson's have *elevated* levels of dopamine activity in the brain's anterior cingulate area, an area that manages risk assessment.

Chapter Fourteen

PD symptoms: Location, Location, Location

This chapter takes a detailed look at the symptoms of Parkinson's disease. It describes the exact locations and physiological changes related to those symptoms, and also how their locations caused a revolution in my understanding of Parkinson's disease.

By the late 1990s, I had seen several people recover from "incurable" Parkinson's disease. Like everyone else in medical school, I had been taught the never-proven and ultimately wrong theory that dead brain cells were the cause of Parkinson's disease. I couldn't imagine why or how the healing of foot injuries was bringing dead brain cells back to life. But the fact remained, when my patients' foot and/or ankle injuries responded to treatment and their Stomach channels started running correctly, the patients "snapped out" of having Parkinson's. I became obsessed with a question: how did healing a person's foot injury or, in one case, a head injury, restore life to dead brain cells?

Every day, for over an hour in the early mornings, I obsessed over this as I walked or ran on the woodsy trails behind my home. Over and over, I played in my mind mental movies of *all* my Parkinson's patients' symptoms, including the new volunteers who were having symptom and personality changes in response to Yin Tui Na treatments but who had not yet recovered.

Western doctors, in defining Parkinson's, had focused on large, overall patterns of rigidity and poverty of movement. I had been more particular. I noted exactly *where* people had rigidity and *where* they had motor poverty: the actual *locations* of specific symptoms. Rigidity and weakness are muscular opposites. I couldn't understand how *opposite* symptoms could result from insufficient dopamine. Furthermore, a decrease in dopamine-producing cells should produce bilaterally symmetrical symptoms. In Chinese medicine, if symptoms are more evident on one side of the body, the doctor should be looking for an injury or trauma that damaged one side of the body more than the other, or even a psychological cause – but not a decreased level of midbrain neurotransmitters.

A *very* small percentage of people with Parkinson's have symptoms that are equally shared over the left and right sides. But most of my PD patients had symptoms that were *all* worse on one side, either left or right – at least in the early days of their syndrome. My earliest patients' first or worse symptoms were always on the same side of the body that had an unhealed foot or ankle injury or surgery. I also saw this asymmetry in people with PD and with pre-PD who were stuck in regular (Type IV) pause from a left-or right-side head injury. I could *not* reconcile all this with the dead-dopamine cell theory.

One day, while running in the woods, after more than a year of puzzling over the question of how foot injuries could be related to dead brain cells, the idea suddenly came to me that I should mentally overlay the *specific* symptom locations of Parkinson's disease from *all* my patients onto a mental picture of a body.

I had a long mental list of symptom *locations* that I'd drawn up from hundreds of hours of talking to my volunteer patients. I divided the symptoms into two groups: rigidity and weakness. I mentally laid out the symptoms over my imagined outline of a human.

I was stunned.

All the symptoms of *rigidity* were located where my patients' channel qi was running *backwards* on the Stomach channel or Large Intestine channel. All the symptoms of *weakness* were located where their channel qi was *missing* on the Stomach and Large Intestine channels. The image was alarming because it was so perfect. All I had done was mentally put two types of dots, one type for rigidity and the other for weakness, on the locations of Parkinson's symptoms. But the *sum* of both types of dots looked as if I had drawn the full lengths of the Large Intestine and Stomach channels…and *none* of the other eighteen channels: the other ten Primary and the eight extraordinary channels. I saw *why* the symptoms of Parkinson's develop *where* they do: something was deeply aberrant with the Stomach and Large Intestine channels. The PD symptoms developed in response to the aberrant channel qi flow.

What follows in this chapter is a word-map of the symptoms of Parkinson's. You can see what I saw in my mind's eye *and* start your own self-diagnosis process. You'll revisit this chapter when confirming or disproving your own diagnosis of Parkinson's.

No two are alike

When perusing the following list of Parkinson's symptom *locations*, remember: no one person with Parkinson's will necessarily have *all* of the symptoms described in this list. At the time of diagnosis, a person may have only a few symptoms. The symptoms of Parkinson's disease usually develop gradually. At first they may even be intermittent. Then again, some of the symptoms might begin years, even decades, prior to an official diagnosis of PD. Others symptoms might *never* appear in a given individual. No two people with Parkinson's have all the same exact symptoms. Usually, a given symptom will be more severe or will have appeared earlier on the side of the body where *other* symptoms also first appeared. To drive this point home for some specific symptoms, I'll include the letters SSFA: Side on which Symptoms First Appeared.

Asymmetry

Due to the resonant properties of electrical currents, an electrical pattern that manifests in one of the bi-lateral (either left or right) Primary channels will eventually be "echoed" by the *other*-side channel. At the same time, the healthy-side channel will help to moderate the channel with the problem so that the electrical problem does not become as severe as it might have. [1]

When a person develops irregular channel qi flow and maybe symptoms on one side of his body, the other side of his body might slowly or rapidly develop almost-matching symptoms. This is why a person with PD might eventually develop backwards-flowing channel qi in *both* Stomach channels even though the foot or other injury was

---

[1] "Injury information spreads throughout the body. Beyond the wound site, undamaged organs show bioelectric knowledge of damaged counterparts," says Dr. Michael Levin, cited previously on p. 6 xxx.

In a young tadpole with one leg removed, a scan of the electric charge in the wounded leg show an area of increased "action potential" (you can think of this as increased "resistance" or build-up of charge) at the cut edge of the truncated leg. The opposite, *uncut* leg shows an area of increased action potential at the exact same location, paralleling the increase on the injured side. You can view this at: https://oshercenter.org/oc-event/grand-rounds-endogenous-bioelectric-networks-regenerative-medicine/

only on one side of the body. Ramifications of this basic electrical principle in living systems are discussed in the book *Tracking the Dragon*.

However, the five percent of PD patients with *only* Type I PD (not combined with Type II) or those with Type IV from a center-head or spinal injury might have *symmetrical* symptoms. They might *not* have a "side on which symptoms first appeared."

An exception to the rule

The side on which symptoms first appeared is *usually* the same side of the body that has the more *immediately* obvious unhealed injury. However, exceptions abound. For example, one patient presented with a puzzling situation. When he was around six years old, his *right* foot was cut off in a hay mower accident. It was successfully sewn back on. His PD symptoms were all on his *left* side.

I eventually found out that he had been lovingly consoled and coddled with regard to the foot injury. However, when he was a few years older, he underwent a surgery in hopes of restoring some movement to his numb and immobile right foot. Tendons were removed from his *left* leg and transplanted into his right foot. His right foot did not gain the hoped for mobility, but his *left* leg became quite rigid after the tendons were removed. Before and after the left leg surgery he was firmly instructed by the nurses and the surgeon, "Don't cry," "Be a *big* boy; don't make a fuss," etc.

The left side of his body first developed Parkinson's symptoms, not his right side. If he closed his eyes, he was unable to imagine himself having a left side of his body. He *could* imagine himself having a right side. It's not always the *obvious* or well-remembered injury that makes the major contribution to Parkinson's disease. It's just as likely, or even *more* likely, to be an injury that the patient doesn't even remember, doesn't remember correctly, or at least doesn't remember *prior* to starting treatment.

Using this chapter's information

If you think you might have Parkinson's disease, you might want to put a check mark beside any symptoms on this list that you have noticed in your own body. In the following chapter on *diagnosing* Parkinson's disease, information from this chapter about the symptom locations will be useful, helping you to either confirm or disprove a diagnosis of PD.

Key to the symptoms list

○ The hollow circle indicates Parkinson's symptoms recognized by western medicine.
• The filled-in circle indicates Parkinson's symptoms that are fairly common, or at least not uncommon, but which are often unknown to western MDs.
Letters preceding the symptoms refer to:
A = muscle atrophy, weakness, or numbness
R = rigidity or tension
P = pause (symptoms characteristic of pause mode)
SSFA – Side of the body (left or right) where Symptoms First Appeared

Symptoms on the Stomach channel

Part 1: Energy flow over eyelid, cheek and lips

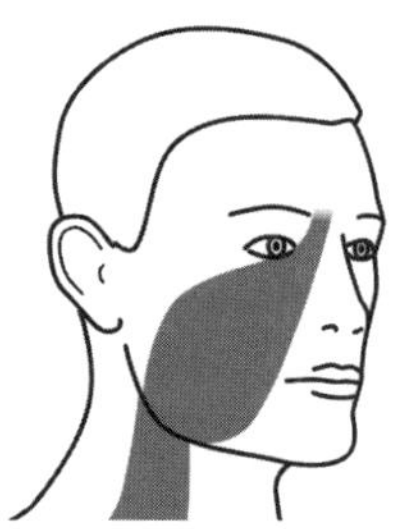

Fig. 14.1
Normal Stomach channel:
Energy is running *down* the face

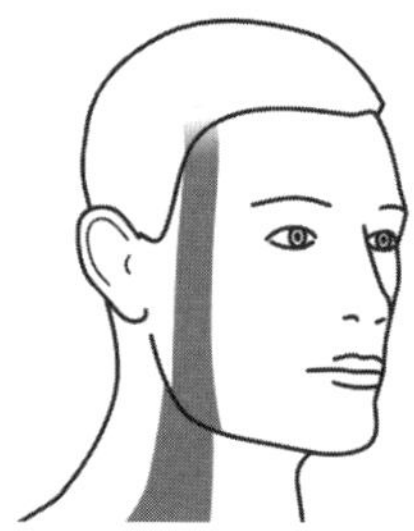

Fig. 14.2
Stomach channel on pause:
Energy is flowing *up* to the side of the head.

Please note: a branch of the Stomach channel runs over both upper and lower lips, circling the lips before rejoining the main current. The drawings do not include this branch because it makes the artwork too cluttered. When on pause, this branch around the lips does *not* flow.

Stomach channel symptoms on the face

○ A . (Reminder: A = atrophy) Minimal or slow eyelid blinking; sagging lower eyelid. This symptom, and nearly all of the face symptoms, are usually worse on the Side of the body where Symptoms First Appeared (SSFA), and are caused by atrophy or numbness. In this case, the exposed part of the eyeball on the SSFA will appear larger than the other eyeball due to the sagging lower eyelid exposing more of the orb.

• A. Overuse of the eyebrow and forehead muscles – which *do* still have normal electrical flow (from the UB channel) – to portray facial expressions. This is a compensatory behavior due to lack of sensation in the cheek and eye muscles. This can sometimes lead to deep grooves in the forehead muscles.

• A. Sinusitis, various problems with the sinuses, including severe snoring and even sleep apnea. These symptoms are caused by a somewhat collapsed soft palate, an area normally activated by the internal cheek portion of the Stomach channel qi. (Not shown in diagrams.)

• A. A sensation as if the roof of one's mouth is sinking down into the mouth at the back of the mouth, as if the bones with the sinus cavities are collapsing downward inside the face.

o A. Seborrheal skin on the side of the nose or cheeks: fungal growth in the skin in these areas due to poor blood circulation due to absence of channel qi.

o A. Loss of sense of taste or smell.

• A. A feeling of deep cold inside the SSFA cheek and eventually in both cheeks.

• A. A groove on the face running from the side of the nostril to the side of the mouth due to atrophy of certain cheek muscles, usually worse on the SSFA.

• A. When attempting to smile, a flatness in the "apple" of the cheek (the muscle that bulges outward along the top of the cheekbone during a smile).

o A. Inability to lift the corners of the mouth when smiling.

• Inability to *realize* that the facial muscles might not be actually moving when consciously attempting to smile. This lack of proprioception is due to numbness in these muscles.

My face in April, 1998, a few weeks after permanently turning off pause mode. The smile is now effortless but the long-weak right-side cheek muscles are still sagging quite a bit.

Note how the saggy lower eyelid on the right side makes that eye look larger or "more open." Also note the flat cheek and groove on the right side of the face alongside the nostril and side of the mouth, as opposed to the round "apple-like" cheek muscle on other the side. I'd had the deep forehead grooves for years.

Prior to recovering, my face had resorted to an expressionless, even dour look unless a conscious, strong effort was made to generate a temporary smile.

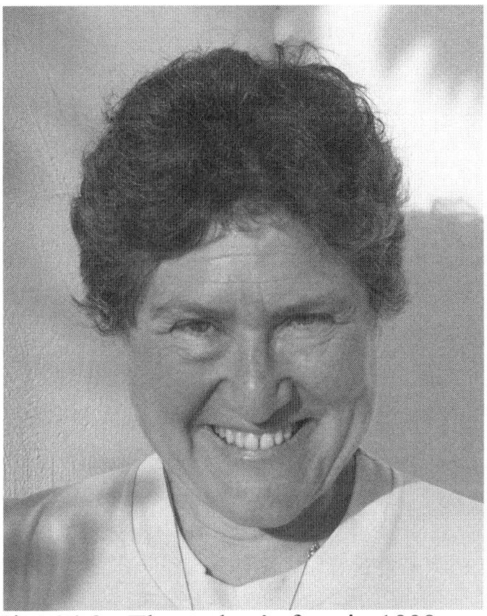

Fig. 14.3 The author's face in 1998

o Following a successful conscious smile, the face might quickly revert back to a stony expression.

• A. Poor lip control; numbness of the lips; unawareness of food clinging to the lips.

o P.(P = pause) Poor swallow reflex, causing drooling and "choking for no reason. "

• P. Teaching oneself to consciously exhale before putting food in the mouth and maybe even keeping up a slight exhalation so long as any food or fluid is in the mouth, in order to avoid a tendency for food to slide down the airpipe when chewing. This often begins many years prior to diagnosis, due to increasingly inhibited swallow reflex.

o P. Aspiration pneumonia from food going down the airways and into the lungs.

This ends the facial and swallow symptoms. Note that, except for the inhibition of the swallow reflex, a midbrain-driven, neurological characteristic of pause, all the other symptoms were caused by an *absence* of subdermal currents, a *lack* of channel qi: atrophy, weakness, and/or numbness – *not* rigidity.

Part 2: Energy flow over the torso and legs

In this section, as the list travels from the back of the jaw to the top of the center of the foot, notice that all the Parkinson's symptoms are characterized by tension and/or rigidity (as noted with an "R"). As before, the *hollow* bullets are symptoms recognized by western medicine. The *filled* bullets note common Parkinson's symptoms of which many western doctors are unaware.

• R. Pain that comes and goes in the back lower molars on the SSFA. This pain in the lower back teeth, either chronic or intermittent, usually has "no reason," according to dentists' exams. One of my PD patients said that her back lower molar on the SSFA "had no root at all." Her dentist had *never* seen that before in a patient.

As mentioned earlier, the lower back part of the jaw is the location of the shunt at ST-6 that sends *backwards*-flowing channel qi up to the side of the forehead, preventing it from flowing backwards over the face to the point between the eyebrows. Chronic pain or weakness in the roots or the physical structure of the lower back molars can be the result of long-term absence of healthy, parasympathetic flow through the ST-6 area.

o R. Spontaneous rigidity and painful spasming on the sides of the throat for no apparent reason, causing choking or coughing from "nothing," choking or coughing from saliva, choking easily when eating.

o R. Hunched posture, head pulled forward due to rigidity in the sternocleidomastoid muscles of the neck.

o R. Choked off voice, soft voice from rigidity in the throat muscles.

o R. Difficulty turning the head from side to side due to rigidity in the neck muscles.

• P. Either a "cast-iron" (numb) stomach or a hypersensitive one with tendency to nausea. Both are due to vagus nerve inhibition, a characteristic of pause.

o R. + P. Orthostatic hypotension (low blood pressure, insufficient blood supply to the head, especially when standing up from a sitting position).

This may be due in part to the pressure on the carotid sinus in the neck. The tight, rigid tissues of the neck press on the carotid sinus, sending a constant, false "high pressure" signal to the carotid sinus. The body might correspondingly lower the blood pressure. This symptom, orthostatic hypotension, is also commonly associated with adrenaline insufficiency as well as being associated with pause.

Many people with Parkinson's are proud of their low blood pressure, never realizing that it is a part of their Parkinson's pathology.

• R. Discomfort, even a feeling of suffocation or panic, if doing an activity in which the arms must be raised over the head for more than a few seconds: for example, while taking down a shower curtain or getting plates down from a high shelf. This compression sensation over the heart is due to the rigid muscles over the chest.

• R. Pain or tingling between the shoulder blade and the spine when trying to sit up very straight with the shoulders back (scapulae pulled *medially*) for any length of time, especially on the SSFA. These muscles on the back are accustomed to being pulled *laterally* by chronic rigidity in the muscles of the chest along the path of the Stomach channel, often combined with the absence or decrease in UB channel qi down the back.

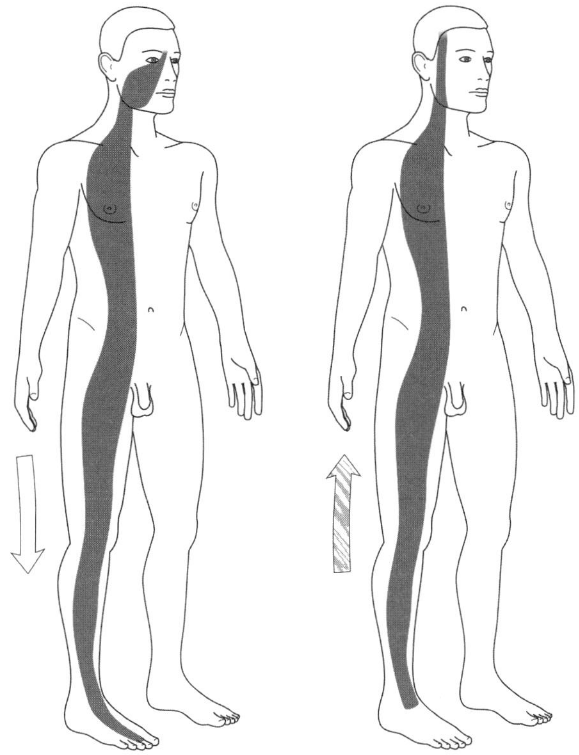

Fig. 14.4 Stomach channel in parasympathetic mode / Stomach channel on pause

○ R. + P. Constipation of a type that usually doesn't benefit from laxatives. This constipation is a normal part of pause. Along with a "cast iron stomach" or chronic low-grade nausea, the intestines might not move very well when on pause. In pause, not only the swallow reflex but the *whole* digestive system is somewhat shut down. A person who is on the verge of death shouldn't have much of an appetite. In long-term pause, a person might have little appetite *or* might feel the need to eat constantly, maybe from anxiety, without ever feeling satiated. Either way, his digestive system is not using normal appetite cues and normal peristalsis (squeezing/pushing movements of the stomach and gut).

○ R. Difficulty turning over in bed at night, or turning from the waist, due to muscle rigidity along the path of the Stomach channel on the torso.

• R. In some women, decades prior to the diagnosis of Parkinson's, *extremely* deep, skin- and deeper tissue-ripping, pathological abdominal stretch marks occur during pregnancy from an utter failure of the skin to stretch normally.

One of my PD patients, many years *prior* to her diagnosis with PD, had experienced failure of the uterus to expand during her second pregnancy, necessitating an early Caesarean section for a baby of low birth weight. Her first child had been carried to term in a fully expanded uterus.

• R. Pain in the groin along the path of the Stomach channel, seemingly for "no discernible reason," especially on the SSFA, due to rigidity along the groin part of the Stomach channel and micro tearing of rigid tissues during movement.

• R. Lack of hair on the legs along the Stomach channel, especially on the SSFA, even if the rest of the leg has a normal hair pattern. This is a symptom of chronically backwards-flowing current. This is a hair-follicle variant of the muscle rigidity and cellular lock-down that occurs when channel qi runs backwards for a long time.

• R. Extreme hardness in the anteriolateral muscles (Stomach channel area) of the upper and lower leg. Many people with PD point with pride to this wooden section of the thigh, assuming that its hardness is supremely toned muscle. However, the inability to *relax* these muscle groups suggests woodenness and rigidity rather than healthy tissues.

• R. A sensation described as "woodenness," "weirdness," "buzzing," "emptiness," "something irritating under the skin," "something not right" in the Stomach channel part of the legs. These feelings can be constant, but they might especially be felt at the end of a long day of standing. They can sometimes be associated with restless leg syndrome.

o R. Festinating gait due to inability to sustain automatic repeated lifting of the rigid thigh. In healthy people, the automatic leg-lifting movement is regulated by the alternating left-right pulsing of the Large Intestine channel, which drives the arm swing. The LI channel qi flows to the head and up to Yin Tang. At Yin Tang it converts into the *opposite*-side *Stomach* channel: the right-side LI channel becomes the left-side Stomach channel, and vice versa. The channel qi of the two connected channels drives the alternating right-left arm swing / leg lift in the thigh muscles on the path of the Stomach channel. Thus, the leg stride is coordinated with and driven by the opposite-side arm swing.

o R. Difficulty in moving sideways or turning to the side while walking.

• R. More difficulty in turning to the SSFA than in turning to the other side.

• R. Cogwheeling (jerkiness or "ratchety" behavior during rotation) in the ankles. The "cog" occurs because of rigidity at the point where the Stomach channel traverses the ankle. If the adjacent Gallbladder (GB) channel is also running backwards (not uncommon if a foot, leg, or hip injury is on the path of and is blocking GB channel qi flow), an extended ST-and-GB channels cog from rigidity might occur where the nearby Gallbladder channel traverses the ankle. Like most symptoms, cogwheeling is usually worse on the SSFA.

• R. Taking the stairs two at a time, or experiencing relative ease during stair climbing. Because the muscles along the Stomach channel don't work, many a person with Parkinson's will use the muscles in the sides of the legs or the backs of the legs and buttocks, along the GB or UB channels, to hoick himself powerfully up each stair: he places a foot on the next stair and then powerfully straightens these muscles, causing his body to rise. These muscles are *not* on the Stomach channel and are still functional.

Also, the task of stair-climbing seems to trigger a call for increased norepinephrine. This pleasant, subconscious surge of power leads many people with mild Parkinson's to opt for climbing stairs two at a time instead of one. Once the top of the stairs is attained, the "emergency" is over. The normal stride – a forward motion rather than a leg-straightening motion and one that requires use of the anteriolateral (along the Stomach channel) thigh muscles, *together* with the immediate drop in norepinephrine, might cause the stride to almost immediately revert back to its usual shuffle.

• R. Walking backwards. The still-normal functionality in the muscles of the buttocks and backs of the legs contributes to a person with *advanced* PD stepping *backwards* following a strong mental instruction to "move the legs!" The muscles along the Stomach channel cannot respond, but those on in the leg portion of the UB channel, muscles that *can* still move, do move: and the person finds himself walking backwards.

This ends the list of jaw to top-of-the-foot symptoms. Note: the symptoms were all caused by rigidity or else were characteristic of symptoms that occur during pause mode.

Part 3: Energy flow over the top of the foot

In the following section, from the top of the foot to the toes, all the symptoms will again be characterized by atrophy, weakness, or numbness, except for a few symptoms that are directly related to injury itself or a channel short-circuit.

o A. Foot drop (toes seem to drag along the floor, foot doesn't lift up off the floor easily, feet "stick to the floor").

- A. Misshapen feet or toes.
- A. Veins on the dorsum of the foot do not fan out over the toes, especially on the SSFA. Instead, the veins might eventually form a *loop* just distal to ST-42 (at the center of the foot). This is an indication of very long term lack of electrical energy in the middle toes.)

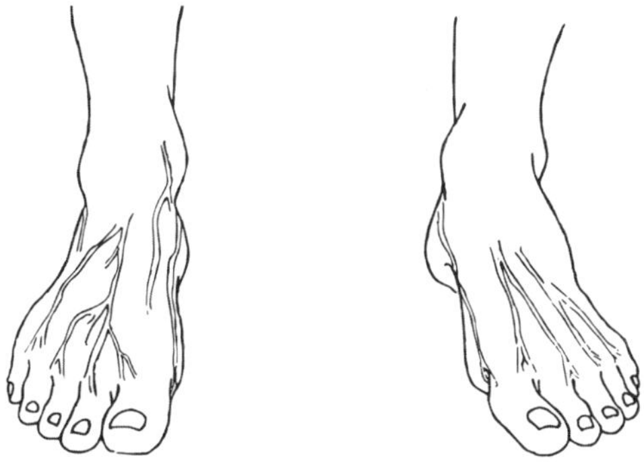

Fig. 14.5 Healthy veins on the feet

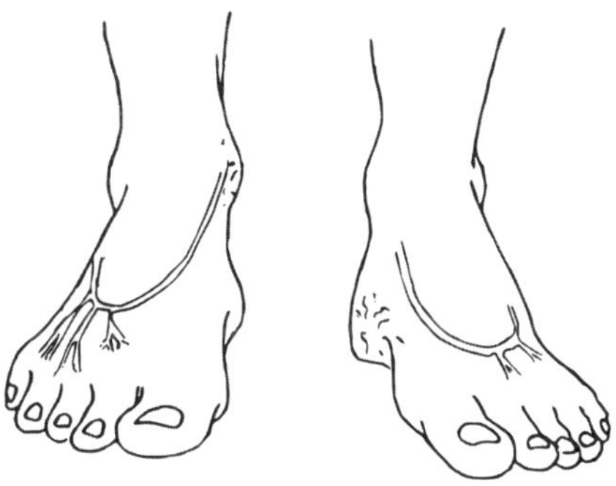

Fig. 14.6 Looping veins and staining on the medial ankle, worse on the SSFA

- Severe vascular irregularities, varicosities, and skin staining may occur on the medial ankle – on the Kidney channel – especially on the SSFA. These are caused by Stomach channel current spilling over into the Kidney channel because of injury blockage or pause-related channel qi stoppage at Stomach-42.
- P. A sensation of tingling or buzzing that comes and goes in the medial (inner) ankle – an area on the Kidney channel. This ankle sensation can be so strong that one may be prompted to pull down the sock and stare at the ankle, looking for the source of the irritation. The cause is a short circuit that occurs when the blocked Stomach channel flows medially into the nearby Kidney channel, causing symptoms of excess amperage in the Kidney channel.
- A. Tendency for cramping in the *sole* of the foot due to no muscle function in the opposing muscles on the *dorsal* (top) side of the foot.
- A. + P. *Toes* curling under the *sole* of the foot due to numbness and atrophy in the opposing muscles on the dorsal side of the toes. Also a characteristic of pause.

- A. Severe bunions and other displaced bones. This can be due to unhealed injury as well as muscle atrophy.
- A. Pale, grey or purplish, cold feet or toes.
- P + R. Smaller foot on the SSFA. Pause can cause a retraction in the plantar (*sole)* foot muscles *plus* there might be protective muscle tension/immobility around an incompletely- or un-healed injury. The foot on the SSFA might be from one half to two full shoe sizes smaller than the other foot, due to muscle tension protectively holding a foot injury in place. The foot very often lengthens out in response to Yin Tui Na therapy and/or in response to turning off pause.

In my own case, about two weeks after turning off pause, my own right foot suddenly went completely limp. It wouldn't bear *any* weight for about half an hour. The foot felt as if the bones inside were moving around on their own, reassembling themselves into new positions. Later that day, as strength returned to the foot and it was able to fully bear weight again, I noticed my right foot had increased by a full shoe size and suddenly matched the length of my left foot. I had received no Yin Tui Na treatment, but I had recently turned off self-induced pause.

- A. Toenail fungus due to lack of circulation and numbness, especially in the three medial toes.
- A. Foot smell. People with Parkinson's almost always have a very specific "dusty and rancid" smell emanating from their feet. This comes from the fungus growing in the toenails and under the skin of the feet, sometimes growing as high up the leg as the thigh. This is not technically due to atrophy, but is due to poor circulation in the feet. In healthy people, the ever-present fungus lives on the underside of the toenails and fingernails. This fungus causes the pretty "white part" on the underside of the nails. Healthy circulation and immune response in the fingers and toes prevents the fungus from getting into the nail bed and from there, into the tissues of the hand or foot. In people with PD, there is little or poor circulation or immune function in the toes. Because of this lack, the fungus can invade the nail bed and the areas of the skin that have poor circulation.

The smell can be quite pervasive. I can always detect the lingering smell when I've had a PD patient in my office. Then again, I have a painfully acute sense of smell. Possibly it's a compensation for my extremely poor eyesight. Some doctors have published articles marveling at how some people, usually women with a keen sense of smell, sometimes referred to as "super-smellers," can diagnose Parkinson's by the smell. They are smelling the fungus in the toenails and feet. [1]

---

[1] Women tend to have a much more acute sense of smell than men. The first woman recognized as able to diagnose Parkinson's by smell was the wife of a man with PD. Researchers have mistakenly assumed that the smell is a chemical produced in the sebum of people with Parkinson's. Yes, the smell is present in the sebum (oil in certain pores of the skin) on the sides of the nose and on the back. In research literature it is described as a "musky" smell. As noted earlier in this chapter, sebhorrheal (fungally infected) skin on the sides of the nose can be a symptom of PD. Sebum glands provide habitat for the nearly omnipresent fungus that can thrive just under the skin in people with poor blood circulation. But if you want a really *powerful* whiff of the smell, have a person with PD take off his shoes. I learned so much about Parkinson's by examining patients' feet.

Most neurologists *never* have a patient take his shoes off. If they did, we might have had a cure for Parkinson's long before now. But as one neurologist in my hometown (known by her

- A. Distinct toenail ridges that run parallel to the white moon of the toenails, instead of normal ridges that run the *length* of the nail.
- A. Inability to separate the 2nd and 3rd toe. Many patients assured me that *no* one can separate their second and third toes, even if they were able to separate the 2nd and 3rd toes on their healthier foot. After pause turns off and the foot heals, the patients are able to easily spread their toes on the side that previously could not.
- A. Numbness on the medial side of the big toe proximal to the ball of the foot (acupoint SP-3), or poor response when a needle is inserted at SP-3. Needling this point to a depth of a quarter of an inch *should* be breathtakingly painful in a healthy person. The *skin* of a PD patient might have mild sensory awareness, but normal sensitivity in the *subdermal* tissues is lacking. Because their *skin* still has some sensory function, patients often insist that there is no numbness in their feet. In the early days of my research, to test for numbness in people with Parkinson's, I needled the SSFA at this acupoint. I warned the patient that he might be numb in this area. The patient usually responded smugly to the needle insertion, "I'm not numb! I felt that." Then, I needled the healthier side. The healthier side is usually *much* less numb. When the needle went in, the patient might scream out in pain while an electrical jolt traveled through his foot: the normal, healthy response to needling at this particular acupoint. When he caught his breath, the patient usually said something like, "What did you just do?!

  I would gently reply, "I did the same thing on both sides. This side of your body *isn't* numb on the inside." I no longer do this test. I now *know* that this numbness situation *does* exist in most people with Parkinson's. So there is no reason for painful tests.
- A.+ P. Lack of proprioception in the feet and toes.

  Proprioception is the ability to feel the location and actions of a body part without looking at it. For an example of poor proprioception in advanced Parkinson's, a person might not be able to know where his toes are once they are hidden from view by his socks. This can make full insertion of the feet into the shoes very difficult. One patient in early recovery told me excitedly, "Did you know you can actually feel where your toes are inside of your shoes?!" He had previously insisted he had *no* numbness in his feet.

The Large Intestine channel

In parasympathetic mode, the Large Intestine (LI) channel runs from the tip of the index finger to the area between the thumb and index finger (LI-4, where the Parkinson's tremor is most likely to start up), up the arm to the biceps, to the shoulder, up the side of the neck, over to the other side of the face and up to the point between the eyebrows, the acupoint named Yin Tang. From Yin Tang, the current of LI channel qi changes name and is called the Stomach channel.

Under the name of "Stomach channel," the current flows back down the face, neck, and torso, and all the way down to the toes. As noted earlier, the right-side LI channel becomes the left-side Stomach channel, and vice versa. The flow of channel qi in

---

patients as The Dragon Lady) declared with regard to her patient's recovery from Type II PD, "There's no way that the feet have anything to do with the brain!" For more details on the diagnosis by smell research, see: https://www.scientificamerican.com/article/a-new-way-to-detect-parkinsons-by-smell/

the LI channel, flow that continues into the *opposite* side Stomach channel, drives the coordinated arm swing and opposite-side leg lift while walking or running.

On pause, if the *Stomach* channel flows *backwards* up the neck to its cross-over intersection with the neck points of the LI channel, the LI channel might also begin to flow backwards. The LI channel qi then flows backwards in the lower neck, arm, and forearm, as far down as the wrist.

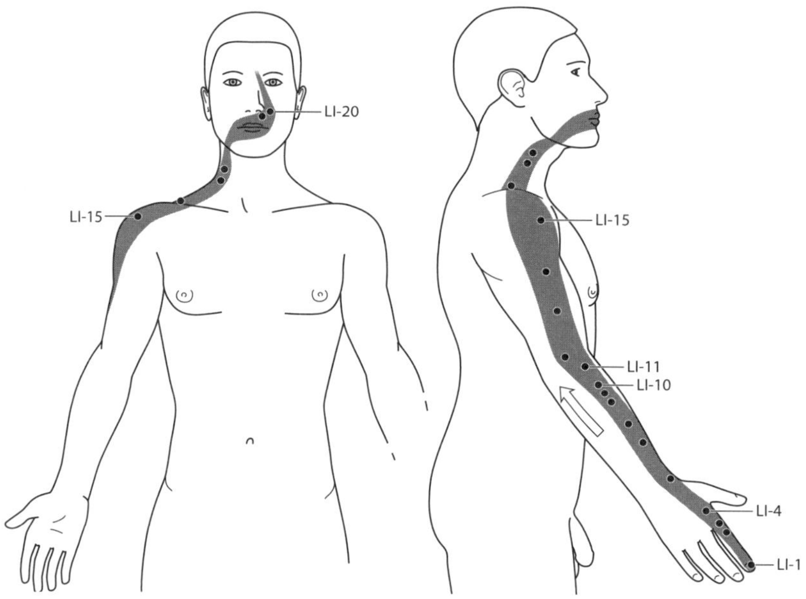

Fig. 14.7 The path of the Large Intestine (LI) channel in parasympathetic mode.

At the wrist, the backwards-flowing channel qi might then flow out into space, in the same way that the UB channel qi flows outwqward from the neck when on pause. If the LI channel qi flows outward at the wrist, the hand portion of the LI channel, (the index finger, and the muscle between the thumb and index finger) will have an absence of channel qi. The muscles in this area will eventually atrophy.

When the Stomach channel qi is running backwards as far up as the neck, then at the point of intersection of the LI and Stomach channels on the sides of the neck, some of the LI channel qi might join with that of the Stomach channel and get shunted up the side of the face to ST-8.

If this occurs, then, from the base of the jaw upwards, there is no channel qi flowing along the facial part of the LI channel. There is no energy in the lips, the sinuses or in the connection of the LI and Stomach channels at Yin Tang, on the forehead. This means that the system that *usually* drives the arm swing/ leg stride coordination ceases. It might still work partially, but only to the degree that an emergency override for pause is in place.

When the LI channel qi is impelled to flow backwards, causing rigidity in the neck, upper and lower arm, then the wrist stiffness and the bent arm position characteristic of Parkinson's kicks in.

Part 4: Energy flow up the arm and over the face

- A. Weakness in the index finger muscles.
- A. Atrophy in the muscle in between the index finger and the thumb. A healthy hand should have a plump muscle (the adductor pollicis) at LI-4, the muscle on the back of the hand that bulges out a bit when the thumb is brought close to the index finger. In Parkinson's, this muscle is often *greatly* atrophied due to the utter absence of channel qi.

o A. Tremoring in the index finger. The index finger is often one of the first places that an obvious tremor occurs. It occurs in this location when the adductor pollicis muscle becomes practically useless due to years of atrophy.

The tremoring of idiopathic Parkinson's is *driven* by what's called "static" in the brain's thalamus and sacrum. Tremor *manifests* in body parts that have become extremely weak, dissociated, or atrophied and therefore are no longer under subconscious motor control.

o A.+ P. Lack of proprioception in the finger(s) and hand. When putting on long sleeves, it may be impossible to know where the hand is as soon as it becomes hidden from view inside the sleeve.

o R. Cogwheeling (jerkiness during rotation) at the wrist. The "cog" is located where the Large Intestine channel flows over the wrist muscles. If the adjacent Triple Burner channel, which runs parallel to the Large Intestine channel, extending up the back side of the arm from the middle and fourth fingers, is also inhibited or flowing backwards, then the "cog" zone might extend from where the LI channel traverses the wrist over to the place where the Triple Burner channel traverses the wrist – an inch or so parallel to the LI channel, moving *towards* the little finger side of the hand. Cogwheeling is usually worse on the SSFA.

This symptom is one of the few localized points that neurologists examine when trying to make a diagnosis of Parkinson's. They know that a person with Parkinson's might exhibit cogwheeling at the wrist, but from my experience, they have no idea *which* specific segments of the wrist rotation are rigid in people with Parkinson's disease, and they certainly haven't been taught why.

o A. + R. Micrographia: small, cramped handwriting. This is due to both the rigidity in the muscles of the wrist and arm and the atrophy and numbness at LI-4 and in the index fingers and very often other fingers, as well.

o R. Rigidity in the muscles that lie just under the Large Intestine channel, from LI-4 up to the front of the shoulder. The rigidity in these muscles pulls the forearm up into a bent elbow position and, on the neck, pulls the neck forward.

o R. Inhibition of arm swing. This is due to rigidity in the muscles mentioned above and the pause-driven inhibition of the movement-imagining area in the brain.

o R. Pain from tension and rigidity in the biceps muscle and/or pain from tension and rigidity at the front of the shoulder.

o R. Rigidity in the neck muscles that lie just under the Large Intestine channel. This tightness pulls the neck forward and also compresses the blood pressure-regulating carotid sinus, which lies just under these muscles.

o A. Lack of smile. Like the Stomach channel, the Large Intestine channel normally crosses over the lips and supplies energy and sensory perception to the lips, but on pause, it is absent.

o **A.** Diminished sense of smell. The healthy Large Intestine channel qi flows up the sides of the nose and helps regulate the sinuses and sense of smell. On pause, this channel qi is absent.

o **A.** Seborrhea along the side of the nose due to chronic absence of Large Intestine channel qi alongside the nose while on pause, causing reduced circulation and therefore reduced immune system access.

Unexpected illumination

So there I was, walking in the woods, mentally organizing all my patients' specific symptoms by location. When I suddenly saw a *map* of the symptoms of Parkinson's, I came to a standstill. I still recall the exact spot. I was on a section of the trail that traverses the north side of the hill. I was surrounded redwood trees and ferns, still dripping from the morning's rain. The glen was in deep shadow and utterly silent. I stood there, staring at my mental map.

My mind's eye was looking at a map of the Stomach channel and a map of the Large Intestine channel. The body has a dozen Primary channels plus eight other channels – but all the *physical* symptoms of Parkinson's were on just these two.

In my mind's eye, I could see that *most* of my patients' symptoms were located on just *one* of the channels: the Stomach channel. The few symptoms that were not on the Stomach channel were on the Large Intestine channel.

Again, patterns of rigidity or of numbness in specific areas will be set in motion if channel qi is flowing backwards or is missing, respectively. The channel qi flow patterns that I had already felt in my patients' Stomach channel qi explained *perfectly* their face, neck, torso, leg, and foot symptoms of idiopathic Parkinson's.

The backwards channel qi flow patterns on their arms' Large Intestine channels fit with the arm symptoms of Parkinson's, as well.

I hypothesized that, if a person has backwards-flowing and missing Stomach channel qi and backwards-flowing and missing LI channel qi in certain portions of these channels, his body would eventually *have* to have symptoms that look exactly like the symptoms of Parkinson's disease.

Suddenly, the idea arose that maybe I didn't *need* dead brain cells to explain the symptoms of Parkinson's. Maybe the weird, backwards and/or missing flow of these two channels could account for all the symptoms of PD!

Even so, I wasn't ready to take the radical step of completely ignoring the dead dopamine cells theory, even though that theory had *never* explained most of what doctors saw in people with Parkinson's.

As mentioned earlier, a dopamine insufficiency should cause *body-wide* poverty of movement (slowness or limp immobility), not limpness in a few specific spots on the feet and face. And I was to see, later on, when patients recovered, a short-term dopamine insufficiency for motor function makes a person *limp*, not rigid, so long as the person's thoughts are predominantly in parasympathetic mode.

I suddenly saw the symptoms of Parkinson's as a glaringly obvious expression of what was going on electrically. Neurotransmitters might or might not have anything to do with where the Stomach channel was running backwards or was missing. That might not matter at all. Instead, the Stomach channel's *electrical* behaviors – in and of themselves – would *necessarily* trigger the symptoms of Parkinson's. The *symptoms* of Parkinson's, regardless of the underlying cause, were primarily driven by the body's sub-dermal electrical system – not by neurotransmitters.

As an aside, in Chinese medical theory, it is recognized that neurotransmitter release is triggered by the flow pattern of channel qi at any given moment. The physical and structural systems in the body are driven primarily by the channel qi system, and not the other way round.

For an analogy, your computer is driven by the electrical behaviors on its hard drive. These behaviors then create images on the computer screen – not the other way round. The *images* on the computer monitor (the screen) don't determine the circuitry in the hard drive. Of course, if you *touch* the screen, the static on your finger might alter the electrical signals in the drive. But the pictures themselves do not inform the software: they are created by it. The electrical drivers of the body, your "software," your channel qi, direct the ever-changing chemical events and physiology in the body. [1]

My first few Parkinson's patients all had an injury at the foot/ankle end of the Stomach channel proper. When it healed, the Parkinson's went away. Clearly, there had been no dead dopamine-cell problem.

I concluded that not only could everyone with Parkinson's be cured by simply having their foot injuries fixed, but it even made logical sense! I was wrong, of course.

Turns out, there are several ways to get the Stomach channel qi running backwards. Also, the foot injury, in and of itself, hadn't actually been the problem. The root problem was that the person had mentally dissociated from the injury so that it locked down and never healed. *Or*, as I later learned, maybe the person was stuck on pause. Or using self-induced pause. Or using self-induced dissociation.

I didn't understand this at the time. I *did* understand that the hands-on healing modality that I was using worked by bringing a patient's attention to the site of an unhealed injury. I *didn't* realize that people can instead/also be stuck in pause mode, which could cause the same channel qi flow patterns that I was seeing in my patients with foot injuries.

The Stomach channel can run backwards in response to *lots* of triggers. I didn't know that, yet.

I was very uneasy with my new hypothesis about Parkinson's. I felt that I still had to address the famous "lack of dopamine." I didn't yet know that researchers in the upcoming years would discover that there *wasn't* a significant lack of dopamine, at least not when a person was first diagnosed. I hadn't yet read the research proclaiming that the dead dopamine cell theory had *already* been proven wrong.

So I kept pondering how this Stomach channel behavior could affect dopamine levels in the brain or maybe "kill" those dopamine-making cells.

I started observing what else was going on in my patient's other channels as the channel behaviors shifted and even reversed in response to recovery and partial recovery. I

[1] Dr. Michael Levin, footnoted earlier on p. 6 and p. 160, refers to the bioelectric networks (routes of channel qi) as "the software of life." These networks "make the decisions over large-scale systems." These networks determine which aspects of DNA will express, and how cells will behave. "All the systems in the body are embedded in a field of [electrical] information coming from all the other cells."

started observing the channel behaviors in *all* my patients, not just the ones with Parkinson's.

No channel theory in the schools

As mentioned earlier, this was a drastic departure from my training in school. Channel theory is illegal in China. This was reflected in the curriculum of all the schools in the USA when I was in school. No one, anywhere, was being taught channel theory in the schools, even though channel theory could still be dug up from the old classic books by using archaic translations instead of using the modern, government-approved translations.

In my case, I stumbled across channel theory on my own, partly because I've always been able to feel the currents of channel qi in other people and partly from my work with Parkinson's patients, where it was obvious to me that currents were running backwards, of all things. I had always assumed that everyone else felt these currents, as well. After I started telling colleagues that the Stomach channel was running backwards in my PD patients, my colleagues all asked, "How can you tell?" I didn't believe them, at first, when they all assured me they had never felt anything moving under the skin of their patients.

But I wasn't the only one talking about channel qi. The late, highly celebrated Dr Wang Ju-Yi, after he was safely in the United States, taught channel theory in post-graduate, continuing-education classes for acupuncturists. I was fortunate enough to meet several times with Dr. Wang in 2006. When we first met, my hope was that he could refer me to a school in China where I could go to learn more about this subject. He explained to me over lunches, with the brilliant and congenial Jason Robinson translating, that channel theory had long been illegal in China and there was no point in my going there. "You will no longer be sent to jail for espousing channel theory. But it doesn't matter because no one in China is even *interested* in channel theory anymore."

No dead dopamine cells?

People's recovery from PD in every case, no matter which type of PD they had, corresponded to the termination of the pause-type channel qi patterns and the resumption of the normal, healthy blend of parasympathetic and sympathetic mode patterns. Because of this, I gradually became certain that by exploring channel phenomena I would eventually come up with a fairly complete hypothesis of not *only* what was going on in people with Parkinson's but *also* why some of the electrical aberrations in the foot *might* also bring about brain changes. The brain changes included those that might be related to inhibition of dopamine release for motor function *and* inhibition of dopamine release for certain mental functions that are related to the Parkinson's personality.

By the way – I did not yet know that backwards-flowing Stomach channel qi was also characteristic of *pause* mode. I didn't discover that for almost fifteen years, while trying to figure out why so many patients got stuck in the weird behaviors of partial recovery.

I didn't even know that I was exploring a field of Chinese medicine that had a name: channel theory. I only understood this some years later, after meeting Dr.Wang. Then, going back over previously obscure translations of older Chinese books about medicine, I saw that so many of the "mystical" incomprehensible passages were simply references to channel theory and to the constantly changing, nearly infinite variations in human channel qi behaviors: the behaviors of *Se Mai*, the paths of "lightwave" energy, the paths of electrical energy. Also, colleagues whose native or learned Chinese language skills were vastly superior to my bumbling efforts generously assisted me in my research.

Even though I didn't yet know all this in those early days, as I stood in that fogged-in, silent, dripping redwood grove, looking at a mental picture of all the symptoms of Parkinson's disease sitting along the paths of only two channels, I felt that I might have stumbled across something to do with Parkinson's that ought to be shared. So share I did.

Sharing the information

Shortly after sharing this discovery with a few colleagues, I had my first article accepted by the *American Journal of Acupuncture*. From 1972 to 2002 this was the most widely read and respected peer-reviewed English language journal of Asian medicine in the world. It was the only journal in the field considered diligent enough to have its articles included in the USA's National Institutes of Health search engine. My lengthy hypothesis article was divided in two and published in the Fall issue of 1998 and Spring of 1999 (volumes 26 and 27).

The editor was brilliant and taught me so much. She told to me go slowly, cautiously, in spite of my excitement. She warned me, "If you have *one* error in your findings, if one of your footnotes or citations is incorrect, even if *all* the rest of it is verifiable, people will latch onto that one error and you'll never get respect in the field ever again. There is big money that doesn't want your hypothesis to get traction. You have to be able to support every single word that you publish."

At the same time, with much help and excited support from a few colleagues and a patient who was a lawyer and who knew about starting non-profits, we founded the Parkinson's Recovery Project, a non-profit organization dedicated to disseminating information about Parkinson's disease from an Asian medicine perspective. I started up a website, PDrecovery.org, to asked if other acupuncturists or physical therapists could replicate my results by doing Yin Tui Na on the foot and ankle injuries of people with Parkinson's disease.

As mentioned earlier, I *did* get feedback from acupuncturists – some saw their patients recover. Others got caught up in the nightmares and tragedies of working with patients who were taking anti-parkinson's medications. Others had patients who developed the symptoms of partial recovery.

Some days it seemed as if every new email sharing insights from a health practitioner or patient contributed to the daily roller coaster of hope and consternation and also brought new questions. Since that time, the research has continued pretty much non-stop, resulting in the information in this book in the year 2020 *and* the realization that most people with Parkinson's, given enough information, don't need to work with a health practitioner at all. Most acupuncturists and physical therapists have not studied enough in this obscure field of channel theory to begin understand the forces at play in people with the various types of Parkinson's disease. If you've read this far in this book, you already know way more about channel theory than most acupuncturists in China or in the west.

But that's OK. For most people with PD, recovery is pretty much a do-it-yourself or a do-it (do Yin Tui Na)-with-a-friend proposition.

Beginning the process of diagnosis

This chapter serves as a starting point for self-diagnosis. If you think you might have Parkinson's disease, go back through the list of symptoms and see how many of these symptoms you have. If you have even a few of the symptoms that are located along the Stomach and/or Large Intestine channels, even if they are mild, you might very well have early stage idiopathic Parkinson's disease.

Then again, if all your symptoms are clustered at just *one* place on the Stomach or Large Intestine channels, and *especially* if that location corresponds to a recent injury or surgery, you might not have Parkinson's. If all of your symptoms are located somewhere *other* than the Stomach and/or Large Intestine channel, and you *don't* have symptoms on the Stomach and Large Intestine channels, then you very likely do *not* have Parkinson's, despite what your MD might have told you.

The diagnosis process will be explained in greater detail in the next chapter. For now, having read this chapter might help you start thinking about and paying more attention to exactly what is going on in your body and *where*.

Chapter Fifteen

Diagnosing Parkinson's Disease

This chapter explains how to make an accurate diagnosis of idiopathic Parkinson's disease. Before figuring out what *type* of Parkinson's disease a person has, it is important to determine whether or not a person actually does have Parkinson's. After confirming that the person in question *does* have Parkinson's, the *next* two chapters will help determine what *type* of Parkinson's it is.

A western diagnosis of Parkinson's: the four traits

Western doctors are trained to look for four "cardinal" (main) physical traits in order to make a diagnosis of Parkinson's disease. The four traits are: poverty of movement (diminished speed and power, and difficulty initiating movement), rigidity, tremor, and postural instability.

To merit a diagnosis of Parkinson's disease, a person must present with symptoms in three of the four cardinal traits. If a person has symptoms in only two of the four traits, he might still be diagnosed with Parkinson's so long as postural instability is not one of the two *and* he has more than one location for the two traits. For example, if he has rigidity in two parts of his body and slowness and/or weakness in two aspects of his movement but no tremor, he can still receive a diagnosis of Parkinson's disease.

Although the general public often thinks of tremor as the primary or definitive symptom of Parkinson's, many people with Parkinson's do *not* have a tremor, but do have rigidity and poverty of movement. And many people who *do* have tremor do not have Parkinson's disease.

The four traits

1) Poverty of movement, sometimes called "bradykinesia":

The term poverty of movement includes symptoms such as slowness, weakness and atrophy, the difficulty or even inability to *initiate* movement, such as going from not moving to moving, lifting the foot off the floor, getting up off a chair, or raising the lips in a smile. The term poverty of movement can also include soft voice, small, cramped handwriting referred to as micrographia, and constipation that does not respond to laxatives.

From the days of James Parkinson's 1817 treatise on what he called the "the shaking palsy" all the way up to the beginning of the twenty-first century, the phrase "poverty of movement" has been used to describe the many physical inhibitions of Parkinson's.

Starting around the beginning of the twenty-first century, the term bradykinesia is sometimes used in place of "poverty of movement." Bradykinesia literally means *slowness* of movement. It only refers to reduced *speed* of motor function.

No doubt some person who didn't understand why the more descriptive phrase "poverty of movement" was originally used got his doctoral degree or at least got an article published when he offered the argument that the word "bradykinesia" was more modern or more technical or more derived from Greek, and therefore better. Call me a stickler, but I continue to use the broader and more *accurate* term "poverty of movement."

The term "akinesia," which means literally "without *any* movement" is even newer and hotter in the Parkinson's world – and even more inaccurate – than the term bradykinesia. Some doctors now refer to people with significant poverty of movement as having the less accurate term "akinetic Parkinson's."

Akinetic PD means the same thing as Parkinson's or idiopathic Parkinson's, but the focus is on the poverty of movement aspect. A person who obviously has PD but who doesn't have tremor or for whom tremor is only a mild symptom might be diagnosed with "akinetic Parkinson's" even though he *can* move, albeit slowly. The drug treatment and expectations for "akinetic Parkinson's" are the same as for idiopathic Parkinson's because, despite the different *name*, it's the exact same syndrome.

2) Rigidity: This trait, also referred to as stiffness or tightness, is usually assessed based on rotating the patient's wrist while feeling for cogwheeling or "ratcheting" as opposed to a healthy, fluid, circular movement in the wrist rotation.

3) Tremor: The tremor of Parkinson's is usually a "resting" tremor. A resting tremor kicks in when the affected body part is *not* being used: when the body part is resting.

At least in a patient's *early* years with tremor, the tremor might cease while the affected body part is being actively used. Many people with PD first notice a come-and-go resting tremor in the index finger. The index finger taps against the thumb, in a motion referred to as "pill rolling." Eventually, the tremor might be active in a body part even when that body part *is* moving. Also, although the pill-rolling motion is the most common place for the tremor to begin, it *might* start elsewhere. Also, no matter where it *starts*, within a few years or a few decades *all* the limbs and even the chin might tremor.

Even when the initial tremor is located in an area other than the index finger, it's behavior will be similar to that of the index-finger tremor. The tremor is rhythmic, it occurs in areas with subtle muscle atrophy, and at least in the beginning, it is a gentle, come-and-go *resting* tremor. Over time, the tremor can increase in duration and intensity. It might momentarily worsen even further in response to fear or even anticipation of stress. The resting tremor does not require that the entire body be at rest – only the muscle group in question. For example, people whose PD tremor begins in the *leg* might first have noticed it when standing up in front of a group to deliver a talk or read a paper. The person is being active, in a sense, but the *walking* muscles are *not* being used: the walking function of the legs is "at rest."

The people I've seen whose tremors first appeared in their legs have had hip injuries or other problems such as scar tissue causing blockages on their *Gallbladder* channels in *addition* to having blockages on their Stomach channels and/or being on pause. The injury can be treated with Yin Tui Na, the scarring with acupuncture.

4) Postural instability: poor balance, including falling or walking backwards. Walking backwards when trying to get the body to walk forwards is usually a symptom of fairly *advanced* PD. However, frequent falls, often attributed to "clumsiness" can be an *early* symptom of Parkinson's.

People with PD cannot move *quickly* enough to make the countless subtle balancing corrections in posture that healthy people make with every step or torso movement. This increasing inability to balance in a timely fashion can lead to increasingly frequent falls and stumbles. Also, people with Parkinson's are somatically detached from their physical movements: this means a person might *think* he is moving his leg the necessary distance, when in fact the leg might be moving much less.

The falling associated with Parkinson's can also include "festinating gait." This occurs when the leg stride suddenly begins decreasing in length in mid-stride but the person, who is still walking, has enough forward momentum that his torso keeps going forward even though his legs are taking tinier and tinier steps. Eventually, his torso, and his center of gravity, have moved so far forward relative to his legs that he falls forward onto his face. If his arm movements are slow and/or rigid, he cannot use his arms to protect his face during his fall.

Most people with *early* stage Parkinson's do *not* experience festinating gait. Oppositely, the falls from losing balance and the foot shuffling due to failure to fully lift the foot off the floor while taking steps might appear early on, maybe even *before* an official diagnosis of Parkinson's.

Another aspect of "postural instability" can be the light-headedness that a person with low blood pressure might experience when going from a sitting to a standing position. People with Parkinson's often have low blood pressure. If they stand up too abruptly they might experience a "head rush" (light-headedness) and lose their balance.

The characteristic "look" of Parkinson's disease

Some experienced doctors are also on the lookout for what is called the "Parkinson's look" in posture and/or face in order to back up a diagnosis of Parkinson's disease. The *postural* "look" might include a tendency to hold the head forward with the shoulders slightly raised, causing the bottom of the ear lobes to be closer to the *front* of the shoulders. The bones of the neck might eventually develop a reverse curve. The shoulders might be pulled slightly *forward*, as well as being slightly raised. The person might be slightly bent forward at the waist. The arms might tend to stay crooked at the elbows instead of hanging limply at the side. These are all aspects of a modified fetal position: the pause position.

The *facial* "look" of PD is sometimes called an expressionless or "masked" face. The expressionless mask might temporarily drop away if the person is making a conscious effort to smile. The masked face can include a failure of the cheek muscles to rise, thus failing to lift the corners of the mouth and/or failure of the upper lip to lift while trying to make a smile.

When diagnosing, some doctors *don't* consider whether or not a person has any aspects of the "look." And some patients are able to temporarily hide or override the symptoms that contribute to the look while in the doctor's office, when a higher level of emergency behavior – more norepinephrine – kicks in.

The "look" in and of itself does *not* constitute a basis for a diagnosis of Parkinson's. For example, a person with severe depression who does *not* have Parkinson's might present with slumped shoulders, hunched posture and expressionless face. And some people with PD (usually Type II or III) *never* develop a severe facial "look." Then again, for some people with Parkinson's, loss of smile might be one of the first symptoms

– although a person is unlikely to see a neurologist just because people around him are increasingly telling him to "Smile more!"

In addition to the four cardinal traits and the look, a doctor might have been taught to look for lack of arm swing or lack of coordinated arm swing/ stride. Even if a patient is *able* to consciously generate an arm swing, the arm swing might stop as soon as the patient stops concentrating on it. Also, the patient might have a hard time coordinating the left-side arm swing with the right-side leg stride, and vice versa.

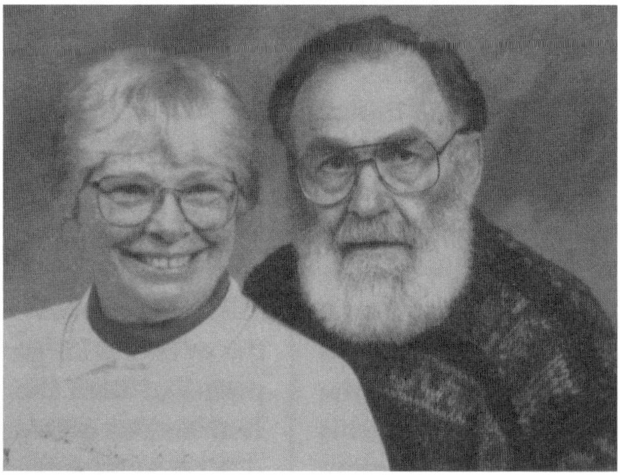

Fig. 15.1. The man in this photo, diagnosed with idiopathic Parkinson's twenty years earlier, was beaming as brightly as possible in this portrait that they took for their annual Christmas card.

In addition to the long grooves running from his nose to the sides of his mouth, his head is pulled forward, bringing his earlobes to a position in front of his shoulders.

He was a retired Lutheran minister. When he was diagnosed with PD, his parents were relieved: when his previously radiant smile had disappeared a few years earlier, his parents assumed that he had lost his faith. When they learned that his flat, expressionless look was "merely" Parkinson's, they were relieved.

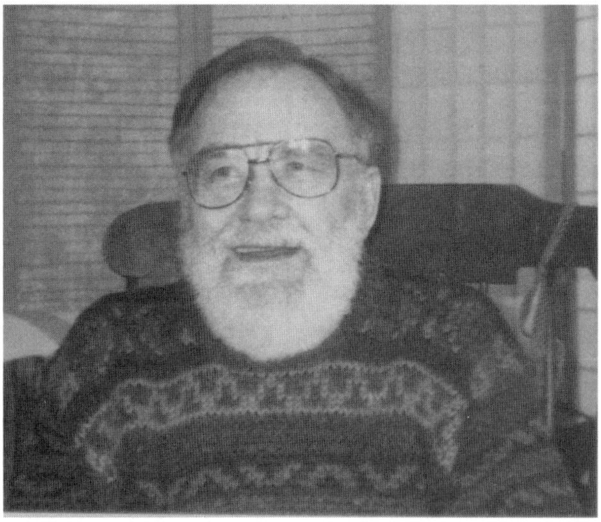

Fig. 15.2 In this photo taken three years later, after recovering from Parkinson's, the muscles in his cheeks bulge out when he smiles. The corners of his mouth move upward during smiling, more on the right than on the left. His right lower eyelid is no longer sagging. His neck is straighter, so that his earlobes are positioned higher and farther back relative to the tops of his shoulders.
(Photos used with permission.)

A few other things a doctor might look for

An MD might also consider the patient's soft voice or, if the patient mentions it, episodes of "spontaneous" choking. In the previous chapter, the symptoms marked off by a hollow bullet are symptoms that are recognized by MDs as being associated with

Parkinson's disease. However, most of these symptoms are *not* usually used to make the original diagnosis. The diagnosis is made on *generalities* about the four cardinal traits. Once the diagnosis is made, then if/when a patient mentions some of the hollow-bulleted symptoms, the doctor can say, "Oh yes, that symptom sometimes shows up in people with Parkinson's.

No test

There is no medical test - no lab test or brain scan test – for Parkinson's disease.

In the late 1990s, doctors hoped that the new brain scans such as PET and functional SPECT scans would be able to confirm or deny a diagnosis of Parkinson's. These scans show the uptake of radioactive dopamine. The thinking was that people with Parkinson's would have less dopamine uptake because dopamine-using cells were supposedly dead.

For diagnosing PD, however, the scans' potential didn't pan out. Many patients whose doctors were certain they had PD showed normal levels of dopamine uptake. Other people who were perfectly healthy showed dopamine uptake behaviors in the brain that appeared to be deficient. There was *no* consistent correlation between a brain scan observation of dopamine uptake and a person's physical symptoms of Parkinson's.

In 2011, DaTscan was approved for diagnostic testing. This is a type of SPECT scan: a scan in which a radioactive tracer is injected into the bloodstream and makes its way into the brain. In the brain, the tracer molecules indicate the level of dopamine *transporter* molecules that are active at a given moment. In syndromes such as PD, multiple-system atrophy, para-supra-nuclear palsy and other situations, including coma of extended duration, *fewer* transporter molecules appear active in the vicinity of the striatum. However, this test does not confirm or deny a diagnosis of Parkinson's disease, per se. It only shows if there's a pathological shift in the number of dopamine transport molecules being released in the brain. In a person with Parkinson's, the transporter molecules have probably been present at a greatly reduced level for decades, since whenever the channel qi started running in the pause patterns. Release of transporter molecules is *supposed* to decrease when a person is on pause.

If a person with some PD-like symptoms tells you, "I was given the medical tests for Parkinson's and I don't have it" or oppositely "...and I *do* have it," either he doesn't understand that there is no such thing as a definitive test for PD or he was misled by his doctor. A doctor's diagnosis of Parkinson's is an *opinion*. There is no *objective* test.

Obviously not Parkinson's disease

Many a person with only stiffness, or with just tremor, has shown up at the doctor's door fearful that he has Parkinson's, when it is obvious to any experienced diagnostician that the person does *not* have PD.

Tremors in particular are associated in the public mind with Parkinson's disease. But tremor can be caused by many *non*-PD health problems, or by medications, or can have a genetic component (familial tremor).

Most neurologists are trained to be on the lookout for very specific symptoms, such as a pill rolling resting tremor, cogwheeling in the wrists, motor slowness and/or a weak voice. However, because many of these symptoms can be a part of other, non-

Parkinson's syndromes, doctors can disagree with each other on whether or not a given person actually has Parkinson's disease.

As mentioned earlier in this book, the Elldopa study used six Parkinson's specialists to vet each person used in the study, and ended up having so little unanimity of diagnosis that they finally agreed to use in the study those people for whom *half* the specialists gave a diagnosis of PD.

Vagueness of the four cardinal traits

As any neurologist knows, many syndromes (collection of symptoms) have at least two of the four traits and are *clearly* not Parkinson's disease. For example, many people who have had a stroke have both rigidity and poverty of movement but do *not* have Parkinson's disease. Brain changes from stroke *can* usually be observed with a brain scan. When a neurologist orders a brain scan, it is to rule out stroke or tumor, not to confirm PD. Some people with heart disease have a tremor and poor balance. They do not necessarily have Parkinson's disease.

Also, many people with Parkinson's disease do *not* have tremor. Depending on what literature you read, the percentage of people with PD who do *no*t have tremor ranges from fifteen to thirty five percent.

Again, no two people with PD develop the same symptoms or develop them in the same sequence. These ambiguities and lack of an objective test can make it hard for a doctor, working from a mere book description, to make a certain diagnosis of PD until the condition has become somewhat advanced.

What doctors might easily miss

1) Other *locations* of rigidity: although doctors are trained to look primarily for "cogwheeling" in the wrist, even if that cogwheeling is not yet obvious rigidity might already be present in an inability to turn the neck from side to side, in chest oppression due to rigidity in certain chest muscles, and tightness in *specific* arm and leg muscles.

2) Tremor: Some MDs who are not neurologists or PD specialists might think that the tremor of Parkinson's is *only* the index finger / thumb tremor. This is not correct. Although the tremor of PD *might* start in the index finger, it might also start in other fingers, or in the arm, leg, foot, hip, or even chin. Eventually, it might manifest in *all* these areas.

3) Difficulty in initiating movement and poverty of movement: some patients, when asked about difficulty in initiating movement, might tell the doctor they don't have this problem. They say this because they have come up with tricks that enable them to "get started."

For example, a person might have cleverly taught himself to slap himself hard on his leg, creating a fleeting moment of pain and "emergency" behavior, every time he needs to stand up from a sitting position. Because he has taught himself this trick, he will proudly tell the MD that he has no difficulty initiating movement.

In the same vein, a person with Parkinson's who has difficulty in getting up from a chair might nevertheless tell his doctor that he has no movement problem because he *can* easily go up stairs, maybe even taking the stairs two at a time. Going up stairs activates a short-term release of emergency mode behavior in most people with PD, so most people with PD who have trouble traversing a doorway without slowing down or even stopping might still be able to take the stairs two at a time. Because he can take stairs two at a time, a patient, thinking of his "superior stair climbing ability" and ignoring his flat-floor shuffle or difficulty in getting up from a chair, will tell the MD that he has no movement problems. This is why it's usually a good idea for the spouse or close friend, if any, who *has* seen the full spectrum of movement problems at home, to accompany the patient to the doctor's office.

I am reminded of a non-PD patient whose tongue, pulse, and other Chinese medicine diagnostic measures suggested that the patient was constipated. At every session, he was asked, "Are you constipated?" He forcefully replied no. After half a dozen sessions, when asked yet again if he was constipated, he burst out, "Why do you always ask that? With all the laxatives I take every day, there's *no way* I could be constipated!" *Without* the laxatives, he was severely, painfully constipated, but he didn't think he needed to admit this to a doctor because he'd found a workaround for it.

In the same way, many people with PD answer their MDs' questions with answers that are speciously, technically, correct, but not helpful to the doctor who is trying to make a diagnosis.

These communication problems can arise for several reasons: the reluctant patient doesn't actually *want* to be sharing with the doctor but the *spouse* made the appointment anyway; PD symptoms might be minimized at the doctor's office because the stress of being "examined" or "judged" causes the norepinephrine override to kick in temporarily, masking many of the motor symptoms; or the patient is trying to avoid a dire diagnosis so he is intentionally not forthcoming, or is even misleading, about his symptoms.

These situations can lead to an MD having to ask extra questions but even then getting only half-truth answers.

Because there is no lab test for PD, doctors can only make diagnoses based on what they see and what their patients tell them. The doctor is not trained as a psychic. If the patient is not forthcoming, the doctor cannot not know what all the symptoms actually are and might miss some key diagnostic points.

Symmetry is possible

Some people with PD have symptoms that are symmetrical, the same on the left side and the right side. One patient that I saw had the poverty of movement and rigidity symptoms of advancing Parkinson's and his neurologist had correctly given him a diagnosis of PD even though he had *no* tremor and his symptoms were perfectly symmetrical.

The patient and I figured out that his PD was due to symmetrical foot injuries. He had been working at a construction site twenty years earlier when the support under him fell away. He fell three stories and landed on both feet. His supervisor came up to him and said, "If you report this as a worker's comp injury, you're fired."

Both feet and both ankles had been equally compressed and broken. His symptoms were completely symmetrical. He had the classic "look" of Parkinson's – with no tremor. He had Type II PD – it was from unhealed injuries and the injuries were *symmetrical*.

I recently got an email from another person with PD who had symmetrical injuries and no tremor: burns on both ankles. He emailed me to say he had recovered, and mentioned his injury symmetry/ no tremor situation.

If someone is looking to do more research on the relationship between injury symmetry and no tremor in idiopathic PD, this might be a fruitful avenue for further inquiry.

Variability: another factor

In most people with idiopathic Parkinson's, the symptoms vary: they ebb and flow, usually depending on mood, activity, *anticipation* of feeling good or bad, or maybe even depending on time of day. Symptoms might be worse when stressed or anxious, and decrease a bit when relaxed or on vacation.

Oppositely, symptoms of stroke or other types of brain damage might cause rigidity and/or poverty of movement *but* these symptoms are *not* variable, nor are they expectation dependent. Symptoms of stroke appear suddenly. Symptoms of PD might appear gradually, over years, but on any given day their *severity* might fluctuate from one minute to the next and certainly will vary over the course of the day.

If one or more of the symptoms that you noted while doing your assessment vary over the course of the day, that increases the likelihood that you have Parkinson's disease.

The brain spin

One symptom not yet mentioned might occur, usually just once or a few times, decades prior to the onset of Parkinson's disease. Not everyone has this symptom, but if you recall something of this sort, it can add further weight to a diagnosis of Parkinson's.

What I call "the brain spin" is a situation in which you suddenly find yourself perceiving everything around you shaking or spinning violently. You might need to grab at a passing refrigerator or doorway to keep from falling. It can feel as if the *inside* of your head was taken over by a whirlwind. There might even be a sense of briefly blacking out.

In my own case, I was seventeen years old, in excellent health, had recently induced pause in myself, and was walking across the laundry room. The room spun around violently. A roaring sound filled my head. I grabbed the sides of the washing machine and clung for dear life. A moment later, I was fine, but the experience was absolutely unforgettable.

I suspect this event occurs when the Stomach channel qi that builds up at ST-8 on the forehead finally breaks through its normal pathway and short circuits into the nearby Gallbladder channel. If this short circuit only occurs on one side of the body, the SSFA, the powerful asymmetry introduced into the brain system might be able to create the sensation of spinning inside the head – which is exactly what it felt like, to me and to many others.

Many of my patients remember one or a few fleeting incidents like this. There are variations, of course. One middle-aged PD patient remembers that, around age twenty, he had several incidents. Each time was immediately preceded by a metallic taste in his mouth. It was "a dizzy sensation…like my mind/spirit/soul was trying to float out of my body. It lasted about 15 seconds and sometimes felt as if it came in waves. It happened about three times over a period of six months."

The metallic taste in the mouth can be set in motion by the Stomach channel flowing backwards. Some people get the same strange taste in the mouth when the Stomach channel runs backwards just before vomiting. The feeling of "leaving the body" is most often set in motion by a blockage at the back of the neck, one that blocks the upward flowing Du channel and the downward flowing UB channels. All of these channel behaviors can occur during pause, or when the backwards-flowing current from an injury (pseudo pause) finally builds up enough momentum to set these pause-mode type channel qi variations in motion.

Another older patient, back in his early twenties, had been riding his bicycle along a country road when his brain spun and he felt as if he'd lost consciousness momentarily. When his mind cleared, he was a *considerable* distance farther down the road, with no clear memory of how he got there. He had never told anyone about the highly memorable episode. To himself, he had always jokingly referred to it as "my abduction by aliens."

None of my patients had ever told anyone else about their weird brain spin moments when the brain or the consciousness seemed to become briefly "unhinged."

If you recall such an event, even though it was years or decades earlier than the appearance of your overt symptoms of Parkinson's, it might help lend even more certainty to your diagnosis of PD.

Feeling the channels: the acid test

To really cement your diagnosis, have a friend learn to feel channel qi. The free, downloadable first chapter of *Tracking the Dragon* teaches how to do this. Most people can start to feel these currents over the course of an all-day workshop. On average, people can become very good at detecting even subtle patterns of channel qi flow after about twenty hours of practice. Many of my acupuncture students have been able to notice channel qi flow patterns in just a few hours although they tend to not trust what they are feeling until they've been practicing it over the course of several weeks.

If a person has Parkinson's, even if the symptoms are still very mild and intermittent, the Stomach channel on the upper and lower legs will either be flowing backwards, rapidly moving back and forth, or be imperceptible. All these manifestations of aberrant channel qi flow are considered variants of "flowing backwards." The Stomach channel qi flow over the face might be missing on at least one side of the face, on the side where symptoms first appeared. Stomach channel qi will be missing from ST-42, on the center top of the foot, down to the second and third toes. These channel qi patterns can be present in people with pre-Parkinson's even if the PD *symptoms* are still in the very early stage *or* if there are not yet *any* MD-recognized PD symptoms.

The Ren channel might be hard to detect, but that can happen in response to a person being nervous about the results of the channel qi test, so you can ignore the Ren channel behavior in terms of diagnosis. On the other hand, *if* the Ren channel is flowing perfectly normally all the way up to the lower lip, you can certainly rule out Type I and Type IV Parkinson's disease, though one of the other two types might be present.

Finally, in *most* people with Parkinson's, the Du channel will *probably* be standing still or moving rapidly back and forth. Even if the *torso* portion of the Du can be visualized by the patient as flowing or can be felt flowing by a friend, it will want to stop at the base of the neck, just above Du-14. In *most* cases of Parkinson's, the Du channel will *not* flow up into the neck and head unless the patient is working to force it to temporarily do so.

Exceptions to the above Du channel variations might occur in the five or six percent of people with Parkinson's who have *only* Type II or *only* Type III PD. If a person has the requisite number of physical symptoms of Parkinson's to qualify for a diagnosis of PD and has backwards-flowing Stomach channel qi *but* has *normal* flow in the Du channel, his symptoms of Parkinson's are probably due to an unhealed injury, surgery, or scarring (scar tissue is non-conductive), creating a blockage along the path of the Stomach channel. This is discussed in depth in chapter seventeen.

Ruling out drug- and toxin-induced parkinsonism

In Parkinson's disease, the channel qi flows in the pause mode patterns. In drug- and/or toxin-induced parkinsonism, it does not. It is possible to have *both* idiopathic Parkinson's and drug- or toxin-induced parkinsonism. In this case, the person's channels *will* be running in the pause patterns.

Most people with idiopathic Parkinson's disease have symptoms that vary *noticeably* in intensity throughout the day, or even come and go. Symptoms might appear or might intensify when doing activities in which a person feels he is being judged or observed: for example, symptoms might be much worse during public speaking or eating in public. Oppositely, symptoms might decrease significantly or even temporarily stop while on vacation. They might ease off altogether when singing, dancing, or doing something deemed "good." Symptoms might diminish momentarily when performing some activity that creates a brief burst of "emergency behavior," such as going up stairs.

Notice whether or not the symptoms in your case vary depending on mood or activity. If they do *not* vary, if the symptoms are fairly *steady* and *consistent* over the course of a given day, even though increasing in severity over the months and years, the problem is unlikely to be PD. The problem *might* be one of brain damage: parkinsonism from drugs or toxins – or possibly a stroke, multiple system atrophy, parasupranuclear palsy, or some other syndrome... but *not* idiopathic Parkinson's. If the symptoms appeared practically overnight following exposure to drugs or toxins, the likelihood is very good that the problem is drug- or toxin-induced parkinsonism – not Parkinson's disease. However, the opposite does not hold: a person *might* develop drug- and toxin-induced parkinsonism years, even decades, following exposure.

Many of the commonly prescribed drugs for depression and anxiety, as well as street drugs such as methamphetamine, can cause "tardive" (delayed onset) parkinsonism many years after exposure to the drug, even if the drug use was of short duration and/or ceased many years earlier. The dopamine-enhancing antiparkinson's drugs have also been shown to cause tardive, drug-induced parkinsonism. If you read carefully the list of adverse effects on either the thin-paper warning that comes with many drugs *or* on the internet when doing a search for "adverse effects" plus the name of your drug, you will read that tardive tremor and other tardive symptoms of parkinsonism can be adverse effects for many mood-altering drugs, including dopamine-enhancing antiparkinson's medications.

If symptoms vary based on thoughts, moods, or time of day, even if not to a large degree, the person might have any of the four types of Parkinson's disease. The *more* one's symptoms *vary* depending on mood and circumstance, the *more* likely it is that the person has Type I PD.

If *variations* in the appearance or intensity of symptoms occur during the course of a day or over a few days, the person probably does *not* have *only* drug- or toxin-induced parkinsonism, with emphasis on the word "only." But if he has a history of drug or toxin exposure and his symptoms are variable, there's always the possibility that he *might* have *both* parkinsonism and Parkinson's disease.

In very early stage idiopathic Parkinson's, one's symptoms might be very insignificant, and *quite* variable - even going away for hours or days at a time. While at this early stage, many patients have told me something like "It's OK with me if I don't recover from Parkinson's: my symptoms are so mild." or "…are so intermittent." These people don't understand that nearly everyone with PD starts out with fairly mild symptoms. However, if a person does *not* recover, the symptoms *will* worsen over time, and eventually can become quite severe, especially during times of physical, mental, or emotional stress. At some point, the severity of the symptoms can itself become a major source of emotional stress, so that a spiraling worsening of symptoms kicks in. Even so, in these cases a person still might notice that symptoms diminish when he goes on vacation, when loved ones come to visit, or when he relaxes at the end of the day.

Noticing whether or not a person has significant, mood- and emotion-based variations in symptoms is primarily used to rule out cases of *only* drug- and toxin-induced parkinsonism. Again, a person might have both idiopathic PD *and* parkinsonism.

As a side note, if a person is taking antiparkinson's medications, his present observations of daily symptom variations will be pretty much worthless in terms of diagnostics. If he wants to determine if he actually had PD prior to starting the medications, he will have to try to remember if his symptoms had mood- or situation-based variations before he ever started taking the drugs. *Since* starting the drugs, he probably has drug-induced parkinsonism. The symptoms might now be quite variable over the course of the day, but that might well be a response to the timing of the dosages.

Some examples of drugs and toxins that can cause parkinsonism

Methamphetamine is one of the drugs that can cause brain damage with just a few usages, leaving in its wake brain damage that can cause symptoms of drug-induced parkinsonism many years, or even many decades, later. For example, American pilots during WWII were required to take methamphetamine so that they could stay awake for super-human durations. An MD friend of mine who works with American military veterans told me that, prior to the 1990s, the vets he worked with had Parkinson's disease in the same low per-capita numbers that are typical for aging Americans. However, as the WWII ex-pilots in his care approached their 70s, nearly *all* of them developed tremors and other symptoms of parkinsonism. He learned from them that pilots had been required to take methamphetamine in order to stay awake during their extended flight hours during the war. Their brain damage didn't show up until nearly fifty years later.

Agent Orange, a defoliant used in the Vietnam War, has been officially recognized by the Veterans Administration (VA) as causing tardive Parkinson's disease. It doesn't, actually. It causes tardive toxin-induced parkinsonism.

At present, the treatments for idiopathic PD and toxin-induced parkinsonsism are exactly the same (dopamine-enhancing drugs), so it doesn't matter what the VA calls it, according to the MDs that prescribe for it. But when doctors begin to accept that idiopathic Parkinson's disease is a treatable condition, doctors will need to become more discerning, differentiating between idiopathic PD and toxin-induced parkinsonism.

Psychogenetic parkinsonism

Mention must be made of another type of parkinsonism: psychogenetic. Some people, in response to a terrific shock such as the unexpected death of a loved one, will suddenly manifest all the symptoms of moderately advanced Parkinson's disease: rigidity, faint voice, poverty of movement, and even tremor. In these cases, the person's physiology has lurched into a high degree of pause mode. This is physiologically appropriate if the person is highly traumatized. If he/she feels so physically destabilized that the body responds as if it's hovering on the verge of imminent death, he/she might immediately or within a few days show symptoms of pause. *However...* unlike people with idiopathic Parkinson's, the person with *obvious* symptoms of pause from psychogenic parkinsonism is *not* using a norepinephrine override. If there's no override, the symptoms of pause from physical or emotional trauma will be *immediately* obvious.

Because these symptoms resemble those of Parkinson's but eventually clear up on their own, over a few days or a few months, this syndrome is called "psychogenic" Parkinson's – a gentle way of expressing the sneering medical opinion that "If it goes away, then it wasn't really Parkinson's: it was just caused by your imagination," or even, "it was all an act."

The fact is, *most* cases of idiopathic Parkinson's start in the mind and are the result of a decision. They are truly "psychogenic."

Self-induced, Type I PD, the most common type, is the result of a person deciding – often for very good reason – that he was safer or better off if he commanded himself to be numb, thus causing himself to behave as if he were on the verge of imminent death or dealing with a severe emotional shock. In these cases, the symptoms of pause *don't* show up right away because the immobility of pause has been countered with a forceful mental command that activates the norepinephrine override: a purely *psychological* effort, an example of "mind over matter."

Ironically, what MDs call psychogenic parkinsonism is a form of Parkinson's that is *not* psychologically induced. It is related to Type IV PD, genuine biological pause mode: a biological, *automatic* response to a body-destabilizing, life-threatening trauma.

The only difference between Type IV PD and so-called "psychogenic parkinsonism" is that Type IV *doesn't* clear up on its own. Type IV PD, like the other three types of PD, is considered "real" rather than psychogenic because it *fails* to clear up on its own. Ironically, if a patient's case of pause mode *does* clear up on its own, as pause is *supposed* to do when the risk of imminent death has passed, it is dismissed as "psychogentic parkinsonism" and the patient is considered to be a mental case.

In Type IV PD, the person had been using a powerful norepinephrine override to keep going. His symptoms of PD only show up when that override begins to lag.

Again, psychogenic parkinsonism is triggered by a severe shock or trauma that is *not* modified with a norepinephrine override: hence the immediate, obvious, symptoms of pause mode.

Diagnosing yourself

Start by going through the list of symptoms in the previous chapter. I suggest you go through this list with a friend or spouse.

Many patients have assured me that they don't have a given symptom such as soft voice or reduced facial-muscle tone only to be contradicted by the accompanying spouse who says, "Oh yes you do!"

For example, many patients have told me that their co-workers are always ignoring them or seem to be hard of hearing. The spouse will interject, "*They* can hear just fine. *You* never speak up, that's why everyone keeps asking, 'What did you say?' "

A person might not be aware that he has a scowl on his face because every time he looks in a mirror, he might make a special, temporary effort to smile.

Many patients have told me that they probably have drug- or toxin-induced parkinsonism and don't want to work on recovering because of something along the lines of "I did a lot of painting/varnishing when I was younger" or "I worked with solvents." In response, the spouse has usually interjected, "No way. You are *classic* Type I Parkinson's!"

When in doubt, believe the spouse or the friend. They are often better observers than the patient.

Make a personalized list of your exact symptoms.

After you have check-marked any symptoms in chapter fourteen that seem familiar, put the check-marked symptoms on a list.

Then add details. Be very specific. For example, if you have trouble holding a spoon in your *right* hand, write that on your list. If you dribble food and/or liquids down the middle of your shirt, write it down. Include on your list the situations that seem to make your symptoms lessen or worsen. Include any of your emotional and mental behaviors that might be significant, or that might seem a bit outside the usual. The goal here is to make as complete a picture of your very own case as you possibly can.

This list might become *very* important when you start to recover.

Down the road, your doctor and your family and friends will very likely be focused on one or two of your most *visible* symptoms, usually tremor and something like a dragging foot or bent arm. They will refuse to even consider that some of your symptoms are diminishing and that ten or twenty of your symptoms are completely gone, because 1) they will be looking at the one or two things that aren't fully healed and 2) they never noticed or knew about *most* of your symptoms – including how you actually felt or weren't able to feel on the inside.

Your list will help you deal with their negativity during your recovery. During recovery, doubt can be a *powerful* force. Doubt stimulates the sides of the brain and diminishes the flow of energy through the center of the brain: reduces dopamine levels for motor function. It's a spiraling pattern that you don't need when you are working on changing your own mental habits.

If you have a thorough list of your own PD symptoms and you are able to start crossing some of them off as well as adding new items such as "I can feel my toes, and I didn't even know they were numb!" this can be a powerful emotional support for you and for the new brain habits of positive thinking that you are working on developing.

People will *not* notice that you feel lighter inside, that you are turning over more easily in bed, have a returning sense of smell, or that you are newly aware of sensations in your toes. They will *not* think it significant that you smile more easily: they will just assume you are in a better mood – finally – and this is something that they do *not* think has *anything* to do with Parkinson's.

Not only might your doctor, friends, and family unwittingly push you into a negative mindset with their comments such as, "Well, you still drag your foot, so you're obviously *not* getting better," but you yourself, your own mind, will be constantly attracted to the comfortable familiarity of saying, "I'm not recovering: I'm just kidding myself."

A person can develop a powerful mental habit of doubt during the years of being on pause. Even after pause turns off, the mental *habits* of pause, the reinforced *brain wiring* you've created that supports negative thinking, might still be well established. Months, maybe years of retraining might be needed before your brain habits are firmly rerouted into something closer to the range of normal positive attitudes. During recovery, doubting that the recovery is real is very common, due to the long-running mental habit of being negative and skeptical.

Your list will be an ally. Even if you are still dragging your left foot, you will see that you have crossed off a dozen or so symptoms, sensations, or lack of sensations that were being caused by being on pause. These small recovery symptoms can help keep up your positive attitude which, in turn, will help increase your dopamine load and hasten other recovery symptoms.

Make your list as complete and detailed as you possibly can.

Do you have Parkinson's disease?

Assessment time

Using your list, see if you have at least three of the rigidity symptoms described in chapter fourteen and if they are in *different* parts of the body. See if you have two, or better yet three, of the poverty of movement symptoms in chapter fourteen, also in different parts of the body. Note if you have symptoms in three of the four cardinal traits, or at least symptoms in two categories in multiple locations even if you don't have postural instability.

Expanding on the above

If you have difficulty in turning your head easily to the side, feel constriction in the chest when holding your arms up for more than a few seconds, and the muscles on the sides of your outer legs feel hard or feel "weird" when you are resting after a long period of standing, that would be three symptoms of rigidity in three *different* parts of the body.

If you notice that one of your eyes is slightly more open than the other because the lower eyelid is hanging lower, and people have been saying, "Smile more!" to you, that would be two symptoms of poverty of movement. A tendency to drool is another poverty of movement symptom, but all three of these symptoms are on the face, and all three might be caused by a stroke or some other neurological problem affecting your face. But if you have additional symptoms of poverty of movement on, say, your feet, such as altered blood vessels in your feet or foot drop now and then, or frequent foot cramping that pulls the toes under, or inability to separate the second and/or third (middle) toe on the side first affected, or *slowness* of stride, or difficulty in coordinating arm swing and leg stride, then you have poverty of movement symptoms in both face and feet: in *different* parts of your body.

1) If you have three or more symptoms of rigidity *and* three or more symptoms of poverty of movement as described in chapter fourteen and they are in various parts of your body, you most likely have Parkinson's disease.

2) If you also have rhythmic resting tremor along either the Stomach channel, the Large Intestine channel, and sometimes in the adjacent Gallbladder or Triple Burner channels, or on the chin, (the Ren channel), a tremor that comes and goes or, in advanced PD, varies in intensity in response to emotion, you very likely have Parkinson's disease.

3) If, in addition to the above, you also have had episodes of stumbling, falling, or whole body "clumsiness," you most probably have Parkinson's disease.

4) If you've had episodes of festinating gait or walking backwards in addition to the above symptoms, you can be as certain as possible of a PD diagnosis based on the *western* understanding of Parkinson's disease.

5) If in addition to having two out of the first three of the above, if your symptoms vary over the course of the day or over several days and/or if you remember a brain spin event, you can be even more sure that you have Parkinson's, based on a broader understanding of Parkinson's than the *traditional* western one.

6) If you answered in the affirmative to two out of the first three of the above *and* your channels are moving in the pause patterns, you can be confident that you have Parkinson's disease according the western understanding of PD *and* the far more objective channel theory understanding of PD.

Do you *not* have Parkinson's?

If your symptoms are all in one location, for example, if your arm doesn't swing and *all* your other symptoms, including tremor, if any, are also on that arm, or if you can't bend your knee following your knee surgery and *all* your other symptoms are also on the leg that had the surgery, you probably do NOT have Parkinson's disease, no matter what your doctor said.

If your doctor gave you a PD diagnosis based on symptoms in just one body part or even two body parts that were both affected during an injury, stroke, or surgery, please see another doctor and let him know that all the symptoms started after an injury, stroke, or surgery.

If your tremor started very soon after starting a new medication and that medication-insert lists tremor as a possible adverse effect, and the doctor said you must have "sudden-onset" Parkinson's disease, please see another doctor – one *outside* of the in-house system of your previous doctor – and let the new doctor know that *all* symptoms began after starting the new medication. The same advice applies if *none* of your symptoms are on the Stomach or Large Intestine channels.

Do NOT tell the second doctor that you have a diagnosis of PD. In western medicine we have a long-standing medical tradition that a second doctor is not supposed to contradict a previous doctor. Even if the first diagnosis is egregiously in error, a second doctor will be very hesitant to contradict the first one unless the first one has expressed genuine uncertainty and is *honestly* looking for a second opinion (rare).

Tell your second doctor about your symptoms *and* any pertinent information such as an injury, surgery, or new drug that *immediately* preceded the symptoms, but do *not* mention anything about having received a diagnosis of Parkinson's disease.

If you have many symptoms of poverty of movement, rigidity, tremor, and maybe some balance issues *but* your Stomach, Du, and Ren channels are moving in a healthy manner even while your friend tests you by saying something scary like "These channels are a mess!" *and* if you can playfully *imagine* positive scenarios and especially if you can *feel* your Du channel qi easily moving up into your neck and head, you almost certainly do *not* have any of the four types of idiopathic Parkinson's disease. You might have drug- or toxin-induced parkinsonism or you might have some other syndrome completely unrelated to Parkinson's disease.

If your channel qi is flowing correctly and vigorously in the parts of your body that are tremoring, you do *not* have a idiopathic Parkinson's-type tremor. Remember, tremor can be caused by many, many problems, including medications, toxins, heart conditions, genetic conditions, a history of anti-depression or anti-anxiety medications, a history of dopamine-enhancing recreational drugs, and so on. Tremor alone does not a Parkinson's diagnosis make.

In summary

If many of your symptoms match up with the description of symptom *locations* that you walked through in chapter fourteen, you probably have Parkinson's disease.

If you have several symptoms in two or three of the four categories of poverty of movement, rigidity, tremor, and balance issues, you probably have Parkinson's disease.

If your channel qi is constantly running in the patterns typical of pause, you probably have Parkinson's disease or pre-Parkinson's disease *even if you have no symptoms or your symptoms are not yet advanced enough to be noticed.*

If you've got PD-type behaviors from all *three* of the above criteria groups: 1) symptoms in the locations described in chapter fourteen; 2) symptoms that match the four traits of poverty of movement, rigidity, tremor, and postural instability (the things your doctor usually looks for); and 3) pause-type channel qi flow, you can be pretty darned certain that you have Parkinson's disease.

If you do have Parkinson's disease...

Good detective work! Continue on to figure out which of the four types of Parkinson's disease you are dealing with. To start that process, you'll first want to learn a bit more about the Parkinson's personality.

Chapter Sixteen

The Parkinson's Personality

In differentiating between the four types of Parkinson's, paying attention to mental attitudes and personality attributes can be helpful. The information about attitude and personality from this chapter will be added to the techniques in chapter seventeen for determining which type of PD is presenting.

Type I PD, Parkinson's from self-induced pause, is associated with the "Parkinson's personality." The other three types of PD, not so much. Being on pseudo pause *can* lead to brain behaviors that lead a person to eventually veer towards some of the characteristics of the Parkinson's personality, but if so, those characteristics might be somewhat mild and/or of recent onset – possibly *not* dating back to childhood or young adulthood.

As you read through this chapter, please don't worry over whether or not you or some other person is a *perfect* match for the all the behaviors described. *No one* is going to have *all* of the personality traits. Just notice if *some* of the personality traits seem to apply.

The following is from the journal *Neurology*.

> "Studies suggest that Parkinson's disease (PD) is associated with a particular group of personality characteristics. With relative uniformity, PD patients are described as industrious, rigidly moral, stoic, serious, and nonimpulsive. In this controlled study, we found significantly less ($p < 0.01$) of a group of traits called "novelty seeking" in PD patients compared with matched medical controls. Patients with low novelty seeking are described as being reflective, rigid, stoic, slow-tempered, frugal, orderly, and persistent: characteristics similar to those in the clinical description of PD patients." [1]

"Novelty seeking" is sometimes described as "playful curiosity" or "inherent curiosity." It is driven by brain behaviors of parasympathetic mode. During novelty seeking, dopamine is released in higher amounts in the striatum and thalamus. This stimulates the midbrain's "reward system." Behaviorally and neurologically, "novelty seeking" is the reason a hen keeps pecking at the ground to see what she might discover, and the reason that computer games or click-bait on social media are inherently compelling, even addictive. The *healthy* mind is compelled towards novelty seeking: activities that increase activation of the midbrain and the release of dopamine, causing contentment and/or a positive-mood upward spiral. In most people with Parkinson's, novelty seeking behaviors are inhibited.

---

[1] "Dopamine-related personality traits in Parkinson's disease"; *Neurology*; Menza MA, Golbe LI, Cody RA; 1993 Mar; 43(3 Pt 1):505-8. https://www.ncbi.nlh.nih.gov/pubmed/8450991 .

The above collection of personality traits reflects behaviors of most people who have already been diagnosed with Parkinson's. Even so, if one looks at the personalities of people in the *decades* before they developed overt symptoms of Parkinson's, some of these traits might already have been present.

Even in the decades prior to their diagnosis with Parkinson's, people who eventually develop Type I Parkinson's were often seen as highly intelligent, reliable, able to focus intensely, and tending towards a strong – and often very narrow – moral compass. They often have a hard time relaxing or even indulging in what might be deemed light-hearted or "foolish" behaviors, such as gazing at clouds or making jokes at their own expense. They *assess* their surroundings rather than feel or resonate with them. Although there are exceptions they are, for the most part, cautious, reflective, and stoic – numb to some types of physical and/or emotional pain…or joy. They tend to *not* be highly profligate or carelessly sensual, in general.

Even *prior* to the appearance of PD symptoms, people with Type I Parkinson's tend to behave *neurologically* – though not necessarily *consciously* – as if they are in a situation that requires constant, *guarded* behavior – the opposite of carefree novelty seeking.

Punctuality and more

In addition to the aforementioned aspects of the Parkinson's personality, people with Type I Parkinson's disease are often pathologically punctual, afraid of making mistakes, or of being judged as doing a "wrong" thing. They tend to avoid passion-evoking physical conflict although they can be prone to exhaustive verbal argument and might have a hard time backing down from a position, once taken. They are often highly judgmental of their own behaviors, as well as the behaviors of others, and somewhat non-accepting of what they call "character flaws" in themselves or others. They are often unable to cry easily. While some *might* be able to cry tears of joy or relief at a movie or on behalf of others, they still might have a very hard time crying from their *own* pain, grief, or self-pity.

For an example of the enormous fear of being un-punctual, *most* of my Parkinson's patients coming to my office for the first time did a test drive to my office the day *before* to ensure that they would not be late when they drove to my easy-to-find office again on the scheduled day. Not *one* of my non-Parkinson's patients ever did this.

Oppositely, the patient with Type IV PD that I described in chapter two was famously late for everything, and always laughed it off.

Many people with Type I PD consider being "tireless" a virtue. Phrases such as "I'll sleep when I'm dead" are often tossed around, and only partly in jest.

During my first year or so of working with people with Parkinson's disease, I gradually became aware that *most* of my patients shared a singular type of personality as well as high intelligence and highly analytical thinking. I didn't yet know about the medically recognized "Parkinson's personality."

Even before I learned about the Parkinson's personality, several of my patients told me that "Old Dr. Dorison," for several decades the only neurologist in my then small town, had often affirmed, "I can never tell my Parkinson's patients anything new. I give them the diagnosis, and the next time I see them they have read up more on the recent findings about Parkinson's than I have." And this observation by highly respected Dr.

Dorosin was made in the days *before* the existence of the internet, back when researching the latest news on a health problem was a lot harder to do, and might involve traveling many miles to a medical school's library or subscribing to a medical journal.

As I met other neurologists, they often confirmed Dr. Dorosin's statement: they thought that their patients with Parkinson's were, in general, better educated and – even in the days before the internet – more inclined to do research about their diagnosis than patients with other types of health problems. Eventually, I found solid research articles on the Parkinson's personality and realized that this was a recognized thing – not just something that I'd seen in my own PD patients.

As for the strong moral compass, I was surprised when the first dozen volunteers I gathered from the Parkinson's support group had a disproportionately high percentage of people with strong spiritual leanings across a wide range of faiths.

Out of the first twelve volunteers, there was a catholic nun, a Lutheran minister, a Unitarian minister, a catholic priest, two practitioners of esoteric (meditation-based) yoga, a student of *The Book of Miracles*, a retired missionary, and a devout Christian with missionary parents. The three other volunteers were not members of any specific church but *all* felt that they held themselves to higher moral standards than most people.

And not only were *all* these PD patients very well read, they *all* had a strong, word-oriented, philosophical bent.

Over the next few years my patient list grew to include rabbis, lamas, swamis, and teachers and adherents representing every major world religion.

The high percentage of people with strong spiritual leanings seemed oddly disproportionate to me, in the early years of my research. But what was *far* stranger was that nearly *all* of my patients had the same, anti-spiritual attitude regarding cultivating an intimate, personal relationship that involved silent or spoken communication with a higher power, a totem animal, a beloved but deceased friend, a saint, God, or some other representative of Universal Love, The Force, or the Divine. They were all opposed to it.

A hands-off relationship with God

The emotionally distant, somewhat intellectual relationship most of my patients had with God or any of the afore-named types of "invisible friends" turned out to be significant.

Most of my patients with Type I Parkinson's, those who went into partial recovery instead of full recovery after their foot injuries healed, had shared with me, during their many hours of answering my fairly probing questions, a very peculiar variant of "spirituality." During their many Yin Tui Na sessions I had eventually asked each of them, "Have you ever prayed or asked for any spiritual help for dealing with your Parkinson's?"

Nearly all of my patients with Type I Parkinson's replied that they did not feel they *should* communicate with God, or the Divine, or the Tao, or with any higher authority, spiritual guide, deceased friend or relative, or savior, with regard to their *own* illness or their *own* problems.

Mechanical prayers, yes. Prayers for others, yes. Words of gratitude, yes. But sharing their intimate worries and especially asking for spiritual help/intervention/insights with regard to their own increasing physical problems, no.

They tended to have deep respect for their isolationist misinterpretation of the old saying: "God helps those who help themselves." Many of my patients expressed this sentiment together with something along the lines of "God is busy running His part of the universe; I'm supposed to be in charge of mine." Or "I don't want to bother Him/Her" or "…make Him/Her feel sad."

Every major world religion was represented in my growing group of patients. Nearly *all* of my patients with Type I PD felt the same way. *Long* before their PD symptoms appeared, they had cultivated this attitude of "*I'm* different from other people: others should confide intimately, constantly, in the Divine but *I shouldn't*."

This attitude of "I should be apart from God" and/or "not waste His or Her time" especially stood out because a disproportionate number of my Parkinson's patients with these sentiments were religious *professionals*: priests, nuns, rabbis, pastors, lamas, rimpoches, and swamis. I also had many patients who were lay people of a wide assortment of faiths, including devout Muslims, Latter Day Saints, Mennonites, and Jehovah's Witnesses. A disproportionately high percentage of my PD patients led lives that revolved around their ultra-strong commitments to their various spiritual paths. And yet they nearly all shared the weird idea that *other* people should talk intimately with and pray to God or someone about everything, including their problems, but in their *own* cases, they should not bother any representative of the Universal or the Divine. Many told me that doing so would upset or worry God or the Divine Mother or whomever, as if by their mental silence their Parkinson's symptoms could somehow be kept secret from the Universal Omniscience.

Those extremely "spiritual" leaders and laity who preferred to not share their troubles with God or a higher power were the patients who were most likely to get stuck in partial recovery if they re-associated with their injuries. Also, despite their devotion to their faith, they could *not* bring themselves to feel biologically or existentially safe.

These patients assured me that they always instructed their parishioners or their fellow followers to talk to the Divine or have some sort of regular communion or prayer engaging with, *sharing everything* with, God or with some higher power. However, they strongly felt that doing so would be inappropriate in their *own* cases. Many even felt that keeping their troubles to themselves and not disturbing a higher authority was a sign of spiritual *superiority*.

The saints and sages of *every* faith have all said that, on the spiritual path, regular communication with the Divine is necessary in order to grow closer to truth, and that it brings great joy. But for most of my patients, asking for help or comfort from God, a saint, or even a beloved, deceased grandmother was considered a sign of spiritual weakness, a *lack* of faith.

This commonality in so many of my patients struck me as so bizarre that it rattled around in my brain for all the years of my research. Not until 2015, when I learned about the research in neurotheology, did I start to see the connection. You will recall, that research found that thinking about a higher power with whom one could potentially communicate leads to increased activation in the striatum. Activity in the striatum, you'll also recall, is inhibited when a person is on pause.

This weird mental attitude, which I noticed very early on, actually turned out to be an additional source of support for my budding hypothesis in 2015 that inactivity in the striatum might also be involved in Parkinson's. This hypothesis, in turn, led to my development of therapies that *directly* stimulate the striatum and so help turn off self-induced pause. Usually, stimulation of the striatum is expectation-dependant. This means that positive mental habits that stimulate the striatum lead to increased activity in the striatum: a upward spiraling of good feeling. Negative expectations decrease activity in the striatum and cause downward spiraling apprehension, fear, and/or rage.

If the striatum is profoundly inhibited, as it is on pause, an empty feeling of being apart from others or even apart from God is the logical result. On pause, with an inhibited striatum, a person not only might perceive himself as being outside of his body, he is also *unable* to stimulate the parts of the brain that are activated when feeling the presence of *or* communicating with intangible loved ones, totem animals, spiritual guides, or God.

I hypothesized that, if an intelligent person finds himself, over decades, *unable* to feel the presence of God or *unable* to have a sense of communication with God, he might very well conclude that he is not *supposed* to feel or communicate with God. He will then alter or adapt any spiritual precepts he has learned in order to accommodate his personal sense of being alone and apart. This could account for the very bizarre conviction among my Type I PD patients that they were not *supposed* to "worry" God with their problems or "waste God's time." They *had* to assume that God wanted them to figure things out on their own because they certainly weren't able to get answers from God when they tried to…because their striata and thalami were turned off…*because* their brains were predominantly running in the pause pattern.

Commanding oneself to be numb enough that pause mode kicks in creates a brain electrical behavior in which a person is physically *unable* to feel somatically connected to or resonant with himself and/or others. He might have a *logic*-based conviction of emotional attachment to others, or a strong *intellectual* sense of a connection to God or some aspect of the Divine. But the healthy, somatically *feel-able* sensations that come with connection and resonance will not be available. A person on pause might even feel apart from the universe, or unable to access somatic awareness or somatic feelings from memories of loved ones who have passed on.

Commanding oneself to be numb creates electrical behaviors in the brain that greatly inhibits intuitive communication and the ability to silently *converse* with loved ones.

This sense of separation from essentially everything *makes* a person feel unsafe. You cannot turn off pause until you can confirm that you are safe. If you intentionally made yourself numb, you *can't* feel safe. You can't even *feel*. If you can't feel safe, you can't turn off pause. A vicious cycle…unless you do some very specific behaviors that allow you to do an "end run" around the instruction to stay on pause. This end run begins with learning to communicate and feel a connection with something, anything. This sense of connection builds as one forces oneself to communicate, however reluctantly, with an invisible, laughing, loving and trusted confidant. This, in turn, eventually wakes up the dormant striatum and thalamus in *spite* of previous instructions to feel no pain.

And so this chapter on the Parkinson's personality is also going to include information about certain spiritual attitudes, as well as personality traits. What makes it even more appropriate for me to include spiritual attitudes is that the people with Type I PD who have recovered have often had a growing, deepening, or even an abrupt, transformation in their spiritual or relationship attitudes that coincided with or *immediately* preceded their recovery via what I call the epiphany. [1]

Culturally-triggered pause mode

In addition to *spiritual* attitudes contributing to or being caused by pause mode, cultural attitudes can also be a factor. In certain cultures, people who can activate pause mode on command are highly regarded. In general, cultures in colder climes are more likely to encourage or approve of emotion-repressed self-control than cultures in warmer, more equatorial regions.

---

[1] Here are some epiphany examples culled from news articles (These people were *not* my patients. I learned about each of them online.): Ricky Peterson had steadily worsening Parkinson's for eight years. He had been praying for years in his usual way, asking to be healed from his Parkinson's, but his symptoms continued to worsen. During a prayer session at the tomb of an Australian catholic saint, Mary MacKillop, Peterson suddenly felt a *personal* relationship with the saint. He stopped his previous style of prayers and switched over to silently *talking* with the deceased Mary MacKillop. He talked with her about how, from now on, he and she would pray *together* for his healing: they would be doing prayers *together*. When he made this switch, his tremor ceased almost immediately. His other symptoms clearly up very quickly, as well.

https://cruxnow.com/global-church/2018/07/kansan-returns-to-australia-saints-tomb-in-thanks-for-parkinsons-cure/ July 28, 2018.

Florence Diekmann recovered from Parkinson's in response to an affirmation. She started silently affirming to the universe that she was "coming alive." She integrated this constant affirmation with her bible study and prayers. One day, she felt herself actually "coming alive," and then her Parkinson's was gone. I suspect that this person had *only* Type II PD, which can respond well to affirmations.

https://www.youtube.com/watch?v=5KWdZ-2dgZs ; Nov. 23, 2015.

A French nun, Marie Simon-Pierre, was "miraculously healed" overnight, two months after she and her sister nuns had an evening prayer session in which they prayed for Pope John Paul II, who had Parkinson's disease. Marie Simon-Pierre had been diagnosed with Parkinson's four years earlier. After her prayer session, she felt a new closeness to the Pope, which she continued to cultivate. Two months later, her recovery was instantaneous. "I just woke up at four in the morning and jumped out of bed. I was completely transformed." This "miracle" was the first official one attributed to the late John Paul II, and was used by Pope Benedict to move forward with John Paul II's beatification. Beatification is the first step in becoming recognized as a Catholic saint.

https://www.bbc.com/news/world-europe-12192639. January 14, 2011.

In the above two cases that had an invisible friend, the friend had strong spiritual leanings: one was a saint, the other was a pope. But I have seen in other patients who've recovered that it doesn't matter if the invisible friend has a spiritual background or not. So long as the invisible confidant is considered to be a true friend, a non-judgmental friend, a friend that one can *laugh* with, then the loving feelings generated by constantly communicating with the friend can eventually re-awaken the dormant striatum enough to turn off pause.

In *general*, I have seen people have easier and faster epiphanies when the communicant was a parent, grandparent, uncle or aunt, than when it was a religious figure. Many people felt they could not, *should* not, laugh with and tease the spiritual figures that they chose as their confidants. These people found that their PD symptoms continued to worsen despite their silent conversations. Dwelling on a spiritual figure that cannot be laughed with can stimulate the fear and rage centers of the brain, not the striatum. Increased activity in the fear and rage centers can *increase* the degree of pause mode a person uses.

The deliberate use of pause mode might actually be advantageous in some geographical settings. The ability to conserve energy and stifle emotions might be a crucial skill set in lands with extreme cold and unreliable or seasonal food supplies. It might be that, since prehistoric times, people in dangerously cold climes who could self-induce pause mode and thus conserve precious energy had an edge in terms of survival.

To demonstrate what I mean by "conserve energy," mentally picture an elderly British statesman or butler. Next, imagine an Italian politician or major-domo. Which one do you imagine as being a bit hunched over, shuffling, and possibly having a mild tremor? Which one do you imagine being more likely to launch into a loud tirade or burst into song? Which one is constantly expending more energy?

Populations with the highest per capita cases of Parkinson's tend to be in countries that have periods of very cold weather. Equatorial regions tend to have lower per capita cases of Parkinson's disease. For example, for more than a century, since British medical record keeping began, people in England and Scotland were considered to have a high per capita rate of Parkinson's. Oppositely, the *native* people of India were considered to have the lowest per capita rate of Parkinson's anywhere in the world. (Though more accurately, I should probably say "anywhere in the British Empire.")

But the *British* people who lived in India during the British Raj, drinking the local water and eating locally produced food, had the same high rates of Parkinson's as are seen in England and Scotland. Although those Brits had moved from the cold and windy UK to a steamy equatorial region, they brought with them their cultural attitudes and maybe even – I'm guessing here – a long-evolved advantageous (in some cases) genetic tendency towards word-based intensity of mental focus that helped them self-induce pause when necessary and, as a side effect, allowed them to conserve physical and emotional energy. Together with their cultural attitudes and *maybe* also a genetic propensity for word-based, analytical thinking, the British maintained their high per capita rate of Parkinson's disease no matter where they actually lived.

Using pause as a cultural advantage

Historically speaking, so long as the average life expectancy for humans was around thirty-five years, as it was for the last few millennia, or even age fifty-five, as it was at the beginning of the twentieth century, the ability to activate pause mode for self-repression and energy conservation might have been an excellent survival mechanism – with natural selection in favor of people who could more easily self-induce pause, especially if they lived in harsh climates. [1]

However, these days, most of us will live *twice* thirty-five years – some attaining even eighty or even ninety years of age. Being stuck on self-induced pause might *now*

---

[1] The tendency towards stoicism in nordic peoples has often been gently noted, but so far as I know it has not been clinically assessed or genetically evaluated. The humorous book, "Scandinavian Humor and other Myths" by John Louis Anderson is a delightful example. One reviewer wrote, "A sophisticated, loving look at a stoic crowd that actually prefers cold weather, almost always wears suits (Pants, Leisure, or Snowmobile), and doesn't like Food that Hurts." Another reviewer with tongue in cheek wrote, "So funny that you [God forbid!] almost laugh out loud." – he signed his review "An Old Swede".

result in the eventual appearance of symptoms of Parkinson's disease, if a person lives long enough. So it's no longer as *ultimately* advantageous as it used to be to go through life on pause mode, even in the colder parts of the globe.

– In case you're curious, in the late 1990s, the average age for the appearance of Parkinson's disease in the United States was seventy-two. In 2020, it is approximately 60 years old. This does not necessarily mean that people are getting Parkinson's earlier. It is possible that it is being *diagnosed* earlier or more eagerly (and incorrectly), or that better records are being kept, or even that cases of drug- and toxin-induced parkinsonism are now being included in with diagnoses of Parkinson's. For example, Agent Orange, a defoliant used widely during the Vietnam war, is officially recognized by the U.S. Veteran's Administration as causing toxin-induced parkinsonism. These people with toxin-induced parkinsonism are very likely included in the national count of people with Parkinson's. Also, in the past fifty years, the number of people taking anti-depressant and anti-anxiety drugs – most of which can cause tardive parkinsonism, has soared. If the numbers of people with PD now include drug-induced and toxin-induced parkinsonism, that could explain why the numbers are rising and why we're seeing an earlier "start" date on average.

Extreme cold weather on its own doesn't automatically *cause* self-induced emotional inhibition. For example, the French-speaking people in far northern Quebec, in the Lac St. Jean area, are characterized as *highly* energetic and fun-seeking (novelty seeking): "live wires." But they came to Canada a mere five hundred years ago. Genetically and culturally, they are relatively recent immigrés from northwestern France, from the somewhat moderate climate of the Brittany area.

Despite pause mode maybe being used to compensate for severely cold climatic conditions or to support cultural norms, the biological use of pause mode is actually designed to be reserved for emergency, near-death situations. Humans aren't *supposed* to use pause mode all the time, even at modest levels. The use of pause inhibits the dopamine-dispensing reward centers in the brain. In animals and in healthy people, the activation of these reward centers provides the main emotional, or heart-based, "purpose" of living.

The sense of power and self-control arising from being on pause with a norepinephrine override *can* bring short-term satisfaction via some ego-based emotions. But at the same time, being on pause *inhibits* the lasting, effortless, ever-new joy that comes with being literally resonant with others and with the vibrations of the universe.

Modes are nearly always shades of gray: rarely black or white

As mentioned earlier, the human body does not use four *distinct* neurological modes. At any given instant, a person is usually using a blend of the electrical circuitries of two or more modes. Even during the dream and REM stages of sleep, a person is using both sleep mode *and* a bit of either parasympathetic mode or sympathetic mode, which determines whether his dreams are joyful or stressed.

A person in *full-bore* pause mode is unconscious: in a coma.

Most people with *Type I* Parkinson's disease use varying degrees of pause throughout the day, as needed, usually blended with some amount of sympathetic mode, supported by brain norepinephrine, not by adrenaline. Not only are they using what seems to be *varying* degrees of pause, people with Type I PD *might* also be capable of using another *personality* or at least a different *aspect* of his normal personality. This other personality *potentially* has access to parasympathetic mode, if and when a person with Type I PD is feeling exceptionally, although temporarily, safe.

The intermittent, *low* level use of pause in the decades leading up to Parkinson's might be why symptoms take so many decades to become habitual. This might also explain why a person's symptoms might become so severe immediately after receiving a diagnosis of Parkinson's: suddenly, the person might need to use a *higher* degree of pause mode and use it closer to full-time to deal with the relentless emotional pain of knowing that he has Parkinson's – a vicious downward spiral.

In fact, the whole issue of the Parkinson's personality is related to that spiral.

The more a person uses pause mode to deal with his pain or his fears, the more the Parkinson's personality becomes entrenched and expanded. And the degree to which a person uses this personality can determine the extent to which his body uses the circuitries of pause and causes the manifestation of PD symptoms. And as symptoms get worse, fear increases *because* the symptoms are getting worse.

I mentioned earlier that western medical researchers have never decided if the Parkinson's personality is the *cause* of Parkinson's, or is caused *by* Parkinson's. The assumption, I suspect, is that the personality is one of the symptoms of PD, and it's caused by the death of brain cells – an hypothesis that is increasingly found wanting.

My work suggests that the personality is both cause and result of the changes that occur in people with Type I Parkinson's. To a large extent, the personality is the result of being on pause. But the personality itself makes pause mode become more entrenched.

I've seen people recover. I've seen the extraordinary personality change that occurs in the *moments* prior to complete recovery. In people with Type I Parkinson's, the decision to refute the PD personality, often in response to a large epiphany, often occurs a split second before the Parkinson's permanently turns off. And never returns.

In recovered people who have a series of small epiphanies instead of one big one, the personality change is more gradual, and a person might go back and forth, even getting to the point that he can recognize which personality he's using at a given moment.

Therefore, I hypothesize that the Parkinson's personality is not *just* a symptom of Parkinson's, it also contributes to the *cause* and the steady worsening of symptoms.

Again, of the four types of PD, people with Type I PD are the ones most likely to manifest the Parkinson's personality. When they recover, they instantly drop much of that personality and become, in their own startled words, "back to my real self!"

This "real self" turns out to be much less fearful, less inhibited, and less critical of others or self. It is more comfortable being around others and is, in turn, a lot easier to be around.

For example, one recovered patient told me that she suddenly found herself talking un-self-consciously with her co-workers. She always walked every day with a group of them during the lunch break. She had always been careful to listen to each person in turn and then, when she deemed it her turn, she would say something that logically followed the previous speaker. After recovering, she suddenly found herself just saying whatever she felt like, and not worrying about whose turn it was. She was amazed at how much less work it was to be part of a conversation. Her contributions still made sense and were logical, but they were effortless. She wasn't expending any energy "keeping track." She was able to laugh at how labored her previous socializing had been.

For another example, a person I never met who was working from my online books emailed me a few days after he turned off pause. He wrote, "I think I hit full parasympathetic mode the other day…every sense was high, everything I looked at was brighter, aura-like, and boy was I happy. I had never before experienced such a level of joy. The height of it lasted about two hours but for the next two days my wife was trying to figure out what drugs I was on!

"Also, I never cry. Even when my father passed. Until now. I watched "Collateral Beauty" on Saturday night. I must have cried four times, teared up a bit, and belly laughed at the funny bits. This is new to me. It took having to recover from PD to discover I'd had no emotions."

The rapid personality change self-described in the above email, a change that might occur almost immediately when pause turns off, is pretty typical. Of course, the person who wrote the above also mentioned with disappointment that, even though he felt recovered in his heart, his symptoms were only *slowly* starting to ease up and recovery symptoms were just starting to occur. He wondered why, if he'd turned off pause, he still had any symptoms at all. I replied to him something along the lines of "the war might end abruptly but the rebuilding after the war will take some time." His symptoms have since steadily decreased.

His only remaining symptom, as of this writing, is neck and arm pain that he long attributed to PD but which, it turns out, was being caused by a cervical vertebra displacement, one that is responding to physical therapy. Even if a person has Parkinson's, not all his aches and pains are necessarily related to Parkinson's disease.

After a person fully recovers, all the pause-related behaviors, attitudes, and "logical" reasons he might have had for having been anxious, on guard, or wary simply disappear and become, in retrospect, laughable.

Many of my patients with Type I Parkinson's were proud of what they thought of as their hyper-analytical mind-set. They did *not* consider the increasingly anxious and wary personality to be a problem. But the truth is, it's probably the most vicious and deleterious of all the symptoms of PD. Then again, some people with Parkinson's *do* recognize that the mental tension and negative attitude is the worst part of the illness and that it exacerbates all the other symptoms.

The mindset of the Parkinson's personality serves as a powerful force – a steadily increasing force – that helps keep pause mode in place and increasingly entrenched.

The longer a person has Type I Parkinson's, the more influence the Parkinson's personality might have on his mental habits. The longer these mental influences are in place, creating and reinforcing neural pathways in the brain for negative thoughts, the harder it might be for a person to overcome the illogical fears, anxieties, and Blockers that his brain has so carefully constructed. And these mental habits *must* be overruled in order to attain lasting, healthy activity levels in the brain's striatum and thalamus, thus increasing the level of energy flow in the brain portion of the Du channel that gives a feeling of being safe, thus allowing pause to turn off.

Long-term mental habits

The long-term use of pause leads to or increases mental patterns that cause the Parkinson's personality. Over time, the use of the Parkinson's personality creates *habits* of negative thinking that make it harder to turn off pause. Based on what I have seen, the longer a person has had overt symptoms of Type I Parkinson's, the harder it might be to turn off pause. It's still do-able, but the longer a person has had Type I PD, the more focus and work it might take to turn it off. Then again, people with long-term spiritual training in what's called "practicing the presence of God" (constantly imagining the presence of something loving being near to you, communicating with you) seem to have an advantage in coming out of pause once they are willing to take the communication habit to a deeper, more intimate, and more irreverent and playful level, even if their PD symptoms are severe. Also, many long-term practitioners of eastern religions have practiced keeping a feeling of energy at Yin Tang, also known as "the third eye," during waking hours. Even if one is on pause, it seems as if this practice helps prevent or slow the formation of fearful or angry neural habits. You might say this habit prevents or slows the "brain wiring," that supports negative thinking.

Oppositely, those who have *never* before practiced communicating with an invisible friend, keeping mental focus at Yin Tang, or other spiritual disciplines that support midbrain function might really struggle to establish new habits that stimulate the striatum.

Many people with Parkinson's have become fond, and even proud, of their negative, ego-based (sides of the brain) thought patterns. They often think that they are smarter than other people because of their wary and anxious thought patterns or their powerful word and memory skills, and/or their relentless, analytical, internal monologue.

These behaviors are associated with activities on the sides of the brain. Very often, people with these behaviors do *not* want to revert back to any type of thinking that they fear might feel less clever or even "stupid."

In fact, recovery does *not* make a person stupid. It makes a person more at ease, more playful and more joyful with his intelligence. But that concept is incomprehensible to many people in the throes of Parkinson's: being on pause alters the way one assigns values to various behaviors, thoughts, and personality traits.

Even though none of my Parkinson's patients wanted to have the physical symptoms of Parkinson's disease, many, maybe most of them, were deeply attached to the sides-of-the-brain thinking that accompanies pause: they didn't *want* to change their negative, intense, pause-driven thinking. They *liked* this type of thinking. They felt it kept them "smart." They *didn't* like the physical immobility and tremor that is inextricably connected to being on pause and is connected to this type of thinking, but they liked the false illusion that they were cleverer and/or more focused than most.

So long as a person holds firmly to pause-based thought patterns, that person cannot recover from Type I PD. That person cannot surrender to the joyful feelings that arise through the steady practice of middle-of-the-brain thinking: thinking that can be encouraged by mentally *communicating* with a loved one or some loving higher authority or *feeling* the presence of love and friendship within and without.

Surrender

This might be a good place to explain the meaning of the word surrender as used in the above paragraph. Most of my Type I patients, even those with years of spiritual training or study, assumed, incorrectly, that "surrender" means "lie down and die."

In fact, "surrender" can mean "stop fighting," or "yield to the stronger, or the more just, or the 'better' power." Surrender, in this case, means letting go of the mental habit of listening to one's own negative thoughts and instead *choosing* to mentally be communicating with someone or something that brings joy. When one fully "surrenders" to the invisible friend, one chooses to trust the friend, to allow the friend's decisions to stand, and to make this preference for the friend as utter as possible – almost every moment, every thought…at least until one recovers. One is "giving up" or "surrendering" his option of choosing the inner monologue with its negativity, bitterness, or a self-serving, twisted rationality.

Surrender in recovering from PD might involve making a new, *conversational* duologue habit to replace the old internal monologue. For some people, this surrender can occur very quickly, in a matter of seconds. For others, surrender can be difficult. At first, a person with no habit of regular prayer or communication with an invisible friend, who wants to change his mental habits in order to turn off pause, might have to surrender anew every few minutes, in the beginning. But this surrender might become easier over time as the physical and emotional benefits of the surrender begin to manifest in snippets of relaxation and momentarily diminished PD symptoms.

If changing the orientation of one's thoughts doesn't sound much like "surrender," think of the situation as a mental battle: a person with self-induced pause is habituated to choose the negative: subconsciously or even consciously *choosing* to fight *against* the positive.

Some people with PD work like the dickens to stay positive. Some have worked at it their whole lives. Others work hard to *appear* positive to others in spite of their secret negative internal monologue. So many are deeply spiritual – even devoting their lives to being a religious professional. And they can tell you, it can be a *battle* to allow the heart to be in charge and thus turn off the negative, fear-driven internal monologue that is set in motion by the use of self-induced pause. If it's a battle, then war-type terminology such as "surrender" is appropriate.

The word surrender can also mean "stop fighting the world and allow yourself to be loved." Surrender can mean, "let your higher self (heart-guided behavior) actively choose the good and the loving, over and over, even though everything in your ego-driven, habit-loving brain is screaming at you to choose the apprehensive, the isolated, and the negative."

And a battle it is. If using only one's *own* mind to fight one's own mental habits, it will be a losing battle: an individual's brain cannot expect its new, weak, fledgling positive attitude to win in a battle against his long-established, powerful, negative, pause-driven habits. But if a person develops a profoundly trusting relationship with something that he considers to *represent* Goodness or Joy then he can, at some point, "surrender" by choosing to trust the judgment of the invisible friend instead of his own increasingly warped judgment. When he sides with the friend, he opens his heart. His immortal heart, his soul, or you might say superconsiousness, *can* win in a battle against his mere conscious and subconscious negative mental habits. Using the Chinese metaphors of the heart being the King and the mind being the governor, the King will trump the governor every time – if he's allowed to do his job.

Two examples of warriors engaged in battle

An email PD correspondent from eastern Europe wrote to me after more than three years of working on talking to a friend: [When I started talking to my friend] "I did not think it was possible for a person to be in control of his thoughts. Control of the mind is a skill that can be learned? Like new language or martial art? Now, I seem to be able to endure stronger devil attacks [negative thoughts] far more than before. It sometimes seems that there is nothing the mind can throw at me I cannot change for more positive. Only it takes some time and energy."

Previous to doing the exercises for turning off pause, he had never mentally engaged with a higher power or friend. Although he considered himself to be deeply spiritual, he was extremely cynical and his emails were deeply negative. For more than three years he wrote to me at least once a week about his doubts and fears. In the several months before writing the above, he had started noticing that his PD symptoms were going away, and he had gotten to the point that they only returned when he allowed himself to indulge in his favorite hypothetical worry about someday being diagnosed with cancer (his "devil"). It had taken him years to get to his new, positive perspective, and it *had* been a battle. For years, he had sent me emails saying that it was impossible to change how his mind worked, and asking how he could justify a positive attitude in the face of so many terrible problems in the world and in himself, etc., etc. My reply was always, "Good questions. Ask your friend, not me."

One month after writing about his "devil", he wrote an email that amazed me because it was so upbeat and positive: "Allow me to express myself: I believe life gives challenges where, in order to go through, one has to change himself. That's the divine gift, because the thing one had to change is one that he was missing or he was not good at. It is a way that God perfects us. It is part of evolution of life."

In his next email, he wrote, "I have a feeling that my symptoms are reducing faster than before. Every day I notice some new positive detail in movement or recovery symptom. It's becoming a game of little things lately. Little things can make me feel either better or worse. So I pay attention to them. I practice my mind to automatically switch to light (positive) when dealing with something. I've noticed I can feel my body a lot more. Even the small things. I know this is a step in the right direction."

An email PD correspondent from France had been writing to me for nearly three years. He felt that he was deeply spiritual, and wanted his invisible friend to be Allah. He struggled with this relationship, and sent me many questions, while his PD symptoms, already fairly advanced, continued to worsen. He was deeply discouraged. After about two years of this, he added his late father to his conversations with Allah. He sent many dark and worried, even hopeless emails, asking me to tell him what to do.

I always had the same reply: "Don't ask me, ask Allah; ask your father."

The "invisible" relationships began to improve. Nearly a year later, when he sent the following, his understanding was so different: "I asked Allah why I was afraid and sometimes do not leave my ego without resistance. The answer was that I'm afraid if I stop checking that something bad is going to happen. My trust in Allah is getting stronger and I keep going. I have always looked for help from others. Now it is clear to me that I should only ask from Allah. I know Allah is here and takes care of me somehow. I am so far along that my heart opens up quite far. I keep talking to Allah and my father.

"I often feel great joy now for no reason. Since last night I had three short episodes so that my symptoms were 70% gone. It only lasted a few minutes each time, but it was here. My conversations with Allah are getting stronger and stronger and I am getting more persistent in seeking to be near him. Thanks for everything."

"Just let go; stop fighting"

One of the most common answers that my patients received from their invisible friends, in response to asking, "What do I need to do to completely recover?" was, "Just let go." Or "Just stop fighting."

A typical patient follow-up question to *me* regarding that answer has been, "What does that even mean?" When I suggested that this was the same idea as "surrender," my patients almost universally thought that I must be wrong. At the same time, they had no point of reference for understanding what was meant by "Just let go; just stop fighting," something that their *own* brain (via their own heart and the invisible friend) was telling them to do.

This subject is addressed in detail in the book *Stuck on Pause*. For now, "surrender" or "letting go" can be understood to mean "*choose* to think of and talk with your invisible, loving friend all the time instead of *choosing* to dwell on your own negative thoughts that you have so vigorously cultivated." Surrender to the companionship and caring of your loving friend and stop listening to the thoughts you've created that tell you, wrongly, that *you* and your fears are the only things keeping yourself safe.

This sounds so simple. But mental habits can sometimes be hard to break. Depending on how long a person has been on self-induced pause, learning to change mental habits of wariness and instead choosing companionship with an invisible friend might take a few minutes…or a few years.

Semantics

As an aside, some people have objected to my use of the term "invisible" friend. They have said it sounds too infantile, too childish, too close to the idea of an "imaginary" friend. I have considered using some of the other traditional terms for the type of communicant I'm talking about: "form-less" and "body-less." However, these terms are too closely associated with specific religious teachings. Other words, such as "communicant," feel too technical. Using just the word "friend" could be confusing, as I often make references to people "getting Yin Tui Na treatment from a friend," meaning a physical, at-hand friend. Capitalizing the word, making it into the word "Friend," seems to incorrectly suggest an underlying religious association. If you do not like the term "invisible friend" to describe the person, fictitious character, or animal that you can feel comfortable talking to and laughing with all the time, please come up with some term that works for you.

The person who wants to turn off self-induced pause has to turn his back on his own mind, and choose to accept the positive truths that his invisible friend offers: truths such as: "I love you," or "I'm right here with you."

The on-pause mind might try to cleverly counter such statements with "poor me" questions such as "Well then, if you've always been there for me, why was I mistreated as a child? Why are innocent children hurt? Why am I so unhappy?"

My patients have given me the above questions and many, many more as justification for not trusting anyone or anything, including saints, loved ones, or God. Especially God. But this is the pause-brain talking. Most humans, and nearly all animals, are able to go through life experiencing being alive in spite of dangers and risks. People in self-induced pause are essentially pretending to be dead and blaming the dangers and risks of life for their choice.

"Surrender" is a word often associated with religious or spiritual seeking, as in the phrase "surrender to the love of a higher power." For a person trying to turn off self-induced pause, take note: surrender does *not* mean "lie down and die." In this case, it means "choose to develop your relationship with your loved-filled friend instead of giving preference to your fear-driven ego." Surrender means turn your back on the secret sulking or resentment – ignore it! Focus your attention on a friend who can help you move forward, who can help bring you back to life.

The big picture

Here I'm going off on a tangent that might at first seem too removed from reality for many patients, but which has proven helpful to many, many people: *If* a person chooses to embrace the loving comfort of his invisible friend, if he "surrenders" to the thoughts held by that friend and rejects the negative nattering of his own mind, he might eventually find out that his *supposed* mistreatment (which might have contributed to his decision to use self-induced pause) was a manifestation of the perfect universal laws of cause and effect (karma). He might be able to consider the possibility that the soul is immortal and can be reborn over and over, but also that it can carry with it the reactions and memories of previous-life actions. He might recall from high-school physics class that for every action there is an equal and opposite reaction. This includes the reactions that help us decide prior to our conception which parents will best help us move forward or help us work out the consequences of our past wrong actions. If this is the case then, although one's life might be challenging or even terrifying, there is no such thing as ultimate "unfairness."

A person who takes the larger, universal perspective and admits that the universe has laws of cause and effect, and that for every action there is (eventually) an equal and opposite reaction might finally be forced to admit he is unhappy because he is keeping his mind focused like a laser on the things that his *ego* doesn't like, while ignoring the universal truths affirming that everything in this highly interconnected quantum universe happens as a response to some previous action or thought. Things happen for a well-deserved reason – even if we have no memory of what that reason is.

In working towards recovery, what starts out as surrendering to the positive attitudes of an invisible friend can end up being surrender to some unappealing-to-the-ego but ultimately liberating and joy-filled truths about the *ultimate* fairness and loving protection of the universe.

Terrible things do happen to people in this world. The origins of these dark events might be obscured in the fog of *thousands* of past lifetimes. By choosing to focus on the positive, many great souls throughout history have been able to bring seemingly impossible levels of peace and joy to themselves and others in spite of the karma – the perfectly balanced and ultimately fair *lifetimes* of karma – of themselves and others. But they can only do this by choosing to keep their *focus* on that which is uplifting. It's a constant choice, and it might require determined, steady mental re-training for some people.

Using sympathetic mode and an invisible friend

Many *healthy* people can flit back and forth between hosting negative thoughts and celebrating positive ones. They use *sympathetic* mode, not pause, while conjuring negative thoughts. But people with self-induced pause have increasingly *locked* themselves into cusp-of-death thinking – including the idea that they are essentially alone in the universe. Even if they believe that a higher power will show up or be with them at a *later* date, maybe after death, they are, at least for now, alone.

Unless they *work* to counter their well-practiced negative thoughts by using their heart-directed conversations instead of their brain habits, people using self-induced pause don't actually have much of a choice as to how they think. They have commanded themselves to engage in a neurological mode that, as a side effect, keeps them focused on the negatively analytical and the *feeling* of being existentially alone.

In order to feel safe enough that pause turns itself off, a person will need to go to the extreme mental position of consciously rejecting negative thoughts. As powerfully as possible until pause turns off, he will want to embrace a constant, *consuming* relationship with something or someone that represents everything that is loving and is aligned with or is part of the "good" in the universe.

There are lots of names for this "good." A religious person might call it God or a higher power. A Star Wars fan might refer to it as "the Force." A young child might call it a magic friend, an invisible friend, or a secret extra Grandma or Grandpa. One of my patients of Alaskan heritage knew it as Raven. It might be the imagined voice of a pet or an historical or even a fictional hero.

It doesn't matter who it is or what you call it. If you want to turn off self-induced pause, you are going to have to immerse yourself in the positive, the good, and the *playful* to such an extreme degree that your striatum and thalamus will become re-activated in *spite* of your previous mental instructions to be numb or apart from the world.

No Parkinson's symptoms while being "morally upright"

Then again, even though the brain might be increasingly locked into negative thinking most of the time, many of my patients with Type I PD were able to move normally when doing activities that they deemed "good": either moral or safe.

Their variations on what constituted moral or safe were all over the place. This was yet another one of the baffling symptoms of Parkinson's disease that led me to the realization that a mental component was present in most of my PD patients.

For example, some of my patients had no symptoms of PD during sex because sex – for those patients – was always a good thing. For others, sex was an activity that made their symptoms worse because, for them, sex was loaded with moral implications and judgments. For some, watching a movie was always safe. For others, watching a movie caused symptoms to increase because watching movies "isn't really productive" or "of value." One patient could always move perfectly normally when doing laundry even though she was nearly immobile the rest of the day. In her words, "Of course I can move normally when I'm doing laundry. Doing laundry is *always* a *good* thing."

Even as their symptoms of Parkinson's worsened, many people with Type I PD could nevertheless move better or even move perfectly normally while doing or thinking about doing an activity that they had decided was morally without fault: a "safe" activity.

I have already mentioned people with Parkinson's who could move normally when they got home from work, when they laid down in bed at the end of the day, or other situations that were temporary respites from being judged. The "judge" might be the person himself or it might be the imagined judgments of others. In my own case, I could always hear both my mother's critical voice judging everything I did, and my own critical voice judging others. And in many people in partial recovery, the Stomach channel qi in their legs would run perfectly normally while I was telling a joke, and only revert into the backwards-flow pause pattern as soon as I portentously said "Uh oh…"

A person on *normal*, *biological* pause should *not* able to go in and out of pause until the situation has been deemed safe and the person has gone through the steps that turn off pause. This is a biological, physiological *law*. And after pause has been turned off, it should not kick in again until a new, imminently life-threatening event occurs.

But people with *self-induced* pause don't actually have normal pause – they have a self-created hybrid of neurological modes, possibly sustained by what one might technically refer to as the use of two personalities. *One* of the personalities is using pause, on an as-needed basis – which is more and more often.

In the first decade-plus of my research, I was completely baffled by how some people could move perfectly normally while doing something they deemed "morally good" or "not currently being judged" and then revert back to pause schematics and symptoms in the blink of an eye. As mentioned earlier, this type of rapid electrical-current transition or symptom change in response to a thought is considered, in Chinese medicine, to stem from a psychological problem, not a physical one.

This come-and-go phenomenon is just one of the many abnormal behaviors that led to my reluctant hypothesis that people with Type I PD might be using a minimum of two personalities.

This is a huge subject and fully addressing it is beyond the scope of this book on Parkinson's disease. To better understand *how* people with Type I PD can have two or more sets of behaviors, including one with Parkinson's symptoms and another with normal, healthy movement while doing activities that are deemed morally upstanding, please read *Stuck on Pause.*

Again, please bear in mind that no two people with PD are alike. Throughout this book I'm generalizing. When it comes to the personality behaviors, I'm generalizing to a high degree.Also remember that *not* everyone with Parkinson's has the specific "spiritual" attitudes described in this book, but might have some secular variation of them. Also, please remember that that mental postures described in this section are associated with Type I Parkinson's, and not so much the other three types of Parkinson's disease.

A regular Joe

For an example of a person *not* having the Parkinson's personality, consider a patient with PD who was attending our free clinic (which ended in 2003), a clinic that took place in a group treatment setting (a large, open room with seven patients at a time). The patients and spouses all got to know each other fairly well over the many months. The spouse of one patient took me aside after a few months and confided, "I'm not sure we belong here. All the other patients are so intense, so brilliant. My guy is so different from all of them. He's what I call a regular Joe. He's never happier than when he's with friends, manning the barbeque with a cold beer in one hand and flipping burgers with the other."

Her "regular Joe" turned out to have *only* Type II Parkinson's. He had a foot injury from a WWII incident in which an ammunition box was dropped on his foot. Everyone in his platoon except for him died that day. He had not only dissociated from the foot injury, but from the horrors of that entire day. He had never told his wife about that day. He had no *memory* of that day until we'd been working on his foot injury for awhile. After several months of Yin Tui Na treatment on his obviously injured foot, his foot bones moved into their correct places. He suddenly recalled the events of that fateful day in the Pacific Theater of Operations. He went into severe, violent shock and went running out of the clinic, green in the face and screaming. He had to be pharmaceutically sedated for months. But the main point is that he never *told* himself to become numb. He had the normal, biological type of dissociation from his foot injury and from that entire bloody day, a dissociation that cannot go away until a person gets to a safe place. His Yin Tui Na treatment evidently was his "safe place." He also did *not* have the Parkinson's personality, although he most definitely had Parkinson's disease: *only* Type II Parkinson's disease.

The western medical term "Parkinson's personality" is a broad generalization. The description does *not* actually fit everyone with idiopathic Parkinson's disease. Long before I figured out that there are four variants of idiopathic Parkinson's, I had quite a few patients tell me, "My personality doesn't fit the description." And some of them were correct. As it turns out, the Parkinson's personality is most pronounced, if present at all, in people with Type I PD, and also manifests strongly in *some* people with Type IV PD.

Then again,

Many people who felt – at first – that the personality description *didn't* fit eventually decided that, in fact, *some* of the time, they did have some characteristics of the Parkinson's personality.

One of my Parkinson's patients insisted that she wasn't in *any* way numb or stoic, and my describing most people with Parkinson's as being numb to physical or emotional pain did not fit her at all. Also, she said she wasn't *rigidly* moral: she never outwardly criticized others even if they made flawed decisions or had wrong behaviors.

I asked her how she handled stressful situations. She was adamant that she never let herself become numb as a way of dealing with pain or stress.

At our third session, she volunteered, "I've been thinking of how I used to deal with my first husband's driving. When he was angry at me, he would drive very fast, take huge risks. He knew it scared me and it was his way of making me suffer. So I dealt with it by going into a place inside that's completely gray, where I couldn't be affected by anything. Is it possible that what I call the gray place is related to what you call 'being numb?'"

As we talked it through, she figured out that, in fact, she was very good at making herself physically and emotionally numb when her husband drove real fast. And at other times, as well.

In fact, her ability to *always* appear calm and always manifest what she called "grace under pressure" was related to her ability to "go into the gray place" to whatever degree was warranted by the situation. She had always thought of her process of becoming deeply calm (numb) as a sign of her high degree of self-control, maturity, and a spiritual ability to rise above negative emotions.

Only when she saw the relationship between what she considered her implacable poise and her use of various degrees of "the gray place" was she able to see that her constant, utter poise under pressure was in fact related to her ability to become numb. Most of the time, her use of "poise" was milder than that which she had used when her now ex-husband drove too fast. But she eventually figured out that, in every situation of stress, to varying degrees, she dealt with the stress by using pause mode, the mode of near death – not by using parasympathetic mode's joy-filled, radiant feeling of connectedness that helps a person abide with competent tranquility any situation of physical or emotional pain. Nor did she use sympathetic mode, the healthy way to confront fears.

Healthy people do *not* use pause mode as a way to maintain social poise. They use a blend of parasympathetic mode and sympathetic mode to get through the day. Pause is an exceptional mode, one that should only kick in during imminently life-threatening moments – a mode that might save your life but will also inhibit your ability to be fully alive and resonant with joy – the somatic sensations of joy that can only exist when a person feels safe, or at least not on the verge of imminent death.

As for her insistence that she was *not* morally rigid, she came to realize that, even though she was always *outwardly* loving, supportive, and non-judgmental, inside her mind she had a stark sense of right and wrong that she constantly applied in evaluating the actions and motives of others as well as those of herself.

Wrapping up this chapter on the Parkinson's personality, trying to sum things up, most of my Type I patients and some Type IV patients had an increasing *in*ability to relax and enjoy or to easily laugh at themselves. Also, most had a dread and a poor understanding of the idea of surrender.

The following paragraphs share two case study examples to help further illustrate these points. Again, bear in mind that no two people with Parkinson's manifest these personality behaviors in the exact same way.

"...made me what I am today"

One patient considered himself to be a great esoteric, meditating yogi, although he never attended his temple's group meditations nor did he meditate, because he considered that he was above all that.

Prior to meeting this patient, many of my *recovered* patients had mentioned a feeling of profound surrender to God or some higher power during the moment when they suddenly and permanently turned off their Parkinson's. I had not yet figured out how a person could restart his striatum by talking to a friend.

Therefore, I was talking with this new patient about the possibility that "surrender to the Divine" (a yogic phrase that I thought he might be familiar with) might be helpful.

My patient was disgusted at this idea. He sat, rigid and immobile, on the sofa in my office, tremoring violently, held up by his full-time aide.

His voice, long since reduced to the merest of whispers, proudly produced the words, "I'm very successful. I make *way* more money than you. And it's my *refusal* to surrender that's made me what I am today!"

I was deeply saddened by his response and, observing his almost utter immobility and ceaseless, powerful tremor, replied, "I couldn't agree with you more."

Another patient's caregiver told me about her client's pride in being "free from emotion."

"One day, after I drove him home from his evening meditation group and helped him to the door, I noticed that all the furniture was missing from his living room. A note was taped on the banister saying that his wife had left and her lawyer would be contacting his lawyer. She hadn't even told him she was *thinking* of leaving. It was a shocking surprise. I felt so terrible for him, and asked him if he wanted me to stay with him for a while. "He replied so proudly, 'No. I'm fine. This is the third time a wife has left me. I'm not upset. I don't feel anything at all. I've risen above having those kinds of emotions.'"

The caregiver continued, "I think that's when I finally started to understand what you were writing about in your book on Parkinson's."

I provided the above examples of the Parkinson's personality to drive home that people with Type I PD might have a ferocious battle ahead if they think they can conquer their highly honed, well practiced mental stoicism and emotional boundaries by confronting them with a few weak, new, unpracticed thoughts. That would be the brain fighting the brain. The new thoughts *cannot* hope win that battle. The part of the brain with the strongest habits will win that battle every time.

In cases like these, the brain can only be retrained to a state of healthy obedience by the heart. The heart, supported and instructed by the constant companionship of an invisible friend, can, either easily *or* eventually, assume its rightful role in regulating the behaviors of the brain and destroying behaviors that are no longer needed. In Chinese medicine, the King of the body, the heart, is the only one who can rein in an out-of-control "governor," the brain.

A person who wants to turn off self-induced pause must choose to live as constantly as possible in a completely different world from the false one he created when he put himself on pause: he must return to a heart-dominated world inhabited by his invisible friend(s), friends who love and can laugh with him. This person must refuse, over and over, to listen to or engage with his own negative thought habits.

Often, people with Parkinson's do not know that there is any way of being other than the one that they have created in themselves. One patient told me, "A friend took me to a concert and I kept looking around and remarking on what people were doing. At one point she said to me, 'Just relax and enjoy the music!' I have no idea what she was talking about…no idea what she wanted me to do."

Oppositely, another patient, a few days after recovering, left me a phone message saying, "Hi, sorry I blew off my appointment with you today. I found myself sitting on the beach watching the seagulls and I realized I've *never* just sat and watched the seagulls. The sensation of just enjoying the sights was so new and delightful I decided to stay at the beach instead of going to see you. I figured, What the heck, it's not like anyone's going to die if I miss my appointment."

When we met later in the week, I congratulated her on being "irresponsible" for the first time in her life: for choosing spontaneity instead of "sticking to the plan," choosing joy rather than "correctness," for deciding/ realizing that she wasn't, in fact, constantly on the verge of death: wasn't keeping death at bay by being "good."

Although this chapter has wandered far from its starting point of merely defining the Parkinson's personality, it has hopefully given the reader a basis for comparing his own thoughts and mental behaviors with those that are common in people with self-induced pause. This information might be helpful when going through the next chapter, which explains how to determine which *type* of PD a person has.

Of course, each person's manifestation of the Parkinson's personality, if any, will be somewhat unique and personalized. When people create their own mental justifications and behavioral rules, rules that apply only to themselves and no one else, you can end up with a near infinitude of mental and behavioral possibilities.

Trying to capture in one short chapter the enormous range of personality variations I've seen is impossible. And yet, certain themes arise over and over: wariness, anxiety, "don't make waves," a powerful moral compass, a sense of mental/moral superiority, a relentless intensity of purpose, stoicism, poise under pressure via numbness, increasing difficulty in feeling joy or *sorrow*, and a feeling of repulsion towards the idea of surrender.

Many readers have emailed me something like, "I just read your book: have you been reading my mind?" or "I think you must be spying on me!" One wrote, "I never thought anyone could know what it's like inside my mind and body. You've described my most secret thoughts."

I have not been mind-reading or spying. But I have worked with hundreds of people with Parkinson's disease, most of whom had Type I PD from self-induced pause. For that matter, I had it myself. So I do have a general sense of what it looks and feels like, including the personality components. I also learned a lot about what happens to them during recovery, as will be discussed in the upcoming chapters on recovery symptoms.

Getting a good diagnosis can be a crucial step in recovering from an illness. If you are now pretty sure that you have Parkinson's disease and you think you might fit the personality profile described in this chapter, you probably have Type I PD. If you aren't sure about the personality, ask a spouse or close friend. Many patients have told me at a first meeting that they don't fit the PD personality profile at all, causing the spouse to erupt in laughter, "Oh yes you do! You fit it perfectly!" Then again, one spouse was adamant that her husband had Type I PD based on his personality and thought patterns. In fact, he had Type IV. The damage to his cranium from the car accident was so severe that almost no channel qi was flowing through his midbrain. After many craniosacral treatments, when his skull bones repositioned themselves back into correct position, he exclaimed, "I'm blissed out!" He was feeling joy for the first time in years. His real personality was very positive and upbeat. He'd only manifested the Parkinson's personality during the twenty years following a car accident. In the world of Parkinson's, twenty years in the life of a seventy-year old is a relatively short span.

Even if you can't decide whether or not you have some aspects of the Parkinson's personality, don't despair. You can use the tests in the next chapter to determine what type of PD you have.

Chapter Seventeen

Differentiating the Four Types of PD

If you've decided that you or that your friend or loved one does in fact have Parkinson's disease, this chapter will walk you through the steps that I take to determine what *type* of Parkinson's a person has.

The exercises in this chapter are focused on determining whether a person is 1) on pause or 2) has pseudo pause from an unhealed, dissociated injury or 3) both. Figuring out whether the pause or dissociation is *self-induced* or not comes later.

As we go through this chapter, we *start* with the assumption that the person in question has Type I PD, Parkinson's from self-induced pause. The tests in this chapter are used to filter out the 5 or 6% of people who have *only* Type II or Type III PD: Parkinson's from pseudo pause.

Pause and pseudo pause each require very different treatments to get turned off. If a person *only* has Type II or Type III PD, the tests in this chapter will let him know that. If a person has *both* Type I and Type II, the most common presentation, he needs to focus on recovering from Type I. When Type I has cleared up, then he can focus on any remaining physical injuries from which he has dissociated. A case study at the end of the chapter gives an example of this.

Diagnostic test #1: temporarily inducing pause mode

This test has two parts. It can make clear what it feels like to 1) *be* on pause and 2) *not* be on pause. The exercise allows any person to *temporarily* experience pause mode, and feel some of the accompanying physical sensations or lack thereof, as well as feeling some of the mental/emotional shifts that might occur on pause. A friend or family member, if any, who is going to work with the person with PD can also do this test, to learn what it feels like to be stuck on pause.

- If you are *not* already stuck on pause, you will be able to temporarily experience and compare pause and not-on-pause by doing the following exercises.
- If you *are* stuck on pause, you will probably not be able to feel much difference while doing the two parts of the exercise – that's how this exercise is a diagnostic test.

Part A) <u>*Not* on pause:</u>

Close your eyes. Imagine a current moving up your back, from the lowest part of the back up into the neck and head. The current is about an eighth of an inch under the skin and about a quarter of an inch wide. This current follows the path of the Du channel.

Your imaginary current can be made out of anything moveable: light, electricity, wind, water, warmth, coolness, or a tingly feeling – anything at all that you can imagine as moving. Imagine you can feel this energy as it flows easily just under the skin that lies over the spine. Imagine that the energy travels from the bottom, the "base," of the spine, up to the neck, into the neck vertebrae, up the brain stem, and through the center of the brain over to the center of the forehead. Imagine it emerging from the brain at the forehead and flowing down the face, staying just under the skin, down to the upper lip and into the mouth. This is the pathway that the Du channel follows when a person is in parasympathetic mode. If you are *not* on pause, this should be very easy to imagine. You shouldn't have to make any effort.

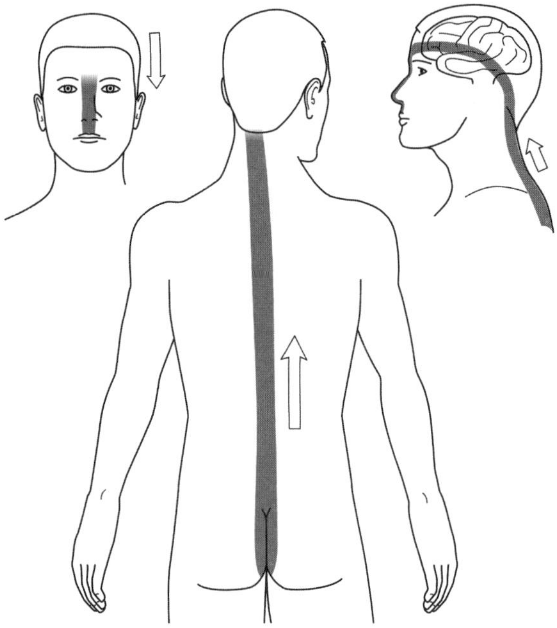

If your immediate response to these instructions was "I can't do visualization," you are probably on pause – either biological or self-induced. But even if you can't usually do visualizations, give it a try.

Fig. 17.1 The Du channel in parasympathetic mode

Part B) On pause:

Repeat the above exercise but *this* time, imagine you are *stopping* the flow of the Du channel at the base of the neck. Do *not* allow any current to flow up into the head. Feel that you have created a holding pattern, a standing wave, in the current that runs over your spine. There might be energy along your spine, but don't allow it to move up into the neck or head.

Maintain this holding pattern for up to five minutes, if you can stand to do it for that long. After about five minutes or maybe even sooner, start noticing the changes in your muscles, your facial expression, and your thoughts. Notice the vague sense of oppression, constriction, or numbness in the vicinity of your heart. This constriction is the opposite of the expansion in the heart area that accompanies joy. Within just a minute or two, your muscles may feel as if they are tensing up a bit. Your arms might even be bending at the elbow, pulling in, becoming rigid along the biceps.

Your facial muscles might be getting saggy, if relaxed, or stony, if concerned. Your thoughts may be wary, and might include notions such as "I *really* don't like doing this" or even "This is horrible; I feel like I'm dying." Your sense of having a resonant area in your chest that expands or contracts with joy or sorrow, respectively, will feel increasingly deadened the longer you keep this up. In this book, this resonance is referred to with several different phrases, including heart feeling, heart awareness, and heart sensations. These terms do *not* refer to heart palpitations, which are the worrisome, tangible sensations of your heart's muscular beating.

As you continue to imagine that no energy is able to move from your back up into the neck, you might want to add a second channel blockage in your neck. Ordinarily, the energy in the back of your head in the UB channels, slightly to the left and right sides of the Du channel, flows from the head down into the neck, and then staying just under the skin, flows down the back torso and under the scapula (shoulder blades).

When on *pause*, the UB channel *usually* cannot flow easily in its usual path down into the torso. Instead, the UB channel usually becomes blocked at the neck, just above UB-11.

Note: the drawing of the Du channel on pause has *no* arrows showing directional movement. For a nice metaphor, we read in the ancient Chinese description that when this stoppage occurs, the Du channel ceases to be a river and becomes "like a reservoir."

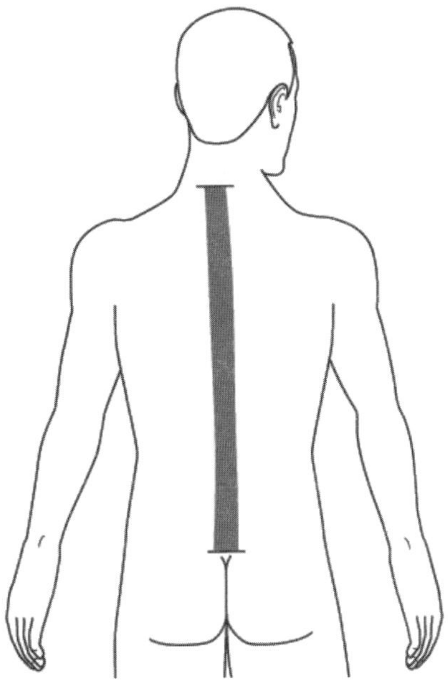

Fig 17.2 The Du channel in pause mode: blocked at the neck

If you want to make the pause-like experience more intense, 1) continue to imagine that Du channel energy *cannot* travel up into the neck *and* 2) imagine that the energy in the UB channel, on the left and right *sides* of the Du channel, *cannot* flow down into your shoulders. Instead, imagine it flowing outward into space from just above UB-11. After a minute or two of this, you might notice that you now perceive yourself as being slightly outside of your own body. A common "outside" location is an inch or so behind the back of the neck.

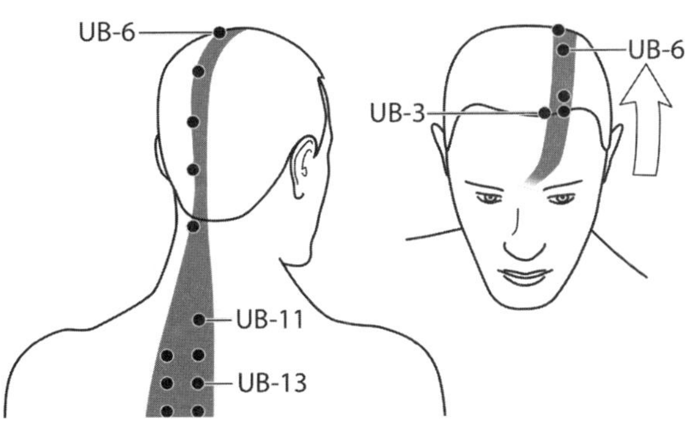

Fig.17.3 The healthy, parasympathetic head and neck portion of the left-side UB channel.

Although it is difficult to discern in this angled pose, the left-and right-side UB channels, after departing from the point between the eyebrows, are just off to the *sides* of the Du channel, and flow from the head down to the toes: flow in the opposite direction of the healthy Du.

The neck blockages of these two UB channels and the Du, along with the increasing rigidity in the body, the oppression in the chest around the heart, and the sense of being outside of one's body are all symptoms of being on pause.

By imagining that energy cannot traverse the back of the neck in either direction, you will be able to make temporary blockages in both the Du and the UB channel. This blocked channel qi behavior is normal during pause mode.

Have you felt for long enough what it's like to be on pause? Let the currents resume moving through your neck and head again.

Please don't worry about getting stuck on pause just by doing this exercise. As soon as you resume the flow of energy through your neck, with both the Du flowing up into the neck and the UB flowing down from the head into the shoulders, all those weird pause symptoms will go away…assuming you were *not* already stuck on pause before you started this exercise.

Assessment

Here's the diagnostic part: if you are stuck on pause, you might not have felt much difference between the physical sensations of part A and part B.

Oppositely, if you could *easily* imagine a current moving up into the neck and head in part A and if it felt good, normal, and even automatic, requiring no mental labor on your part to make the current go into the neck and head *and* if you felt uneasy or strangely inhibited during part B, then you are probably *not* stuck on pause. If you have PD and cannot relate to any part of the Parkinson's personality and are not stuck on pause, then you have *only* Type II or *only* Type III PD. You can move on to the next chapter or stick around and do the next test, if you like.

More details on the Part A response

When doing part A, imagining healthy, parasympathetic current moving up your neck and into your head, if you felt a little giddy at first (an unaccustomed surge of dopamine release that won't last), you are probably stuck on pause. If doing part A made you feel even *more* wary than usual or more vulnerable, or maybe experiencing the thought, "I shouldn't be doing this" or, if you felt a tightening or discomfort, or even the fear of *potential* discomfort, in your heart, stomach, throat or other area, you are probably stuck on pause. If you simply feel "not normal" while imagining energy flowing up your neck and into your head, you are probably stuck on pause. If it takes mental *work* to imagine energy moving up into your neck and head, as opposed to just observing that energy is, in fact, already flowing in this path, you are probably stuck on pause. If you *can* imagine energy flowing up into your head *but* you sense that the energy stops flowing into your head as soon as you stop forcing it, you are probably stuck on pause.

When doing part B, preventing current from going up into the neck and head, if you felt more "normal" or more "natural" or it's "easier" when you *prevent* current from going into your head, you are probably stuck on pause. If you feel more familiar with *allowing* the current to stop at the base of the neck or skull, you are probably stuck on pause.

If you simply could not do the exercise of imagining energy flowing up your neck and into your head, you are probably stuck on pause. If you couldn't feel, imagine, or visualize anything, or can't understand the assignment, you are probably stuck on pause.

For that matter, if you do not know what is *meant* by the words "the resonant area in your chest that expands or contracts with joy or sorrow, respectively," you are probably stuck on pause and may have been for a long, long time. If all the other references to "heart feeling" (an actual, physical *sensation*) or "heart resonance" (an actual, intuitional *sensation*) in this book don't make sense, you are probably stuck on pause. You'll want to focus on turning off pause before you think about dealing with any injuries.

Semantics – an aside

The pericardium is the highly conductive connective tissue around your heart. The pericardium generates and regulates the sensations of heart feelings such as joy, sorrow, and soul-satisfying peace. The heart sensations associated with peace and joy (sensations that are usually elusive to a person on pause) include a sense of vibratory expansion in the chest. This is not the physical expansion of the chest that comes with inhalation. It's a subtle feeling as if the electrical field of influence around your heart has gotten larger.

Feeling peaceful does *not* mean experiencing numbness or drowsiness, as many people with Type I PD wrongly assume. Feeling peace in your heart is a distinct, expansive sensation. It is *not* the absence of sensation. When on pause, *awareness* of the sensations generated by changes in the pericardium is inhibited.

The phrases "open your heart" or "be open-hearted" are instructions to redirect more of your awareness towards the actual *sensations* of electrical, resonance-driven expansion of awareness in the chest driven by increased amperage in the pericardium. By doing so, you expand the number of electromagnetic frequencies with which the connective tissue around the heart can literally "tune in."

If you think that phrases such as "be open-hearted" are used to imply "think good thoughts" or "be nice," you might be stuck on pause. The reason you don't associate heart-feeling phrases with the actual sensations in the chest is because you don't feel these sensations. You may have been going through life assuming that references to heart feeling or being "open hearted" were metaphors or poetic references to being good or kind. They weren't. They were meant literally.

I'll repeat this because this concept can be new and even unsettling – or even ignored – by someone long on pause. I have spoken with many people with PD who told me, "I read every word of your books, except for the heart stuff, which doesn't actually have anything to do with Parkinson's." The subject of heart-feeling *is* related to the subject of self-induced pause. It has to do with feel-able changes, sensations of expansion and contraction, in the heart area. These sensations are driven by the changes in the electrical field around your pericardium that occur in response to thought and mood changes.

Then again, if you have always known that "open your heart" means "tune in to the sense of expansion in your chest as you focus on something joyful," or something along those lines, you are probably *not* on self-induced pause. You *probably* aren't on biological pause, either, unless it is of such recent origin that you still remember what heart feelings are. You probably have *only* Type II or *only* Type III PD: PD from dissociation, not from pause mode.

Diagnostic test #2: outside the body

This test will help you determine if you go through your moments of self-awareness by *feeling* your body from the inside *or* by *looking* at yourself from some location outside of your actual body.

The inside or outside the body test

Close your eyes. Imagine you are walking down a lovely tree-lined street. It's a beautiful day. Birds are chirping. A gentle breeze is rustling the leaves. The sky is blue.

Take ten to twenty seconds to imagine this. Then ask yourself this question: Are you experiencing the stroll from *inside* your body, *feeling* your sensations of walking and *feeling* the pleasant expansion in your heart area as you hear the birds? Or are you numbly *looking* at your body as you stroll down the street?

If you are outside of your body, looking at it, can you equally easily imagine yourself inside your body, experiencing the sensations of stride and well-being from within? If you are *unable* to imagine yourself inside your body, or it takes a bit of work, or it's hard to make your sensory awareness *stay* inside once it's put there, you are probably on pause.

If you imagine that *most* of your self-awareness is inside of your body but one arm or one leg, or maybe your heart area, or some combination of specific body parts are observed from the outside, or maybe your feet are "missing," you might be dissociated from those body parts, but you are very likely *not* on pause. With pause, one usually perceives himself as outside of his body altogether. With dissociation, a person might imagine one or a few specific areas as being inaccessible or viewable only from the outside, but the rest of the body is able to feel that it is inside, rather than outside, the body proper.

If you tend to observe or think of your body as if you are outside of it, looking at yourself instead of *feeling* your existence by using the resonance of your heart (pericardium, actually) as your primary point of reference, you are very likely stuck on pause.

Why do this test?

This test serves two purposes. The first is diagnostic: most people with Type I or Type IV PD perceive themselves as *outside* of their bodies. If you have symptoms of PD *but* are *inside* your body, you probably have *only* Type II or *only* Type III PD.

The other reason I do this test is to help the sometimes resistant patient with Type I PD realize that he is, in fact, using pathological self-perception. Many people with Type I PD are adamant that they have *no* psychological factors involved. Sometimes, the realization that they perceive themselves as if outside of their bodies is just weird enough that they start to *consider* that they *might* in fact have a problem in the mind as *well* as in the body.

Variations on "outside the body"

If, when you speak, you imagine the words being typewritten as you speak or spelled out on the "video screen" of your imagination, you may be stuck on pause.

If you mentally use *words* or *logic* to self-assess how you are feeling instead of checking in with your wordless *sensations* of expansion and contraction in your heart area you may be stuck on pause.

If you move by mentally *commanding* your body to move rather than by enjoying the vibrant or languorous sensations of motor actions that occur automatically and immediately in response to thinking about or *imagining* moving your body, and especially if you don't know what this sentence means, you are probably stuck on pause.

If you have no idea what I mean by "*feeling* your body from the inside" or "heart feelings" you are probably stuck on pause.

Yoga and Qi Gong responses – more variations on "outside the body"

Consider your experiences, if any, with yoga, meditation, Qi Gong, or Tai Ji Chuan (aka Tai Chi). If these self-awareness techniques have not brought you the promised heart feelings of peaceful, expansive joy, you might be on pause. If you have done years of the above practices and have done them without feeling a steady increase in child-like joy and playful sensations of energy flooding the various body parts as they are moved or are focused on, you might be on pause.

If you do the above types of movement or stillness while trying to make your body and/or its movements symmetrical, uniform, mechanical, or "correct," as opposed to noticing and enjoying the pleasant or even thrilling sensations of life force moving around inside you, you may well be on pause.

On the other hand, *if* you enjoy doing these types of self-improvement exercises because they help you turn off your internal monologue and let you savor, *wordlessly*, the heightened awareness of somatic energy in your various body parts, you are probably *not* on pause. If you like doing the yogic "corpse pose" because you love the heightened awareness of energy being released from your muscles and flowing up your spine and into your head and heart, and your increased awareness of somatic resonance with joy in the deep stillness of your body, you are probably *not* on pause. If you do have PD and feel these joys while doing these exercises, you probably have *only* Type II or *only* Type III: pseudo pause brought about by an unhealed or incompletely healed injury from which you have dissociated.

Then again, if you like doing the yogic "corpse pose" because it lets you "turn off" and/or pretend you are numb or dead, you are probably on pause.

Of my Parkinson's patients who have steadily practiced the movement and meditative arts (a surprisingly high percent), most have told me that their decades of silent meditation, yoga asanas, Qi Gong forms, Tai Chi or other "spiritual" movement exercises have *not* led to increased awareness of inner joy or heart resonance. Just the opposite: they have felt less and less joy and/or less heart feeling over the years, despite decades of doing these supposedly "uplifting" exercises.

Also, many of them have said that "corpse" is their favorite yoga pose because it lets them feel *still*, or even numb – the *opposite* of the real purpose of the corpse pose.[1]

---

[1]Vocabulary note: for those who do certain types of Buddhist or Vedic meditation, remember that going into the so-called "emptiness" refers to turning off ego-driven thoughts and constant mental chatter. It does *not* mean becoming *numb* to the joy that vibrates silently behind every atom. The word "emptiness" is a poor translation. "Realm of intangible vibrations of love" or "place of love-filled absence of ego" might have been better choices than the English word "emptiness." I have had Buddhist PD patients, including Buddhist monks and even teachers, whose first language was English, who were stuck on self-induced pause. In *every* case, they had wrongly assumed that the word "emptiness" means numbness, even joylessness!

The English/American language doesn't even have a commonly used word or phrase that means "heart expansion from joy." In English we don't have common phrases that mean "*joie de vivre*" (French) or *kai xin* (Chinese, literally the heart (Xin) expanding in the way a flower bud unfurls (Kai)) – usually translated into English as the insipid word "happy." We don't have an

Only Type II or Type III

If you felt the sensations of walking down the street as if you were inside your body, *feeling* your arms swinging and/or legs striding, you are probably not on pause. If you find the above descriptions of doing yoga or Qi Gong as mechanical exercises laughable or bizarre because you do them for the playful or even thrilling feelings of energy moving around in your body, you are not on pause. If, in Test #1, you could easily imagine Du channel energy going up into your neck and head, that's further confirmation that you aren't on pause. If you also can't relate to the Parkinson's personality at all and even your spouse says "Nah, that's not you," you can be pretty certain you are *not* on pause. If you have PD, it is from pseudo pause causing either Type II or Type III.

The brain's visualizing behaviors

The previous two tests looked at body-wide behaviors. Sometimes it can be helpful to know if an injury or numbness at a *specific* location is unable to heal because of

---

English phrase that means the consciousness of God made thrillingly, electrically manifest as energy and matter. We do have it in Latin: *spiritus sanctus*. Literally, this phrase means "the Sacred breath (of God)," or "the thoughts of God made manifest as vibrations of energy." This beautiful phrase has been very poorly translated into English christian scripture as "Holy Ghost," of all things.

To illustrate the translation challenges, here's an example from signage in India, the homeland of the Buddha and of Krishna and Rama. I noticed, in ashrams in India, dual language signs in Hindi and English at the entrance to some of the meditation halls. The Hindi message had two words. The first word is a verb that can mean "keep" or "stay." (This same verb is used in signs that mean, "Keep off the grass," or you might say, "Stay off the grass.") The second word in the phrase is "shanti," which is usually inadequately translated into English as "peace." These two words together *might* be translated into English as "keep peaceful: stay full of quiet, radiant, joy."

But the signs' translations into English say, "Maintain silence."

The words shanti and silence have utterly different *underlying* meanings. Sweet heart expansion is implied in "shanti." Self-control and rigidity might be implied in "Silence!"

Peace is a dynamic heart-feeling. Many people stuck on pause are not able to access this feeling, or even understand that the word peace can *refer* to an actual sensation: a sensation of expansion or increased heart-attunement coming from the pericardium. Many English speakers who have long been stuck on pause even think that the word "peace" means "motionless," and point to the phrase, "a peaceful evening" as an example. But I doubt the word "motionless" could be applied to the greatly dynamic Jesus, who is sometimes described as a "Prince of Peace."

This footnote is here to point out how hard it is to describe the sensations of heart-joy and heart-peace using English words. Specific words for these sensations *do* exist in other languages.

People who have not experienced heart feelings for a long time – because they are stuck on pause – might have no way of knowing just what they are missing. And if they are English speakers they do not even have a *vocabulary* to explain. Instead, many of my patients have said things like, "I don't even know what the word joy means anymore," or, more simply, "I'm depressed."

Then again, a non-PD patient who only spoke Spanish, when she first felt channel qi resume its flow in her long numbed arm, shared her joy by pointing her finger up and down her arm, over and over, exclaiming "Espirito Santo! Espirito Santo!": God's love made manifest had returned to her arm. At least she had words for it. English speakers do not.

pause or because of dissociation. This can be especially helpful in looking for the location(s) of injury that is keeping *biological* pause in place, causing Type IV PD.

The information in this next section is only an introduction. The subject is developed more fully in the book *Stuck on Pause*. I'm putting this information here, as well, to help explain the diagnostics I use in the upcoming case study.

Determining if a localized area is unable to heal because of pause or because of dissociation is done by *mentally* looking at the locations where injury has occurred or where energy seems to stop flowing.

When trying to visualize unhealed injured or traumatized areas by imagining light and/or darkness inside the body at these areas, the brain tends towards two distinct types of mental images. One type of mental image is set in motion by being dissociated. The other type is set in motion by being on pause.

Dissociation

When a person is dissociated from a body part, if he tries to imagine that body part first filled with light, and then filled with dark, he finds it easier to imagine it filled with dark. The darkness will manifest as being still, motionless, maybe even invisible. The person might find himself saying, "I don't know what I'm trying to look for..."

That's because the brain is saying, as per previous instruction, "There's nothing there."

Pause

If a person is on pause, when he tries to imagine light and then dark in some part of his body where he can't imagine the channel qi flowing easily or his channel-feeling friend or health practitioner cannot feel the channel qi flowing, the person usually finds it easier to imagine that part of his body filled with dark than with light.

However, unlike the deep stillness or invisibility that is perceived in body parts from which a person has dissociated, the areas of the body associated with being on pause will appear to be dark and *agitated.* This imagined visual perception of agitation can take the form of tiny movement, as if the atoms are moving too quickly back and forth. Or as if the capillaries are moving in an agitated manner. Or the perception of movement in the dark area might seem like drifting smoke, or sludge. The point is, there is a sense that something isn't settled. The area is *not* rhythmically or peacefully calm. Again, *unsettled movement* of any type within the imagined darkness is associated with being on pause.

This perception of movement is related to the normal, healthy brain processes for coming out of pause. The first step in turning off pause is assessment. The brain has to pay attention to the injured and/or pause-inducing area. When you bring your attention to or mentally imagine looking at a body location associated with being on pause, your brain tells you that this area isn't settled: it's agitated. This sense of agitation is a call for attention. The sense of agitation is produced in the part of the *brain* associated with that body part, *not* in the actual body part. People with a *missing* limb can feel this type of agitation in the limb that isn't there. Again, the agitation associated with a traumatized body part when doing visualization is actually coming from the brain, not the body part.

This brain behavior is *supposed* to keep your attention on or bring even *greater* attention to the traumatized part of the body, This helps the brain focus on the area, assess it, and move forward with healing, once the life-threatening situation has been stabilized.

People who are *stuck* on pause are mentally avoiding, ignoring, or disregarding these attention-getting brain behaviors. If the traumatized area is still being imagined as agitated even though the physical damage from the trauma has long been healed, it means that the brain is stuck in an avoidance behavior – ignoring the area that is agitated. If the brain is forced to pay attention to the area, it will notice that the area is agitated – still causing the body to be on pause even though the traumatized location has long since stabilized. In terms of treatment, turning off a situation in which a person is stuck in biological pause will begin with focusing on the area(s) that appears agitated.

Assessing motionless versus agitated perceptions at a specific location is a simple way to determine whether a person is dealing with an injury or trauma by using dissociation or by using pause.

Body-wide trauma

Not every pause-inducing trauma is site-specific. Some people go into biological pause while nearly dying from a *body-wide* trauma such as an anaphylactic response to a bee sting, a near-drowning incident, or some other near-death, physical or emotional shock that hits the whole body. In these cases of body-wide trauma, the areas that become perceived as agitated (when imagined) are often areas along the spine: the sacrum, the base of the neck, the brain stem's medulla oblongata, and/or the area of the spine near to the heart.

In some people who are stuck in biological pause, a sense of agitation might be present in an injury-specific site *and* in various areas along the spine and neck.

People who are stuck on self-induced pause have visualizing behaviors similar to those of people who are stuck on biological pause. But if pause was induced in response to emotional, not physical trauma, the perceived agitation, *if any*, might appear at the sacrum, the base of the neck or even inside the head, instead of at some injury site.

The next two sections explain a little more about *why* an agitation situation develops in people on *biological* pause, and how it can be treated, thus allowing pause to turn off.

Paying attention to the agitation

In a healthy response to a trauma, keeping one's attention on the injury site or areas that the brain registers as agitated helps process the injury. The brain can decide whether or not the trauma has stabilized. When it has, if the agitation signal is then turned off, pause turns off and the deepest levels of healing commence in the damaged area.

In animals, a sense of agitation *perceived* as coming from the damaged area induces the animal to lick and rub the injured spot, optimizing blood flow in the vicinity and speeding the healing. Once the sense of agitation turns off, the area can be re-assessed as stable and healthy or at least healthy enough to come back to life. Turning off pause can then occur.

In people who get *stuck* on pause, they haven't yet brought their conscious attention to the traumatized or mentally agitated area, or they're mentally telling it "not now," or they just don't know how to begin going about processing the trauma. For whatever reason, the body isn't able to clear the trauma from this area, and the brain keeps perceiving the area as agitated, and the body stays stuck on pause.

Contrast this with the brain's perceptions of a dissociated area: there's darkness and stillness because the brain's pretending there's nothing there – just like it's *supposed* to do after a significant injury. The dissociation continues until you come to a safe place and then the body can re-associate with the pain or the injury, and start the healing process. Or, the area stays dark and dissociated in your brain because you never find a safe place *or* because you *told* the brain to not acknowledge that body part or the injury.

"You're going to be OK"

Humans trying to stabilize after a pause-inducing trauma benefit from being told by someone, anyone, "It's OK; you're going to be OK." Offering words that confirm "You're going to be OK" is an almost *automatic* human response to someone, even a complete stranger, who is on pause.

Usually, we can hear this "I'm going to be OK" message coming from our own heart. But if we are in a high degree of pause, we might need to hear this from someone *outside* of ourselves. We might also hear it from a stranger, a loved one, or a guardian angel. But we need to hear it from somewhere. Otherwise, we stay on pause. If we have shut down our heart by commanding ourselves to not feel, then we're in a bind – we have no way to initiate the feeling of safety that's needed for coming out of pause.

In surgical recovery rooms, where people are trying to come out from under the effects of anesthesia, patients often cry out, "Help me! Help me!" Even if someone says, "I'm right here, you're going to be OK," which is the correct thing to say, the patient might slide back into the effects of the anesthesia for a while. As he comes to the surface again, he might say, "Help me!" again, having no idea that he's already said it before. This can go on for quite a while. Still, the correct response, every time, is "You're going to be OK." That's what the brain is needing to know. When the body has been on the verge of death or coma, the brain *needs* to be told by the heart, or by the nurse standing by, or by the imagined voice of his deceased pet dog, "You're OK. You're going to be OK." This allows the body to start taking the steps that turn off pause.

Many people who are *stuck* on biological pause were never told that they were alright, or were going to be alright. They weren't given time to fully process their trauma. They were on the verge of death but were jerked rudely back into activity, requiring activation of a norepinephrine response. Pause never got a chance to get turned off.

In working with people who are stuck on *biological* pause, the patient can make use of an imaginary friend. While mentally focusing on the body part that seems agitated, the patient silently asks the imaginary friend, "Am I going to die in the next few minutes from this trauma that happened years ago?" The imaginary friend, speaking truth, will always say, "No. You survived." And then, if and when the patient is finally – usually reluctantly – able to agree with the friend that he is, in fact, alive and no longer at risk of *imminent* death from that specific trauma, while he continues mentally focusing on the area that is perceived as agitated, the patient will be able to go through the steps that turn off pause. Those steps, you will recall, include confirming that the situation is now safe, taking a deep, audible breath, then bobbling the head and shimmying the spine. The agitation will cease. More on this subject is included in the book *Stuck on Pause*.

Then again, if the patient perceives that the area is *not* agitated, if it is perceived as still and motionless, the problem is dissociation. The treatment is very, very different from the treatment for stuck on pause. The treatment involves turning off the avoidance behavior in the brain. More on this subject is included in the book *Yin Tui Na*.

Very few people with PD have Type IV. This introduction to the treatment for Type IV PD was included here to help explain why differentiating between the brain perceptions of "motionless inside" and "agitated inside" can be important, and how an imaginary friend can help in a highly specific way if a person is stuck on *biological* pause. We already discussed the imaginary friend being helpful for self-induced pause. The friend can also be helpful in people with biological pause in the manner discussed above.

I needed to introduce these concepts here in order to explain the upcoming case study. To wrap up this chapter, I'll share a case study where the PD patient was using self-induced pause *and* was dissociated from an injury – although *not* a pause-inducing injury.

Case study: finger on the chopping block

Eight months earlier, I worked with a PD patient over the course of two sessions, a few weeks apart. Now, she had almost completely recovered from PD. About a year and a half before she started working with me, she'd had an accident with a kitchen knife. She'd lost mobility in her fourth finger after the knife had sliced the finger nearly to the bone. The finger appeared to be completely healed, but she couldn't feel or bend her finger. She was a professional pianist. She assumed this loss of feeling and flexibility meant the end of her career. Her doctor wrote off her loss as a permanent disability and told her that cut nerves can't heal. (He was wrong. They can.[1])

I held her finger for a few moments in a Yin Tui Na hold. The finger was utterly unresponsive.

I asked her to close her eyes and imagine she was looking for light, and then dark, in her injured fourth finger. Not only was her fourth finger dark and *motionless*, she said it was impossible to find. It simply wasn't there. This meant she had dissociated from her finger, probably at the time of injury.

Then I asked her to imagine she *did* have a fourth finger *somewhere*, and it was filled with beautiful light. She told me when she was finally able to do this. I asked her *where* the fourth finger she was looking at was located.

She replied with surprise, "It's on the cutting board in my mother-in-law's house!" She opened her eyes and asked, "How can my finger heal, how can I get feeling and flexibility in it if it's still in my mother-in-law's house?" She was utterly surprised that her mind had played this dissociation trick on her because she had always thought she was very much in control of her mind.

---

[1] Dr. Peter Carney, MD, presented findings at the American Academy of Pain Medicine 2020 Annual Meeting (Abstract 421, Feb 29, 2020) that electric cell signaling (similar to the treatments in which acupuncture needles are hooked up to electrical stimulation machines) can reduce or completely terminate pain from painful peripheral neuropathy (PPN). Patients treated with the electrical stimulation "over a 6- to 12-weeks period experienced a 100% increase in nerve density. Pain scores were reduced by 90%, and the treatment was also associated with a 74% improvement in physical funtion."

Carney said, "…we are using physics, not pharmacology, to regenerate nerves…" https://www.medscape.com/viewarticle/926002 .

She was able to restore her finger "back to life" by doing the light and energy exercise for dissociated body parts, an exercise in the *Yin Tui Na* book.

I had first started working with her because of her early-stage Parkinson's disease. She had been using self-induced pause since she was a child, when she was physically abused and kept locked in a very small closet most of the day by her caregiver, a resentful family relation. The abuse lasted from age two to age seven. It ended when her mother came home early one day and discovered the situation.

Because she was still using self-induced pause when she hurt her finger, the finger remained dissociated even after the injury superficially healed. After the normal, automatic dissociation occurred in response to her finger injury, she was never able to "feel safe" enough to turn off that automatic dissociation process. She didn't feel safe enough because she was stuck on self-induced pause. She remained mentally dissociated from her injured finger even after the skin and muscle superficially healed over.

Eight months earlier she had started working on turning off her self-induced pause. She was doing very well. Her Parkinson's symptoms were gone. I had only met with her a couple of times, doing an assessment and then explaining that she needed to talk to some invisible friend. She had done the work on her own. And she had recovered from her symptoms of PD. More importantly, according to her, as a musician, she was able to feel again, both somatically and emotionally. She was going to be able to bring this new sense of heart feeling into her music. However, her finger had remained numb.

The re-association work on her finger was quick and easy. It took one session. Recovering from self-induced pause had taken much longer: nearly eight months. Her invisible friend was her mother, who had died five years earlier from stomach cancer. She worked on developing her relationship with her now "invisible" mother for many months before the presence of her mother started to feel real. After her mother's presence felt real to her, the PD symptoms quickly went away over the next few months.

When she'd been using self-induced pause, her whole body felt sort of numb. Also, she'd been aware that she observed herself as if outside of her body. But even after turning off pause and getting her self-awareness and somatic awareness back inside her body, her *finger* still wasn't a part of her body. Her Parkinson's was gone, but her finger was still in her mother-in-law's house.

The co-existence of both dissociation and pause – or dissociation and *self-induced* pause, in this case – is common. In cases where both are present, it's *always* best to first work on turning off pause, and *then* work on the dissociation(s), if any. Very often, the dissociations will cease on their own when pause turns off. If they don't, the mental discipline developed while turning off self-induced pause will make it easy to turn off any lingering dissociations.

Chapter Eighteen

Wrapping up the diagnostics

The diagnostic tests in the previous chapter should have been be approached with the assumption that the patient *most* likely has Type I Parkinson's: Parkinson's from self-induced pause. It is also *highly* likely that the patient has *both* Type I and Type II Parkinson's disease.

The tests in the previous chapter were designed to tease out the very few people with Parkinson's who have *only* Type II or *only* Type III.

If a person does have enough symptoms to have a diagnosis of Parkinson's but he can easily imagine energy traveling up his spine and into his head, if temporarily stilling his Du channel makes him feel weird and different, if he *feels* as if he's in his body, and if he doesn't have most aspects, if any, of the Parkinson's personality, he probably has *only* Type II or Type III PD.

Only Type II or Type III PD

If you've determined that you have only Type II or Type III PD, you will want to mentally imagine you are looking around in your body, paying close attention to areas that might have been injured. When you find an area that is easier to imagine as dark, and that darkness is motionless or invisible, you'll want to have someone do Yin Tui Na at that location(s).

The most likely locations are the foot and the ankle. However, there might also be injuries elsewhere along the Stomach channel or along the spine, neck and head.

Instructions for this therapy is in the book *Yin Tui Na*, available for free download at PDrecovery.org or for purchase in hard copy at JaniceHadlock.com.

As for differentiating *between* Type II and Type III, that diagnosis will come after the treatment has started. Start the treatment with the assumption that the problem is Type II PD. *If* the problem is actually Type III, *self-induced* dissociation, it will become apparent during the course of treatment because the dark and motionless area will move around evasively. This is explained in the Yin Tui Na book. The few simple steps needed to destroy the *self-induced* dissociation are fully explained.

Everyone else

For everyone else, the Parkinson's disease is *primarily* due to being on pause. Whether it is self-induced pause or normal, biological pause doesn't matter yet. Whether or not there is a foot, ankle, or spinal injury that is *contributing* to the flow of pause-type channel qi, that also doesn't matter for now. That will get sorted out later. Either way, go to the book *Stuck on Pause* and use that book to determine which type of pause you have and learn how to treat it. If you are like *most* people with Parkinson's, you are using self-induced pause *and* you have some body parts from which you've dissociated.

Pause has to be treated first. Before any dissociated injuries are treated, pause must be turned off.

Repeat: pause has to be treated first.

After you come out of pause – and you will know when it happens and the book goes into detail describing how you will know – *then* you can start working on any body parts that are still dissociated and seem dark and motionless inside when you mentally imagine looking around inside your body.

Most people want to start by getting rid of their dissociated injuries. They assume that this will be easier and quicker than turning off self-induced pause. Yes, it will probably be easier and quicker. But if you do this there is a good chance you'll be left with a body and *mind* that is using parasympathetic mode for the body part that has healed *but* … the brain will still be using pause mode for the rest of the body. The resulting subconscious confusion, mental schism, and sometimes, rapid and profound worsening of PD symptoms and anxiety is called partial recovery. It can be far more painful and debilitating than just having Parkinson's disease.

First, turn off pause mode.

Resistance to the very idea of a mental component

Moving on to a completely new topic, why did I bother writing up *two* tests and a description of the Parkinson's personality, since all we usually need is Test #1 in order to determine is whether or not the patient is on pause?

Many of my patients have been powerfully opposed to the idea that their mind is contributing to their symptoms of Parkinson's disease. They have *not* wanted to think that they have dissociated from some body part *or* are using self-induced pause.

Some have told me they prefer to have an incurable illness for "no reason at all" than consider the humiliating possibility that their own mind is playing a role in their sickness. So many patients have told me, "It's perfectly respectable to have Parkinson's disease. It's *not* respectable to have a mental problem."

The reason I've included *two* tests and a description of the Parkinson's personality is that together, they can help a reluctant patient realize that he does, in fact, have Parkinson's, *and* very likely it's self-induced Parkinson's, *and* that this is related to mental processes.

As mentioned in the previous chapter, the test that might first shake up a patient's complacency and sense of being in control of his own mind is the "walking down the street" test. When he realizes that he tends to observe himself from outside the body rather than *feeling* himself from the inside, he might be a bit un-nerved. He might ask, "But isn't it normal to imagine looking at yourself instead of being inside yourself?" My reply is, "Sure it's normal, if you are using pause mode. Otherwise, no." This reply is often met by a concerned look in the patient's eye and a long silence.

The patient is suddenly confronting the possibility that maybe his mind *is* behaving in a way that is not quite "right." This conclusion is based on his *own* experience during that test, not based on some doctor's external assessment or opinion. So many people had told me that the official, medical, written descriptions of Parkinson's symptoms don't actually match up to the pathologies they feel *inside*. Many have told me they didn't believe their doctor's diagnosis for a long time. But the quick tests in the previous chapter can help a patient start to recognize his own pathologies. He might even begin to accept that there *might* be a mental component to his own Parkinson's symptoms.

A bit of history

For historical reasons, western culture has long considered health problems that have a mental component to be less "real" than purely physical problems, and even somewhat shameful, as if mind-activated problems indicate a lack of high morals or self-control, or even a fall from grace.

If you're interested in how and when this attitude developed, please look up the details on René Descartes vs. the Pope on the mid-seventeenth century legal decision on the question of physical versus "spiritual" (including mental) illness. The outcome of the papal decree was that, under the threat of ex-communication, doctors agreed that they would study and care for the physical body *only*. *All* mental/emotional issues would be considered spiritual problems and as such would belong to the realm – and the income stream – of the church.

Thus, mental issues became *legally* separated from medical study. The results of this decision linger, still influencing western insistence on the separation of physical and mental health. In eastern medicine, no such separation exists. *Prior* to the church's spat with Descartes, practitioners of western medicine were familiar with the idea of a connection between emotional, mental, and physical illnesses, as you'll read about in the case of St. Teresa of Avila, in chapter twenty.

The fact is, nearly all illnesses have a mental component. Even the *rate* of healing from an injury or illness can be influenced by mental attitudes and habits. The degree to which a person is physically sickened by physical and/or emotional damage or stress depends to a large extent on mental behaviors, including learned and/or cultural behaviors, that might seem completely unrelated to the illness.

Even in these modern times, some patients feel the burn of social disgrace if their syndrome turns out to have a mental component. And people with Parkinson's often *chose* the mental behavior that landed them with PD, making it seem even more shameful – though shame should have *nothing* to do with it. People who, at some point, chose to go through life on pause made their decision in the face of powerful, sometimes life-threatening physical and/or emotional pain. They are survivors who, in order to survive, forced themselves to into pause. There is no shame in that.

Do not ever think less of yourself if it turns out that you put yourself on pause or dissociated from some problem or body part. It is a perfectly human thing to do.

As mentioned earlier, *not* every human uses dissociation or pause in response to trauma. Most people don't even have the necessary degree of mental focus and self-control to execute these mind-controlling self-commands.

Even if you have made choices that led to dissociation or being stuck in self-induced pause, doing so is *not* an indication of a poor moral compass. It *may* be an indication of a relatively high intelligence and/or a very high degree of mental self-control. It may be a *misguided* intelligence, driven by fear-based commands rather than wisdom and intuitive awareness of ultimate, universal safety, but a *strong* and *focused* intelligence, nevertheless.

Then again, if you find yourself wanting to *justify* and continue clinging to the darkness that you have created inside yourself, you *might* also desire to comfort yourself by insisting that dissociation or using pause is what *everyone* does in the face of trauma. This is not the case.

Many people who are traumatized do not dissociate or use pause. Many can imagine bright light even in terribly injured or smashed-up parts of their bodies, even if they are in a significant deal of pain. Some might even automatically imagine angels getting in there and healing the injury. In fact, holding, massaging, asking others to hold or massage or even imagining light or miniature loved ones inside a painful area are some of the more effective ways to reduce the pain and accelerate healing in any type of injury – slight or severe. Some people just know, intuitively, to do this: they *embrace* the traumatized area once they are safe – they don't pretend that it doesn't exist. A decision to dissociate or go into pause mode was a choice. Very likely it was a *necessary* choice at the time or at least seemed like one.

It might also be a culturally determined choice. When I was in college, I banged myself badly on a kitchen cabinet. I quickly turned to my blond, caucasian housemate and said, "I'm fine, don't worry, I can ignore it."

She looked at me as if I were hopelessly stupid. "You know, in China, they teach you to pay attention to a place that's injured, so that it will heal more quickly."

I replied, "That doesn't make any sense at all! Why pay attention to pain?" Decades passed before I learned what she had been talking about.

If a person cannot even imagine paying attention to an injured body part, it might help him to think of it as paying attention to a little child who has been injured and/or scared. The injured body part can be held and physically and/or mentally coddled by the rest of the body, as if the injured tissues are a helpless, beloved child. This mental approach to being injured is extremely healthy. It can lead to the fastest and most complete healing. This approach prevents lasting dissociation and the temptation to self-induce pause.

Even in the face of emotional injuries, the heart can talk to and give comfort and solace to a terrified or battered mind. By treating the emotional pain as belonging to a helpless toddler – which in fact is a good analogy for ego-based emotional pain – a person can heal more quickly and move forward, rather than staying consciously *or* subconsciously mired in the pain – dealing with it via some hidden or suppressive manner that's causing electrical disarray and mental self-deceit.

How one responds to pain or damage depends on one's personal style in dealing with difficulties. You *can* say that sustaining dissociation or pause for a long time after an injury or trauma is not unusual. You *cannot* truthfully say that *everyone* does it, or that it's always automatic or even helpful. Very often, shutting out awareness of pain is a conscious decision – one that can have long-term detrimental consequences if the pain is not dealt with when a "safe place" opportunity finally arises.[1]

---

[1] I highly recommend reading *Where There is Light*, an extraordinary memoir by Jacques Lusseyran. He was part of the French resistance during World War II. He was betrayed and captured. When he was dying in a Nazi concentration camp, he decided to once again fill himself with light, a practice he started when he permanently lost his eyesight as a lad, a practice that he consciously abandoned when he was taken prisoner as a young adult.

Once again filled with light, he recovered from his almost-fatal illness and fever. He went on to make secret radio communications to allied forces from within the camp. He survived the war even though most of his compatriots in the camp did not. His autobiographical book makes a profound argument against the negative practice of dissociation and the positive practice of literally

However, in my limited experience of a mere thirty-plus years of practicing medicine, I've seen that many, many people, not just those with Parkinson's, do *not* want to think that they have mentally contributed in *any* way to their current health situation.

That's why I shared two tests and the personality assessment in the previous chapters. These can provide extra weight to the idea that the person's brain *is* stuck on pause. This strengthened conviction can sometimes nudge even a reluctant patient to start doing the mental work that might be necessary for recovery.

Case study: denial of dissociation from the gut

Even non-PD patients sometimes *vigorously* resist the idea that they have a mental component to their pain, such as dissociation from some parts of their bodies.

For example, I sent an email to a long-distance patient with severe bowel disease asking him to assess if he might be dissociated from his intestines, or even on pause. I wrote to him about visualizing light and then dark inside, and also sent him some material on dissociation and pause.

He wrote back to me (I paraphrase), "I can dissociate at will, but I usually re-experience the trauma later, when it's safe. For example, I was attacked on the street one night, and I didn't cry until later. But I don't think I *store* trauma.

"I *might* have some degree of injury-based dissociation due to the extreme pain I have experienced in my gut, but my experience of life is not dissociated.

He continued, "It is easier for me to imagine my gut being dark, but I *can* send light through it if I really concentrate. When I imagine my gut, I imagine it *not* in the first person (it's not *me* seeing it). It's as if the gut has a "tiny me" that's sitting inside of my colon, or seeing my colon as though looking at a diagram. However, imagining that I'm looking at it directly, as if it's me on the inside of my body, looking out, is hard when I come to that specific part of my body.

"But I can do it eventually, I *can* send light there from me. Just not easily. Also, it looks like patchwork in there. Some light goes through, but there are some patches that are dark. Maybe those areas are injured or scarred. My problems with my gut started a couple of weeks after a very painful breakup with my long-time partner. But I don't think I'm dissociated from it. I can definitely *feel* pain in my gut. When I visualize the gut and see darkness, it's dark because it's *injured*, not because I'm dissociated. I need *physical* treatment. I do *not* need to change my attitude towards or relationship with my gut."

The person quoted above, like many people, assumed that the dark areas in his gut looked dark because he was actually looking at injured areas. He was not.

He was confident that he was not dissociated because he *could* see light in the area, *temporarily*, *if* he worked really hard at it. Or if some minion worked at it on his behalf. Also, since he could *justify* the darkness as being due to pain, injury or possible scarring, he was sure he was *not* dissociated. He thought he was just the opposite: highly aware of what a mess his gut truly is, and therefore *not* dissociated. He was wrong on nearly every count.

---

keeping oneself filled with light regardless of circumstances. A movie, *All the Light We Cannot See*, was released in 2015. The movie was based on a novel that was based on the memoir. I have no idea if the movie or novel gets the original author's message across. The actual autobiography is profoundly inspirational.

Again, the imagination does *not* see what is actually, physically going on deep inside the body. The relative darkness or light in an *imagined, visualized* body part might have *nothing* to do what is physically happening in that area.

The *mind*, not the health status or injured status of an area, determines whether or not a given body part is going to be easy to imagine and perceived as filled with light, or is dark, or a mishmash, or speckled with dark and light areas, motionless or agitated or, for that matter, looks like a patchwork as seen by a "tiny me" or minion.

I included the above example to demonstrate the high level of resistance to the idea of a mental component that *many* people bring to the diagnostic process, not just people with PD.

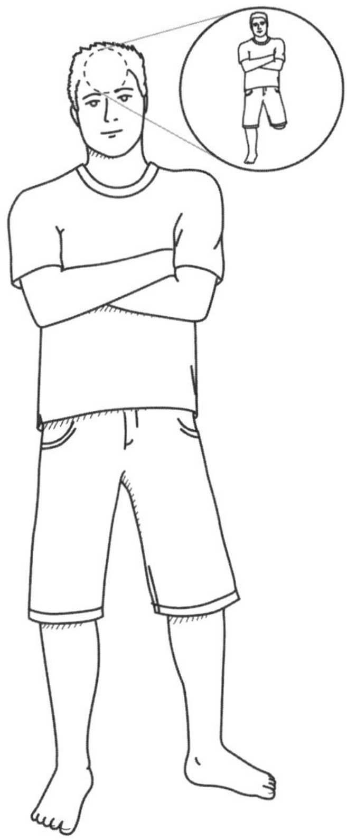

Once the patient is able to see that his mental behaviors are consistent with the mental behaviors of a person who is dissociated or on pause, he might be more likely to do some of the work necessary for changing his brain behaviors.

Until a patient is able to consider that his own mind might be contributing to his health problem, he might prefer to wait passively for the doctor to "fix him" while he, the patient, does nothing.

In treating cases of Type I Parkinson's disease, a patient who is *not* actively working on changing his own mental habits is *not* going to have any *lasting* improvements in his symptoms. No matter how many changes he makes in his diet, his exercise program, his use of ozone or "magic qi" machines, or how many hands-on treatments he gets from doctors, his brain won't change its habits until he takes the reins and practices more helpful mental behaviors. Only the patient himself can do this.

Fig. 17.4 The motionless darkness or "invisibility" you "see" in some body part is your brain's biological, emergency behavior of temporarily ignoring that body part until you are safe *or* obeying *your instruction* to ignore that body part. You actually *do* have that body part. The imagined darkness is in your brain.

Hypnotherapy doesn't work

My patients have discovered that using hypnosis therapy to further cover up their mental cover-ups doesn't work. Hypnosis, in many, maybe most cases, when used to blot out some memory or stop some negative behavior, does *not* actually heal the problem. It masks the problem.

It *can*, in some cases, create yet another level of delusion or avoidance in the brain and can lead to unexpected consequences. It might be helpful to consider that, in terms of brain behavior, self-induced pause is processed in the brain in the exact same manner as hypnosis. In the classical understanding of hypnosis, it is understood that only the person who imposed the original hypnotic suggestion has the authority to *undo* it.

If you think of pause as creating a second personality, and even if that's the personality you now use all or most of the time, bear in mind that you *can't* use the paused personality to turn off pause, to turn off the original self-hypnotic instruction. The paused personality was *created* by your real, original, safe and trusting personality: the personality that can engage laughingly with its invisible friend.

The pause personality is *not* the personality that *gave* the initial instruction. So it can't be the one that turns it off. Your real self gave the instruction. You've got to get back in touch with your real self. Again, that's the self that can talk with your invisible friend, the friend who loves you unconditionally and who can make you laugh.

When a person uses the part of his personality that can communicate with an invisible friend, a personality that can be loved, that finds life joyful and safe - his real, underlying, original personality – he *is* using the personality that created the instruction to be on pause. In terms of self-hypnosis, thd original personality is the only one that can turn off the instruction to "feel no pain" or whatever phrase was used.

Several of my patients learned that neither the paused self *nor* a professional hypnotist will be able to turn off self-induced pause. Your long-repressed original personality, the one that has the capacity to trust and constantly confide in a laughing, loving, invisible friend is the personality that's going to be able to activate the striatum, making you feel safe, and thus causing self-induced pause to turn off.

Another therapy that doesn't work: EFT

While on the subject of therapies that don't work, Emotional Freedom Technique, "EFT," is a technique that consists of tapping on some of the acupuncture points that are channel-shunt locations for sympathetic mode. A few of these shunts are somewhat likely to get stuck in the channel qi's sympathetic route. If channel qi becomes stuck, the person often ends up feeling pain at various places in the body whenever thinking about the old trauma.

By tapping on the stuck shunt locations while remembering the trauma that originally triggered the sympathetic mode episode, one can often retrain these shunt locations to stay in parasympathetic circuitry even while thinking of the past trauma.

I am regularly asked about this technique. As noted by the founders of this technique, this technique does *not* work for situations from which a person has dissociated. It also does not work for self-induced pause, or regular pause. This technique only works in very specific conditions: when some shunt from the parasympathetic path into the sympathetic path has gotten stuck for a long time or is re-activated in response to thinking about the trauma. By turning off the stuck shunt by tapping on it, the person can sometimes turn off the pain associated with the original problem.

A common shunt location treated in EFT is ST-13, on the Stomach channel on the chest (see p. 4). In EFT, this is known as "the painful point." In *parasympathetic* mode, the current running through this point flows down to the toes. In *sympathetic* mode, some amount of this current is shunted *inward* from ST-13, moving towards the heart, to help support the increased heart rate and heart power of sympathetic mode.

Cognitive Behavioral Therapy can *help*

The current over-arching name for *many* types of patient-activated, self-help mental therapies is cognitive behavioral therapy (CBT).

A person doing cognitive behavioral therapy learns to pay attention to his thoughts. He weeds out the thoughts that are contributing to his negative brain chemistry and brain electrical behaviors. He consciously replaces those thoughts with other types of thoughts: positive, striatum-stimulating thoughts that alter his brain's wiring, activating the brain chemistries and electrical circuits associated with parasympathetic mode combined with a healthy, *moderate* level of sympathetic mode.

The core treatment for turning off self-induced pause – learning how to talk to a supportive, invisible friend – is very *normal* and *healthy* behavior. It is also a very specific type of cognitive behavioral therapy.

If you want to learn more about the way most people talk to something outside of themselves, I highly suggest you read a few collections of "Calvin and Hobbes" cartoons. Talking to an invisible or imaginary friend is a main point of that strip. Also, please read *Feeling Good*: *the New Mood Therapy*, by Dr. David Burns, as footnoted on p. 126.

Patients' incomplete knowledge

Completely changing the subject, patients very often tell me, "I know why I put myself on pause in the first place." The patient then gives me an elaborate story of some well-remembered injustice or something "wrong" that happened to him.

In many, maybe most cases, the patient is incorrect. After 1) learning to feel safe and 2) pause turns off, the patient suddenly remembers the *actual* event that caused him to be on pause – it's often something very different, less dramatic, and long-forgotten. The memory only resurfaced because the person had turned off pause. I do listen to what the patient *thinks* is the reason for being on pause, but I'm also not surprised when a completely different trauma is remembered after recovery – a trauma from which he may well have *also* dissociated at the time, and therefore cannot remember it until he recovers.

An example of false memory

Many people assume they need to remember the issue that led them to put themselves on pause. This is *not* the case. A person first needs to feel safe. *Then* he can turn off pause. A person might remember why he started using pause before *or* after turning off pause, but very often a person doesn't remember until he feels profoundly safe.

For example, one patient was certain that he had put himself into pause mode when he was age six, in response to the painful divorce through which his parents were going. He told me about the divorce in great detail and with tremendous resentment.

Less than an hour after his epiphany in which pause mode turned off, he told me that he'd been wrong about why he went into pause. We'll call my patient Bob to keep things straight. Following the divorce, young Bob and his mother were extremely low-income. They ended up living in mom's car. Every night, they parked the car at mom's best friend's house. Mom's best friend was also the mother of a six-year old: Bob's best friend. At some point, the six-year old best friend betrayed young Bob: best friend told all the other children at school that Bob's mother was so poor that they were living in their car. The other children at school were merciless. In response to the humiliation and pain of this betrayal, Bob commanded himself to not be a part of the world: the world was too painful. Bob only remembered doing this *after* he'd turned off pause. He had *not* activated pause mode in response to the divorce – an event that he *did* remember.

Because the brain often *dissociates* from the thing that is so painful that a person is driven to mentally induce pause mode, people very often cannot remember what the actual trigger for pause was. Again, most of my patients, trying to remember what the cause might have been, have come up with something that they are bitter about, but after turning off pause they remembered that the actual trigger for pause was something different, something long forgotten that had been completely dissociated from normal memory or that they had been remembering as "not having been so bad."

Many of my patients have wasted a lot of time and energy, sometimes *years*, trying to figure out their triggering event for self-induced pause before being willing to start practicing the presence of an invisible friend. Others have wanted someone to blame for their use of self-induced pause – another waste of precious time. Please don't waste time trying to figure out what caused you to command yourself to be numb or detached, or who to blame for your pain or your symptoms of Parkinson's. You may well end up dwelling on negative things that have nothing to do with pause. Dwelling on negative events will stimulate your amygdala. It will make you more entrenched in your fear and negativity habits, making it harder to turn pause off.

A surprising number of my patients have been certain that they are on pause because of some *past-life* injury or atrocity. They just *love* to dwell on this unforgiveable memory. Many have told me that they *need* to dwell on this past injustice or unfairness, in order to "process it." Some have spent years *not* doing the talk-to-a-laughing-friend cognitive behavioral therapy that can turn off pause because they are so fascinated with their sad history. They feel they need to explore their tragic past to the fullest before turning towards a new future. While dwelling on past tragedy or on cruel and "unfair" experiences, their symptoms continue to steadily worsen. We now know that the brain is very obedient and its behaviors are habit based. If you practice thinking about some past atrocity, your brain will get better and better about dwelling on the atrocity, as well as devoting ever more brain cells to self-pity, resentment and other negative thoughts.

For that matter, a few patients have told me that they remember having Parkinson's in a past life. And they tend to dwell on the inescapability of worsening symptoms in this life and maybe the next. If you find yourself reluctant to work on changing your mental habits, one question you might want to ask yourself is, "How many lifetimes do I hope to spend having Parkinson's disease?" According to many world religions, if you die with a wrong mindset, a mindset that keeps you on pause, you will have an inclination to resume that wrong mindset in the hereafter or in a next life.

Even death will not alter your consciousness. "My Father's home has many mansions" [1] is a reference to the infinite number of possibilities in which you might find yourself after you shed what Hamlet called this "mortal coil." What determines your "residence" and happiness – or not – in the post-death plane is determined in large part by the mental attitudes and heart feelings you've developed in this one. Those aspects of your consciousness are *not* altered by death. Don't imagine you can "die" your way out of Parkinson's disease.

---

[1] John, 14:2, The New Testament

When *you* create an unhealthy mental behavior, *you* alone are responsible for deciding to get rid of it. But once you are determined to get rid of it, you can ask friends to *help* you, including your invisible friends.

A person cannot turn off pause until he learns to focus the mind on being safe, and being in the present. Brain habits of dwelling on negative events of the past or the imagined future, whether real, imagined, or inflated, *increase* when the brain is in pause mode. Risk-assessment is amplified. Dwelling on the negatives in one's past or in the imagined future *encourages* pause mode-type thinking; pause mode-type thinking encourages dwelling on the negative. A vicious cycle. In my limited experience, this morose or bitter dwelling has *never* helped a patient feel safer, nor has it helped him turn off self-induced pause.

Remember – the whole point of dissociating is that your brain blocks off your memory of the dissociated event. The harder a person tries to remember or dwell on the significant negative events from the past, including the one(s) that triggered pause, the stronger his brain might work at hiding the truth from him (dissociating harder or digging deeper into pause) as per the person's previous instructions – or even creating a new, terrible story line as a distraction.

New research proves that digging relentlessly into past negative events – the old, passé model for Freudian psychotherapy – does *not* lead to healing from these events. Instead, focusing on the negative usually *increases* the amount of brain area devoted to the negative events and increases any physiological and emotional damage from the negative events, whether real or imagined. Please, just move forward with the positive work needed to turn off pause. Forgive the past, whether known or unknown.

In my own case, although I have *always* clearly remembered staring into a mirror and commanding myself to be numb – which felt strangely evil at the time and I had to look away from my own face in the mirror as it changed shape, becoming strangely hard and unfeeling looking – I have never remembered the specific event that led up to my making that dramatic self-command during my high school years. And I don't care what it was. There were so many negative events in my childhood, as in so many persons' childhoods, that possibly the specific event that led me to formally turn on self-induced pause was, in my case, just one small event too many: the last straw. The exact cause doesn't matter. The choice to use pause mode was mine and no one else's. In order to recover, I had to change my attitude and my focus. Not dwell on or try to alter my past.

In case the reader is curious, when I injured my foot at age five I was already very good at not feeling specific pains. I presume I *dissociated* from my injuries in those early days. My stare-in-the-mirror command to not feel emotions, period, didn't come until high school. So I most likely had both Type I and Type II Parkinson's – just like most of my patients.

"I didn't have a choice"

Many of my patients have been adamant that they had no *choice* but to use, and then stay, on pause. I had one patient who insisted that he needed to put himself into pause mode because his father yelled all the time. I asked him about his brothers. Did father yell at them, too?

He replied that one brother dealt with it by leaving home. The other dealt with it by becoming an alcoholic. I suggested that his use of pause was therefore a choice – his brothers had chosen paths other than pause. He became furious with me. He said that he didn't want to drink and he didn't want to leave home, so he *had* to use pause mode, and use it for the rest of his life. He had *no* choice in the matter.

I said that, if he had no choice, then he probably couldn't turn it off, so there was no sense in him working with me. He replied that he shouldn't have to change any part of how he used his mind. Instead, he would recover if I held his foot every week for an hour for the rest of his life even though his foot injury had long since healed up.

His wife and I agreed that this didn't seem to make any sense, and that they would stop coming until such time as he thought he might be willing to change some of his thinking patterns.

Please don't waste time and energy trying to remember or dwell on what physical or emotional injuries you've undergone. Move forward with your life.

Then again, one patient told me he *was* looking forward. The only reason he wanted to recover from Parkinson's was so he could some day "shove his mother's face" in the fact that her cruelty had ruined his life and caused his Parkinson's. If he could recover using my theories, his recovery would prove that his mother had caused his Parkinson's disease. He looked forward to that moment. His greatest concern was that she might die before he could have his victory dance over her. He wasn't interested in learning to connect with an invisible friend or anyone who could make him feel safe. He wanted to stay focused on how much he hated his mother. We agreed that I probably wasn't the right health practitioner for him. He spent a lot of time paying a therapist to do Yin Tui Na on his injured foot. He never did turn off pause mode. And he never recovered from Parkinson's that I know of.

The brain is not clever

I am often asked by patients, "Why doesn't pause mode or dissociation from pain stop when the pain of the injury backs down?"

In general, the brain is not very bright. It does *not* necessarily work in your best interests. The brain is *extremely* obedient. It learns through habit. For better or for worse, it does what you tell it to do. It thinks what you tell it to think. And it does so over and over, until you actively decide to change the status quo: until you stop using your ongoing negative habits by overwriting them with new instructions.

The brain's neurons connect or detach from other neural cells in response to your instructions and habits. The more *often* you *do* something or *tell* yourself to do or think something, the stronger, deeper and faster those particular brain connections, routings, and disconnects become. The brain is *not* the fixed, unchangeable switchboard, established since birth, that we were taught in the 1900s. The brain's connections and areas of elevated or decreased activity change constantly, influenced by thoughts and habits, and by the neurological mode of the moment. The brain's ability to change is called neuroplasticity.

The brain is capable of constant change. It changes in response to changing instructions from *you* and the responses you *choose* to make to external events: your own thoughts, decisions, and mental and physical behaviors during a given event help determine how you will respond *next* time in another event.

If you think the same things over and over, the brain effectively becomes more rigid, more locked in to doing the same thing over and over. Still, no matter how locked in a person's thinking has become, he *can* change his thoughts. It requires self-aware observation of one's thoughts and the *replacement* of outmoded or unwanted thoughts with the new, preferred thoughts.

It's hard to get rid of an unwanted thought. It's easier to train yourself to focus on and repeatedly use a new thought. The old thought will eventually wither from neglect.

A good example of this is the "earworm" phenomenon in which a musical tune gets stuck in your mind and plays over and over. Telling it to stop isn't going to make it go away. *Replacing* the tune with a less compelling melody of your own choosing is the fastest way to get rid of the unwanted tune.

If one of your commands to the brain was a powerful, effective instruction to "pretend some specific pain or problem never happened," you will have to live with the dissociative consequences of that suppression until such time as you execute brain behaviors that serve to turn off your previous instructions – even if you don't remember what they were.

If one of your commands to the brain was "Feel no pain," or "I am not a part of this terrible world," you will have to live with the consequences of that command – self-induced pause – until you make mental changes that allow you to feel safe and at peace in a *neurological* sense.

If dissociated, whether automatically dissociated or using self-induced dissociation, then use the techniques in the book *Yin Tui Na* to turn off the dissociation.

If on pause, go to the book *Stuck on Pause*. If pause mode was *not* self-induced and is just basic pause that has gotten stuck and the original site of injury/trauma has healed, then go through the five steps for turning off biological pause (in chapter one of the book *Stuck on Pause*), while staying mentally focused on the agitated area that was the location of the original trauma. This should turn off pause.

If you are using self-induced pause, the book *Stuck on Pause* has instructions on learning how to turn the striatum, thalamus, and adrenal glands back *on* and thus feel safe and powerful enough to turn off this type of pause.

Chapter Nineteen

Scar Tissue

Before treating *either* pause or dissociation, a person hoping to recover from Parkinson's disease will want to clear up any scar tissue that is blocking the pertinent channels. Scar tissue is non-conductive. If wide enough or deep enough, it can cause channel qi to take a detour, flow into another channel's pathway, or even flow backwards.

The channels on which scarring can most affect Parkinson's are the Stomach, Large Intestine, Du, Ren, and Gallbladder. But large amounts of scarring on any of the channels can cause disruptions in channel qi and should be taken care of. Check the channels for scar tissue and be sure to go all the way to the fingers and toes.

Scars that are not a problem

A small scar, shallow and less than a quarter inch across, will not cause problems: the channel qi can divert around it. Also, a scar that runs *parallel* to the path of a channel will not cause problems.

Scars that might be a problem

If scar tissue runs perpendicular to or at an oblique angle to a channel, preventing the channel qi from following its normal route, it might be disrupting the flow of channel qi.

The most elegant, quick and effective way to breakup scar tissue is with acupuncture. Most acupuncturists are not trained in school on how to treat scar tissue. They do NOT have experience in treating scar tissue efficiently and effectively. Some of them have even been taught techniques that are painful and not particularly successful.

If you are able to find an acupuncturist open to learning something new, please direct your acupuncturist to the website of the Parkinson's Recovery Project. Two chapters from *Tracking the Dragon* that teach how to most effectively and quickly clear up scar tissue are available for free download at www.PDRecovery.org. Click on Publications, then click on *Tracking the Dragon*. Print out the two chapters on treating scar tissue. Share this information with your acupuncturist.

Therapies that break up scar tissue by using physical force on the scarring doesn't clear up the scarring well enough to prevent it from disrupting the flow of channel qi and, if rough enough, might even encourage the growth of new scar tissue. If your therapist isn't willing to learn the very simple principles of using acupuncture needles to break up scar tissue, please look for a different acupuncturist.

If you cannot find an acupuncturist who is willing to learn how to do this job using the protocols in *Tracking the Dragon*, you might be able to rope a friend in to do this simple work for you.

If one person is inserting acupuncture needles into a mutual friend, you might be able to call this an interpersonal activity between consenting adults. You are NOT practicing medicine without a license because technically, you are not practicing medicine. Practicing medicine involves assessment and making a diagnosis. You or your friend won't be doing anything of the sort. You'll just be sticking some acupuncture needles through the scar tissue. This is no more "medical" than piercing someone's ear lobe to make an earring hole.

Acupuncture needles can be purchased online or maybe from your local acupuncturist. You will want half-inch long ("half cun," pronounced "half soon") needles, either a 34 or a 32 diameter. If the scarring is severe, get the 32 diameter. If the scars seem fairly small and shallow, get the 34 diameter. The most common diameter of acupuncture needles, 36, is usually too thin and delicate for scar tissue work: the needles will bend rather than penetrate the scar tissue.

If you are uneasy about doing this to yourself or a friend, please know that MDs are legally allowed to put needles into a patient's skin. You might be able to talk your family doctor into doing scar tissue treatments using acupuncture needles..

Leave the needles in for up for forty-five minutes. Two treatment sessions are usually sufficient to get channel qi flowing through the scarred area.

If you have a friend who can feel channel qi, the friend can check before doing treatments to confirm whether or not the scar tissue is blocking the flow of channel qi. If it is, and someone treats your scarred area with with needles, you can also have the friend check the currents *after* the treatment to make sure that the channel qi has resumed flowing correctly.

If a patient is on pause mode, breaking up scar tissue is the only condition for which acupuncture is appropriate. Almost any other use of needling will make the pause pattern stronger.

Chapter Twenty

Some Tangential Observations

Many of my PD patients felt that the underlying roots of their symptoms or their recovery insights had significant spiritual overtones. Many have told me that our long talks on spiritual or religious subjects were the most important or favorite part of our working together. Of course, no one recovered because we shared stories about some saint or other. Much as people enjoyed the long talks and found them helpful, in the end, they each had to do themselves the work that led to recovery.

In past editions of this book, I rather shied away from an in-depth discussion of the Parkinson's personality and especially from the spiritual aspects that kept arising in paticnt's questions. Since the beginning of my project, I really, really wanted to show that recovery from Parkinson's disease could be an antiseptic, non-mental, non-spiritual, purely objective, biological solution.

However, because *subjective* mental postures, including faulty, negative spiritual misunderstandings, can be significant for a person trying to recover, I'm including in this edition some of the observations that I often shared with my patients but which I have been hesitant to put into print up until now.

Today, I'm writing this hopefully final revision of this book for the people who will be diagnosed with Parkinson's disease long after I am gone. So I'm including a sampling of the "spiritual" facts, musings, and discoveries that my patients often found helpful and/or inspirational.

Of course, a person who is *not* so inclined does *not* need to adopt a "spiritual attitude," whatever that means, in order to recover from Parkinson's. He doesn't even need to understand the biological forces at work behind PD. In most cases, he just needs to kickstart his striatum or re-associate with his foot.

Many people have argued with me that they can't recover from Parkinson's because they don't *believe* in "something *perfect* enough outside of myself that will be willing to talk with me." Bear in mind that some of the fastest recoveries have occurred in people who used a beloved parent, grandparent, or other relative as their invisible friend: not some "perfect" being. These departed parents, cousins, and grade-school friends represented love. Most recovered patients have *not* befriended God or someone "perfect." Then again, one might argue that affection and love are *manifestations* of the Divine, even in an "imperfect," very human form.

Famous people with Parkinson's disease

Many patients have told me that having Parkinson's means that they are a "bad person" or even a "spiritual failure."

If a person is thinking along these lines, I like to point out that many famously spiritual people have had idiopathic Parkinson's disease. I make this point for several reasons. Most importantly, many people in partial recovery have told me that *because* they have Parkinson's, that's proof that they don't deserve to recover or they aren't "good enough" to recover. Please do not indulge in that wrong type of twisted or even circular thinking. That's the Blocker talking.

Many of the great saints and sages of various faiths have had Parkinson's disease. You don't have Parkinson's because you aren't spiritual enough. You *might* have Type I Parkinson's because you *are* quite spiritually advanced and able to tightly control your thoughts and emotions. But… you've maybe taken a wrong turn in response to some dreadful fear or pain even as you got close to the summit of your spiritual searching.

Parkinson's is *not* a disease that occurs because a person is bad or lacking in spiritual wisdom. If I'm going to make a non-proveable hypothesis, I would say that it's just the opposite: Parkinson's disease, in my experience, is most easily set in motion in people with advanced spiritual understanding who've spent *lifetimes* pursuing intense spiritual self-discipline.

The average person simply does not have the presence of mind, the intensity of focus, and the training in this life or a previous one regarding manipulating one's own life force and biological energy to be able to lock himself into self-induced pause. The mental and self-control qualities that are required to effectively command one's self to go through life as if numb and nearly dead are just *not* available to your average person.

The average Joe or Jane, if punched in the stomach, will scream, burst into tears, run away, or punch back. It takes a rare sort of person who will make himself impervious to pain so that he appears to offer no response to such an affront. People with Parkinson's, in general, love to present themselves as unresponsive to pain, and put a positive spin on it by calling it something like "grace under pressure" or "mind over matter."

For *good reason*, they might have learned to "stoicize" their composure. They might have had very compelling reasons, as well as the somewhat rare mental capacity, to make themselves numb to the slings and arrows of daily life. However, in my experience, they also often assume that this graceful or self-effacing composure reflects spiritual *superiority*. On this count, they are incorrect. If that self-effacing graciousness is made possible by the use of self-induced pause mode, the "composed" behavior is being underwritten by fear, lack of faith, and *ego* protection. These negative attitudes might then be justified by creating a skewed perspective, a perspective that claims these behaviors reflect superior spirituality.

Office hours in the Netherlands

Once, after lecturing in Amsterdam and preparing to treat eight new PD patients there on the following day, I decided to do an experiment.

The evening before, I had been reading an excerpt from the somewhat obscure *Yoga Sutras* (yoga teachings) of Patanjali (estimates of its age range from somewhere between the 2nd century BC and the 8th century AD).

I had long been aware that my Parkinson's patients were almost always ready to jump into a philosophical or even deeply spiritual discussion. Even though many of my patients have had an aversion to one or two particular "spiritual" trigger words, words such as Divine, or God, or Love, they were still interested in talking about deeper meanings or spiritual implications of sickness and health – so long as I didn't use whatever words were on their "bad" list. In comparison, when I saw general-practice patients at my school's clinic, the patients almost *never* had any interest in or even a capacity for such subjects. But a disproportionate number of my patients with Parkinson's were unusually sophisticated when it came to spiritual philosophies, and quite verbal about it.

I decided that, as an experiment, I would mention the fairly obscure subject of the aphorisms of Patanjali to each of my Parkinson's patients, none of whom I had ever met before, to see how they might respond.

I opened each patient's session by asking if the patient was familiar with traditional yoga meditation precepts, such as the sutras of Patanjali.

Only a few of them were practicing a formal religion. But as I directed each discussion towards Patanjali's eight-fold path to enlightenment, most of the patients nodded in agreement or even commented, as if familiar with the general idea of the principles. Over the course of the day, I was not too surprised to learn that, not only had a majority of them heard of Patanjali's sutras, they were clearly qualified to discuss them.

But the real shockers came when I asked each of my patients, "Do you feel that, if you are successful in turning off your negative and fearful mindset and if you can successfully surrender to the Divine, you will find yourself attaining Patanjali's eighth and final level of spiritual attainment, therefore "graduating" from this earthly plane and no longer needing to reincarnate? And if so, is that something you fear?"

I actually thought this was a preposterous question, and only asked it because my own thoughts had tended in that direction prior to my own recovery.

Some of the patients were a bit surprised at my asking such a deeply personal question at our first meeting...and nearly all of them answered yes. They feared that making the attitude changes required for turning off pause would mean either the final end of their thousands of cycles of reincarnations or, at the very least, instant death in this life!

I was able to reassure them that, because they were still struggling with the very *bottom*, *first* level of spiritual striving, paraphrased as "Don't do morally wrong things" (similar to the Judeo-Christian ten commandments), they didn't need to worry about hitting the top, eighth level any time soon. As for dying, I had *seen* un-medicated people recover from Parkinson's disease and not *one* of them had died in the process. The only people who died due to recovery had been people who'd been taking the antiparkinson's medications for a significant period of time, and those deaths were due to drug excess or withdrawal, not spiritual transcendence.

When each patient asked me why I considered him/her to still be stuck at the bottom rung, at the first, lowest, level of spiritual attainment, I pointed out that they were enmeshed in fear and mentally living a lie: they were choosing to pretend to be dead (on pause) even though alive.

One of the main "wrong" things a person can do, on the spiritual path, is be fearful. Another is lying. Considered in this light, I suggested to each person that he/she was doing both of these "wrong" things and was more likely to be at the low end of the "spiritual progress" scale, not the high end. None of them disagreed with me.

In fact, they were *reassured* by the idea that they weren't actually on the verge of irreversible enlightenment. They were relieved to learn that, from this new perspective, they were still struggling with the very first level of spiritual attainment, not hovering at the eighth and final level.

Then again, as an aside, many deeply spiritual people who, one might argue *are* on the verge of the highest levels of spiritual attainment, have had Parkinson's disease.

It makes me think that the path to intimacy with Truth or with the Divine is not a straight path with distinct steps, but rather a process in which all the steps are tackled simultaneously, at varying depths. The sense of there being specific, ordered steps might be somewhat academic, helpful mainly when it comes to putting these arcane principles into words and into writing.

Getting back to people with Parkinson's in general, this very high level of verbal philosophical/ spiritual engagement that I could enjoy with these patients fit with what I'd already seen with most of my other Parkinson's patients who had Type I PD.

Spiritual giants with Parkinson's disease

Pope John Paul II

In the 20th century, Pope John Paul II (1920-2005), deeply loved, was known to have idiopathic Parkinson's. In his late teens/early twenties, he witnessed helplessly as Nazi thugs murdered his father in the street. Sometime later he witnessed his mother, and then his sister, being pulled into the streets and attacked, and then murdered by Nazi troops.

He never took antiparkinson's medications because they cause too many adverse *mental* effects. He died of kidney failure.

St. Clare of Assisi

Saint Clare of Assisi (1194-1253), a close friend of Saint Francis of Assisi and founder of the Order of the Poor Ladies (known today as the Order of the Poor Clares), had idiopathic Parkinson's disease. Of course, the syndrome had not yet been given its present name. Her well-detailed symptoms, a perfect match for Parkinson's, are officially referred to by the church as "the Afflictions of St. Clare."

As her symptoms worsened, her immobility became nearly utter. When Francis came to say the mass in the chapel of her domicile (San Damiano, in Assisi, Italy) she would request that the other nuns drag her body across the room to the hole in the floor that looked down on the altar in the chapel below, so that she could see Francis deliver the mass. The hole in the floor has been preserved.

As for her tremoring, in the report submitted to the Vatican after her passing, a report required for her beatification to go forward, her fellows nuns gave high praise: "Her fear of God was so great that her tremoring never ceased."

Clare notoriously celebrated being numb: "rising above pain." She sometimes wore an under-robe that had shards of sharp metal sewn into it, so that her body was constantly slashed and bleeding. Other nuns sometimes asked to be allowed to wear the garment, but they could never tolerate it for more than a few hours. Clare would wear it for days at a time.

Her explanation for this and her other acts of self-harm, including near-starvation, was that "Jesus suffered. God wants us to be more like Jesus."

St. Francis, the spiritual head of her order, was often called in to command her to eat or take a few cares for her body. She usually argued with him, but was then obedient, for a while.

Francis, whose relationship with God was communicative and personal, talked intimately with Jesus every night. He had no interest in self-harm or self-induced suffering in the name of spirituality.

Clare however had a very different understanding of what it meant to "please God." From what we know of Clare from her writings and the writings of her fellow nuns, Clare might have considered having a personal, communicative relationship with Jesus to be taking a liberty. She chose instead to make herself impervious to pain so that she could make her body suffer and thus – to her way of thinking – please a non-communicative, critical God by being more like Jesus.

St. Teresa of Avila

Another great saint that suffered years of increasing immobility is St. Teresa of Avila (1515-1582). Her doctors diagnosed her with a "disorder of the heart," which back in her day referred to an emotional or spiritual problem, not a physical cardiac problem. (The relatively modern idea of the heart playing a role in blood circulation was proposed and proved nearly a century after her passing.)

Teresa's immobility became so severe that eventually the other nuns in her order fed her by dripping sugar water into her mouth. However, after several years of nearly complete immobility, she experienced a great epiphany and completely, instantaneously recovered.

Because she spontaneously recovered from her steadily worsening paralysis, modern doctors have proposed that she suffered from temporal lobe epilepsy – a come-and-go syndrome that does not match her well-detailed symptoms. Although her symptoms were those of Parkinson's disease, PD is officially incurable and yet she recovered. Therefore, doctors have looked at other syndromes for a possible explanation of her Parkinson's-like symptoms and her remarkable recovery.

Following her sudden and complete recovery, she had a tendency to levitate. She was highly embarrassed by these "flights of joy," which came on when she was overwhelmed with bliss from communicating with what she referred to as the "bodyless" and/or "formless" Christ: her invisible friend. She requested that the other nuns hold her down when these flights occurred.

Of course, these manifestations of physical lightness (the opposite of the physical sense of heaviness of Parkinson's disease) got her into trouble with the church authorities. She had to go to Rome so that the Pope could decide if she was bewitched or was, in fact, attuned to God. The pope determined that she was divinely, not demonically, inspired.

After that, her spiritual superiors commanded her to write down the steps she had taken in attaining her profound relationship with the Divine. She described her inner life in her autobiographical writings, *The Interior Castle* and *The Way of Perfection*. She has become known for the intimacy of her conversations with Jesus and with God.

Although arrived at by her own reflections, her understanding of the steps that lead to knowing the Divine matches up fairly closely with the eight-step principles espoused by Patanjali.

Teresa of Avila's influence is responsible for many modernizing changes in the Catholic church, including making it "legal" for Catholics to speak to God in the language of their own hearts instead of being restricted to rote recitation of prayers that were approved by the church fathers.

A famous story about Teresa recounts how, after her recovery, she was traveling in early spring to give a lecture or start a new convent or something: there are several versions of this story, but they all have the same general outline. In all the versions, she had to cross a rising river. She prayed to God that she might *not* fall in the river. Holding her clothes and possessions high over her head, she started to cross. (Some versions have her crossing in a cart.) She fell into the river and got drenched.

When she got to the other side, she shook her fist at the sky and demanded, "Why did you do that to me?!"

A voice answered, "This is how I treat my friends."

Teresa immediately snapped back, "That explains why you have so few!"

I include the above because it shows the highly intimate, loving, and even snappy, irreverent, and teasing relationship that she had with Jesus, her invisible Love, her "bodiless Christ."

As for God's or maybe Jesus's saucy reply that "This is how I treat my friends," that can be understood as a reference to divine assistance in working out the small bits of karmic obstruction that a person might still have, unremembered, from a past lifetime *or* possibly the fulfillment of some long-forgotten prayer that might have been made on behalf of self *or* on behalf of another person: taking a bit of trouble upon oneself in exchange for that other person's health or safety.

Again, notice the loving, laughing intimacy between Teresa and her invisible, her "formless" Christ. They tease each other. They are completely comfortable with each other. They communicate constantly with each other. This type of relationship stimulates the striatum.

The Mahabharata

The hoary Hindu epic, *The Mahabharata* ("The Great War": war between the soul and the ego), said to be several thousand years old at a minimum, contains a chapter in which the evil prince metaphorically chooses to have Parkinson's disease rather than deal with the consequences of his actions.

The point of the overall epic is crystallized in a poem, the *Bhagavad Gita*, in the midpoint of the epic. In the *Gita*, the hero Arjuna, one of the good princes, born of the warrior caste, says he doesn't want to be a fighter. His uncle Krishna explains that we all must fight in this world in order to protect others, perform our duties, and overcome our own negative qualities.

Arjuna replies that he's a lover, not a fighter. He says that the way to God is through passivity. Krishna explains why the laser-like focus on some aspect of God while in the stillness of deep meditation *is* activity, *not* passivity. Also, why sometimes a person, in order to obtain oneness with the Divine, needs to get up off his meditation pillow and engage in the world, even if that means pain and fighting.

In the larger story of the Mahabharata, the evil princes (the evil or ego-driven tendencies in each of us) and the good princes (our innate good qualities) end up on a metaphorical battlefield. After many days of fighting, only one of the evil princes remains. He is Duryodhana, ego itself, the most powerful fighter on the side of evil. All of his brothers, the other, lower evil princes, the "temptations of evil," have been conquered. In the same way, many people with Parkinson's have learned to "rise above" the temptations of the most common vices with their stoic self-control, killing the evil princes of temptation. However, their ego is still alive and fighting – or as you shall see, *not* fighting…but using self-induced pause!

As per the rules of war, the princes and their armies end the daily combat at sunset. They plan to resume battle the next morning after sunrise. However, the next morning, the evil Duryodhana is nowhere to be found! The good princes track him, following his trail across the plains and up into the mountains. And here's where a person with PD wants to take note.

They find Duryodhana in the high mountains. He has smashed a hole in the ice of a mountain lake and submerged himself. The ice has frozen back over. Inside the frozen lake his body is rigid and trembling. He is numb and joyless.

The good princes stand over him and command him to come out and fight like a warrior. Duryodhana replies he will not. He would rather stay there forever, rigid and trembling, than engage in a fight that he, the ego, might not win. (Sound familiar?)

Backing up a bit, Arjuna is the prince that represents one's inner warrior. As noted earlier, in addition to waking up the striatum (striking up a metaphorical "conversation with Uncle Krishna," who represents the All-Loving Divine) some people need to re-awaken the feeling of force and power that flows into the Du channel at the back of the neck. When recovering from Parkinson's, this willful increase in power helps restore adrenal function. The *amount* of power (channel qi) in the body is greatly diminished when a person is on pause. Even in people with PD who keep running or going to the gym, they are using mental commands to keep going. They are not using *adrenaline*, or at least not much, to open the chest and increase heart rate. In people with Type I PD, the adrenal function increasingly diminishes to the point that it must sometimes be *consciously* re-activated after pause is turned off.

In Hindu scripture, Arjuna, the warrior prince, is the metaphorical regulator of the lumbar area ("ruler of the fifth chakra"), the spinal area around the small of the back: the location of the adrenal glands.

This portion of the epic Mahabharata is explaining that self-induced pause mode, intentionally making oneself frozen and apart, like the evil prince Ego, is *not* a "spiritual" option. The spiritual choice is to be like Arjuna: talk with and be guided by someone loving, like Uncle Krishna, while *feelingly* using the fullest measure of one's power to confront evil, no matter how frightful the task.

Now, you can completely dismiss all of the above bits about saints and ancient scripture if you like. I have included it only because many of my patients found great comfort in these bits of information. Many found it helpful to know that the issues they were dealing with were not their own, private, unique battles. Knowing that good, highly regarded people, saints, and even demi-gods in world scriptures have addressed the challenges of life by using self-induced pause instead of by reaching out for help has been enormously inspirational for some. For others, it serves as discouragement: "I can't be like those other people, those "good" people. I'm not like St. Teresa. I don't deserve to recover."

Don't *ever* think you aren't "good" because you have Parkinson's disease, or that you are "not good enough" to recover. If you have these types of negative thoughts about yourself, it might be helpful to consider that the Blocker was a liar from the beginning: a mental behavior created to protect the lies created by the ego.

Modern examples of people with Parkinson's

Moving into modern times and people with Parkinson's who were known not for their spirituality but for their great drive and intensity of purpose (the norepinephrine override), the list includes General Douglas McArthur of WWII fame, U.S. Attorney General Janet Reno, Governor George Wallace of Alabama, U.S. Senator and passionate environmentalist Mo Udall, and China's Chairman Mao Tse Tung.

The above are *not* known for being particularly associated with a spiritual path. Their similarities lie in the extreme *intensity* of their behavior: their ability to sustain being stronger, smarter, and/or more tireless than "regular people": emergency mode behaviors.[1]

Musings on the spiritual aspects

The fact that so many people of recognized spiritual attainment have had Parkinson's might be construed as evidence that having Type I Parkinson's disease means that a person with PD *is* actually getting a bit closer to attaining his spiritual goals. He might still be deeply confused as to the nature of surrender and/or wrongly thinking that he must *all alone* protect himself against a cruel universe or must *do* something in order to find joy or find love or, if you prefer the religious vocabulary, "find God." But still, he might be lifetimes ahead of the average person in terms of the spiritual discipline of life-energy control.

What if the traumatic situation that led to self-induced pause was a spiritual test to see how a person responds to terrible fear or pain? When in the throes of some trauma, did the person trust the universe enough to reach out for a greater Love or Wisdom? Or did he withdraw into isolationist self-protection – a level of mental protection he can create *only* because of years, lifetimes, of spiritual practice? These are the kinds of questions I find myself pondering as I consider my own choices in this life, my own recovery from Parkinson's, and the questions that my patients have shared with me.

Those who have recovered have tended to see, in retrospect, that they made a unhealthy, wrong choice years earlier through lack of understanding or fear. Their learning how to accept help and love from a larger source or an invisible friend has

[1] Adolph Hitler and Michael J. Fox are not included in this section of famous people with Parkinson's because they both had drug-induced parkinsonism, a completely different syndrome from idiopathic Parkinson's.

Hitler was a huge fan of methamphetamine. He used it to give himself "power." His troops were dosed with methamphetamine, giving them the "superhuman" speed and strength for their *blitzkriegs*, their "lightening strikes."

Michael J. Fox, as described in his autobiography, developed symptoms of drug-induced parkinsonism overnight, together with a small group of friends, after they all partied with synthetic heroin. He then embraced the "high" he got from his prescribed antiparkinson's drugs, causing his symptoms to rapidly worsen. People with *idiopathic* PD very often do *not* experience a "high" from their medications. People with drug- or toxin-induced parkinsonism very often *do*.

If you do a search on the internet for "famous people with Parkinson's disease" many of the names that come up are actually people who have received diagnoses of parkinson*ism*, parasupranuclear palsy, and other syndromes that tend to get lumped together in articles on Parkinson's. I recently did such an internet search and the first names that popped up were all people who are known, in research circles, to *not* actually have idiopathic Parkinson's disease, but have other syndromes in the "movement disorder family," including drug-induced parkinsonism.

brought them back to a healthy, *humbled* mindset – and turned off the Parkinson's. To grow in humility is to grow closer to Wisdom and divine Love. And in some cases, but clearly not *all* cases, recovery brought a deeper level of spiritual inquiry or even wisdom regarding how to behave when scared.

Then again, some people's immediate response to recovering from Parkinson's has been looking for a way to capitalize on their recovery and make a cash profit from it even though they've had no idea what they did that caused their recovery. One person (not my patient), after recovering following an epiphany, published a copy of *my* book with a very slightly altered title, under his *own* name, and started a business telling other people how to recover. I had to initiate a lawsuit to get him to cease and desist publishing my copyrighted material under his own name. He was quite hostile towards me, writing, "Hey! Why are you doing this to me? I've got to make a living, too!" He even sold expensive health products for people with PD, products that actually had nothing to do with his own recovery.

Another recovered person (not my patient) who has *no* idea what actually causes PD or how to treat most forms of it charges people with PD a substantial fee just to get his emailed, "personalized" advice. His advice is based on my earlier theories about foot injuries, so he can only help people who have Type II PD, which means when he "helps" other people, he is probably moving them closer to partial recovery – a hindrance, not a help.

So don't worry about necessarily turning into a saint just because you recover. If you were a jerk or scam artist before recovering, you'll still be a jerk or scam artist after recovering. Recovering isn't necessariy going to bring you closer to God or to sainthood, either, although many people felt that it did. After you recover, you'll still be exactly who you were before, but with a new attitude, one that's able to stand up to and engage with life instead of pretending to be numb or dead.

Spiritual responses versus Parkinson's responses

A person who is resonant with Universal Love or with the Divine sees the more profound workings of the laws of cause and effect during injury or emotional challenge – so he doesn't take things so *personally*. When caught up in worldly pains and trauma, a person who is resonant with Universal Wisdom or Love *increases* his reliance on his spiritual relationships, surrendering more deeply to, trusting more utterly, the loving but incomprehensibly vast Universal laws of cause and effect. The inner peace thus attained allows for a calm, even minimized, response to events that might send a less resonant person into the fear and panic of sympathetic mode…or, if capable, into pause.

The result of this feeling safe, and its concomitant impersonal or minimized response or increased surrender might *look* to an outsider as if the person is simply maintaining composure, or it might look like "rising above pain."

But this saintly, bemused serenity has its roots in the exact opposite physics and biology from what most people with Parkinson's assume is "right attitude."

Being fearlessly, radiantly at peace despite the "crash of breaking worlds" is the *opposite* of hiding behind numbness. [1]

---

[1] "Learn to stand unshaken amidst the crash of breaking worlds." According to the yogic saint Sri Sri Daya Mata, this spiritual advice from the ancient *Mahabharata* means, that, "when

For example, St. Francis of Assisi – who did *not* have Parkinson's – was known to absent-mindedly forget to eat for days at a time. He was in such a constant state of union with Jesus, his friendly, laughing confidant – sometimes invisible, sometimes visible – that he once wrote, "Such love does the sky now pour, that whenever I stand in a field, I have to wring out the light when I get home."

One time, returning to his fellow disciples after being out of town for a few days, Francis noted that they were looking weak and glum. He asked what was the matter.

"We want to be more like you, Francis, so we are fasting, like you do."

Francis lovingly explained, "If I am hungry, I eat."

What the disciples didn't understand was that his fasting didn't make him spiritual. Rather, his spirituality, his constant communion with Jesus often prevented him from noticing whether or not he had eaten. His deep calm and joy came from feeling close to and constantly talking to Jesus, not from making himself numb or refraining from food when hungry.

Another example of spirituality that completely baffles most of my Parkinson's patients is this quote from Meister Eckhard: "If He let go of my hand, I would weep so loudly, I would petition with all my might, I would cause so much trouble…that I bet God would come to His senses and never do that again."

Meister Eckhard – who did *not* have Parkinson's – is describing the exact opposite behavior from what most of my Parkinson's patients think of as spiritual. He is talking about making a ruckus in order to keep God *tangibly* near, even if it means acting like a naughty child.

My patients, for the most part, are trying to cultivate the *appearance* of saintliness by showing the world a stern grimness or maybe a gentle numbness – either way, a non-responsiveness to pain and affront. They are doing this by *suppressing* their emotions: they are sedating themselves into silent martyrdom. They are *not* joyfully choosing to focus on the Divine despite ongoing negative events.

Like the followers of St. Francis who wrongly thought they could win spirituality by starving themselves, most of my Parkinson's patients have been trying to present what they think is a spiritual front by inhibiting their feelings. They command themselves to behave in a manner that they think *mimics* the outer appearance of great saints and sages. But all the while, they are secretly feeling horribly apart from anything divine, or they are even feeling "unworthy."

Notice that I say pretending to be *apart* from God is the problem. Being *angry* at God is not necessarily a problem. Being angry and expressing it vigorously and fearlessly implies a relationship. Oppositely, thinking that one is apart from God or the rest of this interconnected quantum universe is indulging a fallacious, sulky, ego-based fantasy. The modern research in quantum pairing tells us that every bit of everything is connected to everything else. If you are nursing a mindset that says you are apart or inherently different, you are literally wrong. This wrong attitude can make you sick and keep you sick.

---

things become difficult, that is the time to rush to God's feet, to cry to Him within, to demand as His child that He help you." *This* is how a person remains "unshaken" at his core: he *goes* to his core, to his most trusted friends, to his heart, for help.

http://yogananda.com.au/dayamata/daya_mata_purpose_of_tests.html

By the way, if my use of the word "God" is offensive – as it well may be, and for good reason, for some people, – please substitute the word Love or Universal Consciousness or some word or phrase that you like. Even if your past religious training has taught you to distrust or even hate and fear the concept of God, I hope you can still believe that there is such as thing as Love in the universe. And whatever you call that concept, you need to have a relationship with it – not be apart from it. For example, imagining that you are apart from Love, separated from all the love in the universe, is a problem. Being *angry* at Love is *not*. Being angry at Love, or God, or Consciousness, and feeling free to express yourself vigorously and fearlessly to it implies a *relationship* with Love, God, or Consciousness. It's the *relationship* that is going to help you turn your brain's striatum back on if you've gotten stuck on self-induced pause.

Many of my patients with Type I PD have had views similar to those of the body-torturing St. Clare with regard to "rising above pain," being numb to "worldly pain," or being happy to martyr their health for a presumably spiritual cause.

Oppositely, others have considered that the *avoidance* of pain, or good health in and of itself, should be one's prime spiritual motivation. Some of my patients have created extensive, even obsessive diet and/or exercise protocols for their own health. These exercise and food regimens have *not* slowed the progress of their Parkinson's symptoms, although a few people have noticed a brief reduction in symptoms, at first, in response to their regimens: the type of reduction that occurs in response to *any* convincing placebo.

Effective, short-term placebos for Parkinson's include nearly every food and supplement. People have proclaimed their success at slowing Parkinson's with products ranging from filtered water, thiamine, and CoQ-10 all the way to marijuana and alcohol.

However, like all other placebos, the exercise or food regimens and the various magic "spiritual" formulas have ceased to work when the person came up against some new, powerfully negative event that threw him right back into steadily worsening symptoms of Parkinson's disease.

My patients' variations on what constitutes "spiritual" or "morally upright" lifestyle, including dietary and exercise fads, energy machines or Qi Gong machines and other gimmicks, are all over the map. In my limited experience, none of these fads, machines, physical "tricks" or miracle diets ever worked for the long term.

The Type I patients who eventually recovered were those who were able to 1) turn their backs on their nattering negative mindset, 2) cultivate practices that increase the flow of energy through the midbrain: practices such as constantly communicating with an invisible friend, keeping one's mental energy focused at the center of the brain's frontal lobe or Yin Tang and keeping up a steady stream of grateful thoughts plus, if necessary, 3) restarting their adrenal gland function.

Next, let's move away from this chapter's intuitive and un-provable observations.

Let's look at the very objective, physical phenomena that underlie the processes at work in idiopathic Parkinson's disease. Nothing makes the underlying biology of Parkinson's more clear than the changes and temporary symptoms that can occur during *recovery* from Parkinson's.

While the brain scan research I stumbled across in 2015 led me to techniques for turning off self-induced pause, the *most* important findings, the things that pointed me to what actually causes Parkinson's disease, the things that will answer your remaining questions about what Parkinson's really *is*, is the upcoming discussion of recovery symptoms. The utterly unexpected recovery symptoms don't just show what happens in recovery. They reveal what was actually going on in the body during the years that Parkinson's was still invisible.

Working backwards from the recovery symptoms, I was able to figure out what causes the neurological changes of Parkinson's disease, and from there I could understand why people were recovering, or not, in response to various therapies.

Hang on to your hat.

Chapter Twenty-one

Recovery Symptoms: An Introduction

The greatest proof that my patients had recovered from Parkinson's, as opposed to having been "misdiagnosed," was their recovery symptoms. These bizarre symptoms took all of us by surprise. We could not have predicted these weird physical behaviors that, in the end, made perfect sense and even brought about a better understanding of the processes that had been in place during Parkinson's.

After people with Parkinson's turned off pause or pseudo pause, nearly all of them experienced the same unexpected, counterintuitive, and even bizarre physical events and specific emotional changes. In the early days of the research, these events were as much a part of the puzzle as the symptoms of Parkinson's disease. Although the *exact* details of these events varied from one patient to another, there was an overall similarity in the symptoms they reported.

My very earliest PD patients didn't know each other. This was good. The probability of research "contamination" from patient-to-patient was unlikely. Also, since my hypotheses as to the cause of Parkinson's disease were not yet formed when the first patients recovered, there is no way that I or a patient could have correctly guessed at what recovery symptoms, if any, might occur. I was as baffled as the patients when one recovering patient after another manifested wholly unexpected symptoms that are the opposite of Parkinson's, after turning off the electrical current behaviors that I know now are typical of pause mode. I named these events "recovery symptoms."

The recovery symptoms ended up being some of the most important phenomena for shaping my ideas about Parkinson's. Together with my deepening understanding of channel theory, the recovery symptoms provided the proofs that my patients had *not* been misdiagnosed. They had, in fact, had Parkinson's. The recovery symptoms also exposed the physiological processes of Parkinson's that are *not* in any way related to dopamine or the lack thereof.

"What the heck?"

The very first patients, the ones I named "the pioneers," expected any improvement from Parkinson's to be pleasant. They assumed that recovery, if that was indeed what was happening, would consist of steady, linear improvements in motor function. They assumed as well that any benefits would take the form of a "return to the past." In most cases, this would have meant a return to the previous way of life: high pain threshold; strong will power; command-based movement.

What actually occurred did not fit anyone's expectations. Every one of the pioneers was shocked by the unanticipated, seemingly negative, collection of new, short-term symptoms that occurred as their long-dissociated injuries began to heal and/or they turned off pause mode.

But as they began to see the positive flip-side of these sometimes fleetingly painful and/or alarming changes, they started to appreciate that something incredible was going on: they were truly recovering from Parkinson's disease – not just feeling better by masking the symptoms. After all, the new symptoms, though weird, were the exact *opposite* of the symptoms of Parkinson's.

The credo of many pioneers became something like: "I don't know what the heck is going on, but it sure as hell isn't Parkinson's disease."

Introduction to physiological symptoms

Although most doctors think of Parkinson's in terms of *movement* disorder, many *physiological* pathologies of Parkinson's develop through the years that have nothing to do with movement. Examples of physiological changes that aren't movement related include coldness in the hands and feet, numbness in the face and toes, the rigidity of the psoas muscle paired with the looseness of the lumbar quadratic muscles, the frequently occuring backwards curve of the neck, and the fungus growing in the feet and face. These are all conditions that exist whether or not the person with Parkinson's is trying to execute large or small motor function (walking or using the hands).

If a person with PD has numbness in the muscles of the cheek or the lower eyelid, it will be present whether the patient is trying to use those muscles or not. Many of these *physiological* symptoms of Parkinson's disease do not change with mood or expectation: they are caused by physical changes that have taken place in muscle tissue, nerve tissue, blood supply, and brain-to-muscle connectivity during the long years of using pause schematics. These symptoms may *contribute* to the poor performance of certain movements, in the same way that a polio-shortened leg or a smashed index finger may contribute to poor motor performance. But these physiological changes do not *cause* the pause-based inhibition of automatic movement or the tremor. The inhibition and tremor only become obvious when the norepinephrine override begins to fail. The *physiological* changes, the breakdowns in the physical body, have been invisibly worsening long before the obvious motor symptoms of Parkinson's showed up.

The physiological symptoms are *not* improved by taking dopamine-enhancing medications because they are *not* dopamine-related symptoms. They are simply the result of long-term changes in nerve and muscle that are caused by channels running in the pause schematics for the long term. These are the changes in the body that I metaphorically refer to as "war damage."

During recovery, the healing of the physiological damage is the "rebuilding after the war." These healing changes might start to occur automatically as soon as channel qi starts flowing in the healthy, ever shifting blend of sympathetic and parasympathetic circuits.

The list of recovery symptoms

In 1999, in the first edition of this book, I included a list of recovery symptoms that had occurred in my first dozen patients. Because I was concerned that some symptoms were individual flukes, and not characteristic of recovering from PD, I only included recovery symptoms on the list if *several* people manifested them. Once I'd seen a given recovery symptom three times, I included it on the growing list. As the project grew, I kept updating the information on the website, listing additional recovery symptoms as I observed them.

The recovery symptoms were sometimes startling, even alarming. I wanted people to know about the recovery symptoms so that they could 1) be encouraged that they had turned off Parkinson's and 2) *not* be frightened. I wanted people to *celebrate* these weird symptoms, not fear them.

However, I soon found that many patients were using this list as a *required* checklist: if their own recovery symptoms were *not* on the list, they panicked. Oppositely, if a person *didn't* experience *all* of the items on the list, he might become certain that his recovery had stalled.

In some people who had been obviously recovering from *Type I* PD, the panic or worry about stalled recovery *based* on the list of recovery symptoms often resurrected the old Blocker and even some of the old Parkinson's symptoms. After all, even after turning off pause for good, a person can always *choose* to re-activate it, especially if he hasn't yet resumed using sympathetic mode – the *correct* mode for dealing with fear or rage.

Some patients who were clearly recovering were still always on the lookout for a reason to resume the numbed familiarity of pause mode. A person's variation from the list of recovery symptoms turned out to be a popular reason for resuming anew the use of pause.

Pause mode is *never* supposed to be used casually, as a way to deal with fear, anger, or unpleasantness. Pause mode is a drastic mode. It should only be used for trying to stay alive while on the verge of death. But patients who were not yet comfortable using the adrenaline of sympathetic mode often found it more familiar and comfortable to return to the use of pause mode in response to *any* new negative thought, even after they'd turned pause off completely for some period of time.

This is yet another reason why learning to direct one's silent thoughts to a friend or a beloved somebody is helpful over the *long run* – not just while working to turn off pause. Even after helping turn off pause the first time, the presence of the invisible friend can also encourage the use of *healthy* modes in response to fear, and oppose the reversion *back* to the use of pause mode. Instructions on re-starting and/or learning to use sympathetic mode are included in the book *Stuck on Pause*.

An example of reverting back to pause

In my own case, when I resumed running for exercise after not having done so in a while, I noticed that, when running hard, I was once again "outside my body" and mentally commanding myself to move my legs. This was pure habit. I should have been engaging a higher degree of *sympathetic* mode to support my physical output of energy. I should *not* have reverted to pretending I was on the verge of death. But when I got my heart rate up and was running strong, I noticed that my body-awareness reverted back into that of pause mode. I was once again outside my body, as I had always been since I was young. Because the rest of the day my somatic awareness was now *inside* my body, the strangeness of being *outside* of it while running really stood out.

I was *never* using pause mode any more *except* during running. It was obvious that my use of pause during sports was a *habit*. Not a need. In my younger days I had very consciously used my mind, rather than my somatic awareness, to perform sports. Now, after recovering from Parkinson's and enjoying the novel sensations of being inside my body, I still found myself automatically switching back into a pause mode frame of mind while running hard.

I had to force myself to mentally stay inside my body while running. I had to imagine my adrenal glands glowing and discharging adrenaline, and to *celebrate* the "out of control" sensations of powerful, increased heart rate and animal-like, powerful breathing. It took me a few days to learn to stay in the "modes of the living" instead of reverting back into pause while running hard.

Once a person has learned to use pause instead of the healthy modes, he can easily slip back into pause now and then, due to habit. Adding to this, people who had Type I PD were very often poised to turn pause back on at the least sign of anything new, unexpected or mildly risky. The recovery symptoms were new, unexpected, and *weird* – therefore inherently risky.

Many people reverted back into pause mode in response to recovery symptoms, or *lack* of them, and then stayed there. They would tell themselves that they hadn't recovered, after all – even though their PD symptoms had greatly diminished and they'd already had *some* recovery symptoms.

So, starting with the 2012 edition of this book, I got rid of the recovery symptoms list.

Understanding the mechanisms

Since 2012, instead of a list, I explain what causes the recovery symptoms. If people understand the *mechanisms* involved they don't have to panic that they aren't recovering in exactly the same sequence or manner as other patients. They have more time to enjoy *not* being on pause and slowly learning to use sympathetic mode when they are scared, instead of lurching back into pause at the first hint of variation from the list. Therefore, the following chapters share only a *sampling* of recovery symptoms, together with explanations of *why* the symptoms occur.

Even so, people recovering from Type I PD can still find reasons to panic. One patient who had clearly been having recovery symptoms for a couple of months went into a tailspin with returning PD symptoms when he started having periods of muscle spasm in his back, between his shoulder blades. The periods of come-and-go, brief spasms would last for about twenty minutes. This had been going on for several days. He wrote to me in a panic. I explained that this was a *classic* recovery symptom, as described in the recovery symptom chapters: the hesitant, often spastic, budding return of muscle function for twenty minutes at a time in muscles that had been long been non-functional which were starting to resume function, albeit intermittently, at first. He wrote back that he'd never read about the muscle spasm recovery symptom occurring between the *shoulder blades*, and so probably his Parkinson's had returned.

I emailed him that weakness in the area between the shoulder blades *is* mentioned in chapter thirteen, in the discussion of which muscles become rigid and which become cold or atrophied. My chapter on recovery symptoms gave many examples of come-and-go spasms, lasting for a period of about twenty minutes, over many days, in muscles that had previously been rigid *or* non-functional. The recovery chapter on this subject did *not* specifically mention *this* set of muscles. Even so, this set of muscles *had* in fact been listed in the chapter on muscles that can be affected by weakness during Parkinson's.

As soon as I pointed this out to him, he agreed that his new symptoms did, in fact, match perfectly my description of recovery spasms. But until I was able to direct him to the page where I mentioned this set of muscles, he was convinced that he had new Parkinson's symptoms, not recovery symptoms. He had been in a panic, and a few of his

Parkinson's symptoms had even returned, for the forty-eight hours it took for enough email exchanges to occur showing him that these were, in fact, recovery symptoms.

If everything else I saw wasn't enough to convince me that there's a strong psychological component to Parkinson's, some of my patients' pause-mode reversion responses to recovery symptoms – which are *nothing* like the symptoms of PD, which are the *opposite* of the symptoms of PD – would have convinced me.

The tempo of recovery

With regard to the *physiological* recovery from muscle atrophy, poor nerve function, left-right coordination, and so on, it happens gradually.

Turning off pause might happen in an instant. The inhibition of dopamine release for motor function might be gone in the blink of an eye. But the repair of the physiological damage will take some time. Please remember, there was never a distinct day when a person woke up and *suddenly* had full-blown idiopathic Parkinson's disease. The *physiological* symptoms of idiopathic Parkinson's almost always develop slowly. The physiological recovery also takes time. The time frame varies from person to person. The only generalization I can make is that older people tend to take longer to heal than younger people. But even this is a generalization, and exceptions abound. And I refuse to state at what age a person is "younger" or "older."

Repairing the damage caused by backwards and inhibited electrical flow during the previous decades can take weeks, even months. It will take time to grow new muscle. It will take time to retrain new nerve connections. It will take time to return to full sensory function.

Once you get started on the recovery symptoms, you will be glad that they move along slowly. They can sometimes be overwhelming even at their moderate pace. Recovery symptoms are unstoppable (unless of course, you revert back to using pause mode). They are not always pleasant. At some point, you will be *grateful* that they do not happen all at once, but merely progress as quickly as you can tolerate.

How long will the overall process take? How intense will this be?

The amount of time required for healing is variable, and I will *not* make estimates as to how long it might take for any given individual.

I have had patients whose more obvious physiological symptoms of Parkinson's disease were gone within three to five weeks of turning off pause. I have had other patients who were still noticing tiny improvements in motor function several years after the injury was healed and/or pause turned off, and their symptoms of PD were long gone.

In my own case, for example, within half a year, I assumed I had recovered completely because I had no more PD symptoms. Even so, for years afterwards, I kept noticing small motor improvements.

For example, five *years* after recovering, one day, as I was putting my shoes on, my *right* leg (the leg that had the more severe symptoms) lifted up and crossed itself over the left knee in order to facilitate putting the right shoe on. For nearly all of my life, up until that moment, when putting on my shoes, I used my *hands* to lift my right leg up and lay it across the opposite knee. It was pure habit. My *left* leg had always performed this movement automatically, without even thinking. My *right* leg had always needed a lift from my hands. I was amazed to watch my right leg lifting up and lying itself across my left knee without the help of my hands. This move occurred effortlessly. I hadn't even thought about it. It made me realize that my automatic motor function was *still* improving: still recovering from my years on pause.

No one looking at me or watching me move would have been able to see any symptoms remotely related to Parkinson's. But here I was, five years after turning off pause, still experiencing tiny improvements, now and then, related to *recovering* from Parkinson's disease. So I am not about to offer a reply to the query: "How long it will take to fully recover?"

My swallow reflex abruptly restored itself more than twenty years after I turned off pause. One day I noticed, several times during the day, my throat "caught" something that was about to slide down the wrong way and diverted it into the esophagus. I was so amazed at the sensation, one that I don't remember ever having had before. It was wonderful: I didn't choke or even almost choke. Ever since that day, my frequent choking or almost choking is gone. Again, this spot of healing occurred more than twenty years after I turned off pause and my obvious symptoms of Parkinson' disappeared.

Linearity

In my original list of recovery symptoms, I listed them in the *order* that recovery symptoms had often, but not always, occurred: first, second, and so on until the last.

I learned that, no matter how many times I wrote "recovery symptoms will *not* necessarily take place in this sequence," *some* people, usually ones who'd had Type I PD, panicked if their recovery symptoms were not in the sequence in which I'd listed them. In the early days of this research, I was not yet aware of the powerful, well-established brain habits favoring negativity and imagining worst-case scenarios that many people with Parkinson's, especially those with Type I, had acquired and/or cultivated. This negativity might be the result of a challenging childhood or a pre-natal disposition. And it might have gotten far more entrenched because of living in pause mode for many years. At any rate, a person who embraced negative thinking in general would be likely to respond negatively – even go back into pause mode – in response to recovery symptoms that didn't happen in the "right sequence."

So, in this edition, there are no references to which recovery symptoms *tend* to occur first, second, and last. Toes *might* recover before fingers, or vice versa. Improvement in *sensory* function *might* precede the return of improved *movement* function in some body parts, or vice versa: toes might regain *sensitivity* prior to recovering full range of *movement*, or vice versa; facial muscles might show increased *movement* long before full *feeling* returns to the face, or vice versa. I might have seen that recovery symptoms *tend* to occur in a certain order, but I'm no longer going to *share* that information.

I will just say that the path of recovery is *somewhat* predictable. But recovery symptoms do *not* necessarily follow a straight line. Also, the recovery symptoms are sometimes subtle, sometimes blatant. The *intensity* of recovery symptoms varies from person to person and, in any one person, might vary from day to day.

The organization of the chapters on recovery symptoms

The recovery symptoms that *tended* to occur earlier are discussed in the earlier chapters of this recovery section and the recovery symptoms that *tended* to occur later on are described in the later chapters of this section. "Later on" in the above sentence might mean a few hours or days later or a few months or years later.

Each chapter has an explanation as to *why* these symptoms occur and a few specific examples of what these symptoms might look or feel like. I might also include an example or two of the fascinating ways in which some patients have used the recovery symptoms to mentally convince themselves that they were getting worse instead of better.

I repeat: no two people with Parkinson's have the exact same collection of symptoms. Each person's *recovery* from Parkinson's disease is also unique. The next ten chapters describe the recovery symptoms and the *reasons* behind the recovery symptoms. The chapters are presented in *approximately* the order in which recovery symptoms *might* appear, but there is NO hard and fixed sequence.

Also, as promised earlier, these chapters will show the differences in *perception* of recovery symptoms between people who were fully recovered and those who were stuck in partial recovery. Hopefully, this will help convince people with Parkinson's who intend to recover that they *must* recover from self-induced pause before they work on any injuries along the Stomach or Du channels.

And as you learn about the recovery symptoms, you will also see why the dead dopamine-cell theory of Parkinson's, which only addresses automatic movement inhibition, is *completely* inadequate to explain the physiological changes that occur during Parkinson's *and* during recovery from Parkinson's.

Chapter Twenty-two

Recovery symptoms: Numbness Becomes Pain

Symptoms of numbness vs. rigidity

As you recall, numbness and atrophy is the eventual result of a long-term *absence* of channel qi. Rigidity is a correct response to *backwards*-flowing channel qi. The *locations* associated with these *opposite* types of PD symptoms (numb and/or atrophied *or* rigid and/or tense) were described in chapter fourteen.

Differentiating between symptoms that arise from an *absence* of channel qi versus symptoms from *backwards* flow of channel qi will enable you to make sense of many recovery symptoms.

For example, when pause-type channel qi flow turns off, the numbness and rigidity both begin to melt away. Areas that were previously *numb* become highly sensitive and even painful, for a while. Oppositely, the areas that had been *rigid* become limp, for a while.

Areas that were numb resume feeling

This chapter will address the recovery symptoms that occur in body parts where channel qi flow had been absent or minimal: areas that developed numbness or atrophy and a lack of proprioception. Chapter twenty-six will discuss recovery symptoms in areas that had become rigid.

Often, one of the first changes people notice when pause-type channel qi turns off is improvement in blood circulation in the feet and face: the two areas in which channel qi flow is *diminished* or *absent* during pause mode. The following section will address changes in the feet. The section after that will discuss changes in the face.

Improved circulation in the feet

As the normal blend of healthy parasympathetic and sympathetic channel qi flow resumes, foot color often improves significantly. Blood vessels in the feet often become larger and more visible. Temperature regulation in the feet, if poor, improves.

Prior to turning off pause or starting Yin Tui Na treatment, the skin on the feet of many of my patients was mottled, sometimes purplish, or even a ghastly gray, with no or few distinct blood vessels. If a large vein *was* visible, it often formed a semi-circular pattern on the top of the foot instead of flowing all the way from the toes.

Some patients' ankles had severe staining (dark reddish brown discolorations) or angry, bright red varicosities. After turning off pause and/or re-associating with the foot injury(s), the skin color might become healthier and healthy blood vessels might show up more. The semi-circular vein might develop branches feeding into it from the toes, or a completely new set of healthy veins might appear that fan out over the toes. Sometimes, the dark "staining" lightened up a bit and angry-looking varicosities diminished in size and intensity. These changes sometimes coincided with or foreshadowed an improvement in temperature regulation in the feet.

Warm feet!

After turning off Parkinson's, many patients who'd had cold feet for years deeply enjoyed the novel sensation of having feet that could warm up easily after having been subjected to cold. Long-lasting cold in the extremities that doesn't respond to normal heating methods, also known as Reynaud's syndrome, is not unusual in people with Parkinson's disease.

One recovering PD patient had abject fear of getting cold feet. If his feet got chilled, they remained horribly cold for *days*. When his foot injury healed and circulation in his feet improved, he enjoyed sprinting barefoot along the snow-blanketed walkway out to the mailbox to pick up his letters and then scampering back into the house. He didn't mind that his feet got cold. Rather, he was *thrilled* because, each time, after getting back into the heated house, his feet would quickly warm up again! He said he was as pleased as a child at the novel sensation of his feet getting warm all by themselves after having been briefly chilled.

The return of sensation

A recovery symptom that accompanied improved circulation was the cessation of numbness.

Prior to recovering, many patients insisted that their toes were not numb. As proof, they pointed out that they could feel their toes if they stubbed or touched them. However, their proprioceptive awareness of their toes, which is to say their internal sense of how the toes feel and awareness of where they are located could be *completely* lacking. The three medial toes on the more affected side are *usually* quite numb. During recovery, when feeling returned to their toes, patients learned how extremely numb they had been.

In some cases, the return of sensation in the toes was mildly pleasant. In most cases, however, the return of sensation to long-numbed nerves was somewhat painful. Common descriptions of foot sensations that occurred during recovery from numbness were "tingling," "burning," "pins and needles," and "like the pain during recovery from frostbite."

Frostbitten toes are actually painless – so long as they remain frozen. In fact, they are often "not a problem" until they warm back up. *Recovery* from frostbite, on the other hand, can be quite painful. The return of sensation in the feet after turning off pause can be similar to recovery from frostbite. If one is not aware of how numb the feet are, one might imagine that the feet are perfectly fine. Only when feeling resumes do the prickly sensations of pins and needles appear.

One particular area on the foot tended to experience a very powerful sensation during recovery: the medial side of the ball of the foot, in the general vicinity of SP-3.

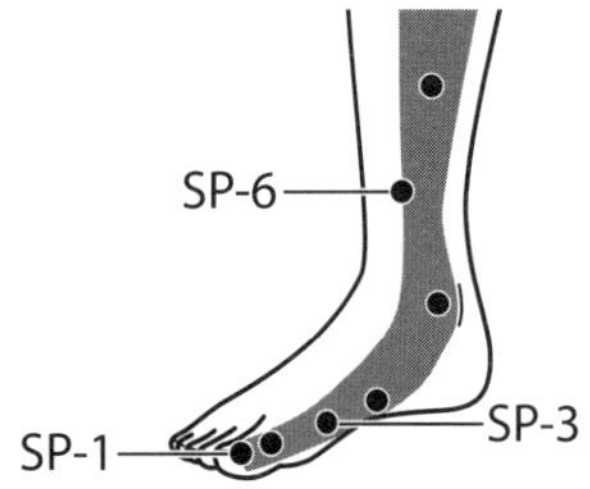

Fig. 21.1 Acupoints on the medial side of the foot, on the Spleen channel

Many recovering patients reported a powerfully strong stinging sensation at SP-3. They said things such as: "I was certain I had a splinter in my foot right there. I took my shoe off six times to try to find the splinter but there was nothing there," or "I thought a bee was stinging me there; I took off my shoe several times but there was no bee."

However, some of the tingling that occurred when the nerves come back to life was less site-specific: the sensations moved around. Many people described the sensations as "ants moving around in my toes." Another description was "someone's dragging a miniature rake back and forth over the top of my foot and my toes for the last two weeks."

The sensations might last for a few hours, or occur on and off for days, weeks, or months. Eventually, when full feeling is restored, the tingling and/or pain ceases.

Variations on the tingling sensation

Some people experience glowing warmth or even alarming bursts of heat instead of or in addition to tingling, spiders, or ants.

Also, the emotional response to the reawakening of foot and toe nerves varies from one patient to another. Some recovering patients found the tingling sensations to be amusing or even thrilling: proof that change was underway. Others were fearful that the pins-and-needles sensations would only keep getting worse, or even that the new sensations were being caused, not by anything healthy, but by cancer, gout, imbedded carpenter's nails, broken glass, or some rare and incurable foot disease. The examples in the previous sentence came from my patients – I am not making up these far-fetched explanations for why the return of sensation in the feet presaged something dire.

Most people *enjoyed* the reassuring feelings of once again having toes. Others found the awareness unfamiliar and even frightening.

As to the intensity, a few recovering patients told me that they were so shocked by or fearful of their few, fleeting, stabbing sensations in their feet and toes that they screamed out loud during the more dramatic moments. Others said things like, "It was no big deal," "You got me worried for no reason," and "It's nothing; why did you even put it in your book?"

The descriptions and variations regarding the return of nerve function in the feet and face were different for every person. But I did notice that, in general, people who were more oriented towards cynicism or negativity tended to experience the return of nerve function as painful, or even terrible.

Those people who were more curious than frightened *tended* to enjoy, or at least not mind, the sensations. The sensations of recovery from Parkinson's are merely that: sensations. In the early days of my research, it seemed to me that whether recovery symptoms were perceived as augurs of health or omens of suffering seemed to depend entirely on whether or not a person was in a predominantly positive or negative mindset.

Now, having a fuller understanding of Parkinson's disease, I can say that people with Type I PD were the ones more *likely* to be scared by the return of sensation to their feet and faces. People with the *other* types of PD, and *many* people with Type I, responded to these changes with delight.

In the few cases in which I suspected that bones had been *broken* and dissociated for years and were only just starting to heal, the pain was temporarily excruciating, just as it *should* be with a broken bone. The pain of a broken bone should be powerful enough that the person doesn't use the area with the break until the bones have knit enough to stand up to usage.

Recovery sensations in the face: feeling, taste, and smell

As with the feet, the first changes to the face are often improvements in blood circulation. This can lead to improved color and warmth in the skin. The subsequent tingling, mild stabbing pains, and the sensation of bugs crawling under and over the skin usually comes and goes in short spurts. The spurts might come and go over the course of weeks or months.

Sensation often returns to the face more slowly and mildly than to the feet. But even if the facial sensations are milder, they can be much harder to ignore. Compared to tingling in the feet, the sensations of spiders crawling over the face and under the scalp can be less sharp and painful but far more startling and/or annoying for some people.

People who are more fearful in general were more likely to be agitated by their spiders and spider webs. People who were more curious and grateful tended to feel the spiders were benign, or that the sensations were more like ants or loose hairs, or maybe "little rakes" or "something scratching at me." I suspect that, in terms of nerve function, the actual sensation being transmitted was exactly the same. Whether the transmission was compared to ants, spiders, rakes, or scratching was merely a matter of personal *interpretation*.

When did the tingling occur?

The sensations tend to be intermittent. As with most types of recovery symptoms, these sensations are at their strongest when a person is awake and relaxed – in a relatively high degree of parasympathetic mode.

In *all* people, parasympathetic (conscious and curious) mode and sleep mode is when most healing occurs. This is possibly why recovering PD patients usually noticed the strongest symptoms of tingling or crawling bugs – or *any other* recovery symptoms – during those times when they were relaxing. Very often, people felt their recovery symptoms most strongly while watching TV in the evening or just before falling asleep.

Some patients were worried that they might have recovery symptoms while they were out in public – in the public eye. This almost never happened. It seemed as if, whenever a recovering patient was worried or frightened, the patient's mind switched over to a higher degree of sympathetic mode – as it should when one is concerned or, due to old habits, temporarily switched into pause mode, as it should *not* – and either way, the recovery symptoms temporarily ceased. So don't worry: recovery symptoms will not appear in public *unless* you are OK with it, *unless* you don't mind them so doing.

Numbness of sensory function in the face

In addition to poor muscle function, the numbness and poor circulation in the face from long-term use of pause mode can contribute to diminished senses of taste and smell, as well as coldness and lack of sensitivity in the facial skin, including the lips.

For example, many people with PD dribble on their shirtfronts when they drink from a glass or cup because their lips are somewhat numb. They cannot accurately sense *where* to apply lip pressure to the rim of the glass nor discern *if* they are applying pressure.

Just as with the denial of foot numbness, many of my PD patients denied that they had any impairment of taste or smell or tactile perception in the face. They assured me that their sense of taste and smell was perfectly normal. Others knew that their sense of taste, smell, or tactile awareness was declining or gone, but often insisted that the loss was a normal part of aging.

When recovering patients experienced the full range of healthy sensation that returned to face, tongue, and nose, they often asked me questions like, "Did you know that wet asphalt has a *smell!*?" or "Did you know that different kinds of tea actually taste different?!" These queries suggested that the person's sense of taste or smell had been numbed for a very long time. Some patients admitted that they were once again experiencing common smells, such as the smell of newly cut grass, for the first time in *decades*. When a person is numb, he cannot be a good judge of how numb he is: he may be too numb to know.

For example, one patient confessed to being humiliated for years even prior to her PD diagnosis because she was often told by fellow diners that she had a spot of food sitting on her lip or that she had a "food mustache." Also, she had increasingly spilled drops of her beverages down the front of her shirt. She did not think that her facial skin was numb. Instead, she had assumed that she was a clumsy eater because she ate and drank too *quickly*. Her son had even asked her once if she was able to *feel* the bits of food stuck on her face. She had assured him that she could, even though she wondered to herself how anyone could *possibly* feel a bit of food stuck on the face. After recovering, she was able once again to feel when her facial skin or lips were accidentally decorated with food. She no longer dribbled onto her shirt when drinking.

The duration of recovery symptoms

How long did the increased sensitivity and "crawling ants" go on? The period of *heightened*, excessive sensitivity only lasted until the brain accommodated, or you might say became inured to, the new incoming sensations – a few days, a few weeks, or a few months.

As with recovery from frostbite, the toe tingling comes to an end when blood circulation is fully restored, the nerves are up and running regularly again, and any cells damaged from lack of sufficient circulation have been broken down by the body and replaced with healthy new cells. After that, healthy, conscious awareness of the toes or face is possible. The same applies for people recovering from the numbness of long-term pause mode in *any* part of the body.

The timing and durations of the tingling sensations varied. For example, over a period of days or months, a patient might experience a few *moments* of tingling, followed by a period of calm. Or the tingling might occur a few *minutes* at a time. Or there may be a period of a day or two – or several months – during which the feet or face feel stabs of spiders, ants, or pins and needles for *hours* at a time. Anything is possible. Timing of recovery symptoms has an enormous range, spanning moments to months.

After the brain becomes re-accustomed to getting incoming nerve signals from the feet, face, or scalp, it behaves as it does in healthy people: awareness of these areas only rises to the consciousness when something significant – positive, negative, or otherwise – is occurring in these areas. For example, a healthy person might *not* notice her feet during the course of her busy day working at the computer. But when she's on vacation, she might find herself focusing on the luscious feeling of warm beach sand sifting through the toes.

Some patients, not appreciating this, worried because they'd had *constant, new* awareness of their feet or face for several weeks during the tingling stage of recovery but then that *constant* awareness dropped away. When they stopped noticing their toes or scalp all the time, they assumed the Parkinson's had returned. It hadn't. *Not* noticing sensations in body parts at all times is *normal*. Healthy people *sometimes* notice their feet, and sometimes they *don't*.

Asymmetrical healing

I'm introducing this subject here, in the section on recovery from numbness, but it applies to all the recovery topics.

Many patients noticed that recovery from numbness or rigidity occurred *first* in the *healthier* side of the body, where symptoms were less severe.

If the PD symptoms had started on the left side, the recovery symptoms might occur first on the *right* side. It seemed as if, when the channel qi started to flow correctly and the body started healing all the damaged bits, the parts that were *less* damaged often healed up first. The recovery symptoms on the more damaged side of the body were often more severe and took longer to heal. Sometimes, the healthier side of the body would be completely returned to health and vigor before the side where symptoms first appeared even started to experience the pains, warmth, tingling, and the new movement that indicated a return of circulation and function.

Patients were sometimes alarmed that their "healthy side" was tingling or wanting to move by itself. They assumed, wrongly, that their Parkinson's disease had spread to the healthy side. Considering that the recovery symptoms are the exact opposite of Parkinson's symptoms, this fear seemed illogical to me. But I didn't yet understand that, in addition to the wariness inherent in pause mode, some patients had developed brain habits that were focused more on anticipating *problems* than on anticipating health or joy.

The pleasures of recovery...or not

Whether the recovery symptoms felt like ants or spiders, or sudden awareness of stiffness and rigidity, my patients loved the eventual *results* of these recovery symptoms: return of sensation and function. Even in the earliest days of the project, when we could hardly dare to believe that we'd found an effective treatment for Parkinson's, the pioneers were thrilled at the improvements in their faces and feet. They were also surprised when they began to *feel* the full extent of their PD symptoms – and then felt them going away.

Family members also were usually thrilled to see the return of full facial expression.

A *few* patients grew angry when people suggested that they were now moving better or looking better. Supportive compliments from friends and loved ones were interpreted as criticisms of how the person had moved or looked in the past.

I remember one recovering patient insisting that he'd never had a lack of facial expression: he claimed he had *consciously* refrained from "stupid smiles." He claimed he was emulating the reserved, Buddhist monks that he'd briefly studied with, back in his college days. His face had expressed emotional "reserve;" it had *never* been frozen.

His wife and I did not argue with him. He could not be argued with. Although he was a brilliant professor of sociology, he had the social skills of a three year old – including stubbornness and temper tantrums. He was utterly unable to deal with the idea that he had ever been imperfect – especially with regard to his facial expression.

But the fact was, over the last ten years, his wife's friends had been increasingly afraid of him because he always looked as if he was glaring with disapproval. (He himself had no friends.) After muscle function returned to his face, he was clearly smiling at people once again, even as he continued to assume a mild, pleasant look of unctuous "reserve." Her friends were pleased that he was finally "warming" to them, that he had become "welcoming." His *behaviors* were actually just the same. So far as he could tell, he was still giving her friends the same calculated look of benevolent wisdom. So when any of us expressed delight with his new smiles, he grew angry, even belligerent.

He was very intelligent and witty. I'd noticed in the early days of treating him that, when he told jokes, his facial expression never changed. As he was recovering, his eyebrows, cheeks, nose, and mouth all danced with expression when he told his jokes and witticisms.

After his face recovered full sensation and the ability to move, the only thing that remained unchanged was his inability to admit that he'd ever had a frozen face – or been imperfect in any way.

His severe OCD behaviors including frantic germaphobia, and his stubbornness and temper tantrums were *somewhat* unusual in my experience. In general, my PD patients *tended* to be people-pleasers: careful to not show antagonistic emotions, and careful to prevent anger rising up in those around them: the characteristic emotional-harm avoidance traits of the "classic" Parkinson's personality.

Increased awareness of rigidity and other PD symptoms

Often, along with a cessation of numbness came an increased *awareness* of rigidity in other body parts. This rigidity might have been there right along, but had not been felt. For example, many patients had not realized that their wrists or ankles had been moving in a cogwheel motion until their doctor pointed it out. They couldn't *feel* the wrist or ankle very well (they were numb), so they didn't realize the full extent to which the ankle or wrist was rigid.

While recovering, due to improved circulation and the concomitant return of nerve sensitivity, many patients began to notice that their bodies were far more rigid than they had realized. As one person said, "I can feel my feet better and I'm walking better and faster, but I never knew my legs were so heavy and stiff!"

Another patient said, "I think I'm getting worse. I have a limp." In fact, according to her spouse, she had been limping long before she started to recover. When her spouse reminded her of this, she recalled that, for decades, she had *heard* herself limping, but had never *felt* it before. She only *felt* the limp when her foot numbness began to recede.

No crystal ball

Many patients, prior to entering the program, have insisted on knowing exactly what their own recovery symptoms will be like. Of course, it is absolutely impossible to guess, and I never even tried. There is no way to predict who will experience what during recovery. Some patients were *very* displeased with this lack of predictability.

The symptoms of *recovery* from Parkinson's seem to be as variable as the symptoms of Parkinson's itself: no two patients have the exact same set of PD symptoms, the same time frame for developing PD symptoms, *or* the exact same mindset.

In retrospect, attitude seems to the best predictor of whether or not the recovery symptoms will be fascinating or hellish. An attitude of curiosity and gratitude allows a person to see his recovery symptoms as wonders, miracles: harbingers of recovery from an "incurable" illness. As for the "pain," the patients who felt *safest* noticed *sensations* more than *pains*. Oppositely, those who were in partial recovery, who tended to be more wary, fearful or negative, often experienced their recovery symptoms as being ominous, painful, and/or anxiety-provoking. The extremely wary ones, the ones who were clearly stuck in partial recovery, could not even *consider* that recovery symptoms might be signs of *improvement* – let alone recovery.

Most people who'd had Type I PD had turned off the wary mindset after turning off pause mode for good. But a few found themselves constantly tempted to go back into negative thinking, or even back into full-blown pause mode, complete with a resumption of their Parkinson's symptoms, in response to recovery symptoms.

The variability of recovery symptoms

As noted previously, there was absolutely no cut and dried pattern for the recovery symptoms. Some patients even resumed full feeling *without* experiencing tingling or pins and needles.

For example, one patient's unhealed foot was treated for nearly a year. After the foot healed, over the next many months, she experienced "ants" in the feet and face, and then regained feeling in them. Her facial expression returned. Workouts at the gym helped restore range of movement in her arms. However, she still favored her left knee and hip and she still tremored. I asked her to take a course of homeopathic pills (Arnica Montana). As an aside, she was the only patient for whom I recommended homeopathic medicines. I cannot know if the homeopathic product made a difference or not. This particular homeopathic remedy is reputed to hasten the healing of injuries by drawing one's attention to the injury. After taking the Arnica for about a month at an *extremely* low (and therefore more subtle and more powerful) dose *and* continuing to get weekly one-hour sessions of Yin Tui Na on her knee and upper leg, a mass of bruises suddenly appeared on both sides of her left knee, her left thigh, and her left *forearm*. These bruises were consistent with the foot-in-the-bicycle-spokes, knee-wrenching injury that she'd had at age seven. These bruises went away over a period of two weeks. Three weeks later, she announced, "I can feel my fingernails! They're like wind-chimes!"

Wind chimes? She had never been prone to flights of poetic fancy. Prior to full recovery, most of my PD patients were more comfortable and experienced with analytical thinking than with metaphor or poetry. I had to ask what she was talking about. She explained, "I can feel the tiny weights of my fingernails. I'm aware of my fingertips. It's as if I have ten little bits of weight at the tips of my hands: when I move my fingers, I *feel* them moving, fluttering like the little noise-makers on a wind-chime."

I'm including this example because she never experienced *any* tingling or pins and needles in her *fingers* prior to the return of sensation. Also, there was no specific sequence of events that could have led us to expect a return of sensation in her fingertips following the discovery and healing of a *knee* injury. And she'd *never* suspected that her fingertips were numb. This was before I learned that a foot or leg injury could eventually lead to *body-wide* use of pause schematics.

On pause, the channel qi on the back of the hand is absent, especially in the area of the thumb and index finger. The pause-type, *backwards*-flowing channel qi coming down from the shoulder can flow *out* of the arm, out into space, at the wrist. When pause turned off after her knee injury healed, normal channel qi flow – and somatic awareness – returned to her hands. Although she'd previously had plenty of ants in her toes, face, and scalp, she never experienced *any* tingling or ants in her fingers. More importantly, maybe, her mind was suddenly able to think in terms of charming imagery: parasympathetic mode imagery.

Another sweet, parasympathetic mode-type remark from a patient who regained proprioception and feeling in his hands – even though, prior to recovery, he'd insisted that his hands weren't numb – was, "My fingers have eyes again! They used to get lost in my sleeves because they couldn't see where they were going. Now I can see where my fingers are even when they're inside my sleeve!"

Many people had *no* symptoms of tingling or pins and needles in areas that had been numb. As in the case with fingernails being like wind-chimes, many people went straight from non-awareness to heightened feeling, with no tingling or pain.

An example of variability: a one-off

Only one patient in my experience developed malodoria: a condition in which *all* smells are perceived as foul and nasty. When her foot injury healed but she was still using self-induced pause, she developed malodoria.

In response to Yin Tui Na treatment on her feet, this patient went into partial recovery. She soon became able to once again detect smells. She was assailed each day by whatever the first smell of the day happened to be. For hours, she could not get rid of the stench of that particular smell, and when it finally ebbed, the next thing she smelled would take its place – and would be perceived as equally noxious.

This patient was extremely cynical about the *bona fides* of everyone, to the point of paranoia. This was in the very early days of the Parkinson's Recovery Project, back when we were still working with medicated patients. She was taking a high level of antiparkinson's medications. At the same time that her foot began to heal and the malodoria appeared, her responses to her medications became suddenly violent. She tried for several days to decrease her medication, but found herself addicted and instead started *increasing* her medications. She dropped out of the program and I never heard from her again.

Malodoria is extremely rare. It occurs when a person is deeply entrenched in fear. The "cure" is feeling safe. When in parasympathetic mode, a person usually has a positive or curious response to innocuous smells. The malodoria case was unique in my experience. Most people were *extremely* pleased when their diminished senses of taste and smell returned back to full strength.

Doubting their own experiences

I'm writing about some exceptions as well as the general "rules" because patients need to know that whatever their own personal experiences, even if I *don't* mention them in this book, they should *not* be a cause for worry if they fit the general principle of "the opposite of Parkinson's." I mention this here and will mention it several times because so many patients have insisted on assessing their Parkinson's recovery based on how closely their own recovery experiences match what I've selected to include in my writing.

The reader who does not have PD may think that this is ridiculous: the way to know if Parkinson's is going away is that the symptoms of Parkinson's go away. However, many people with PD are so out of touch with or afraid of sensation in their bodies that they don't have an accurate knowledge of their own symptoms. Therefore, they cannot recognize when their symptoms are changing for the better

In the same way that "a watched pot never boils," a patient who is fixated on a particular symptom might *not* notice that all the other symptoms *except* for the "watched" one are going away. For example, one patient's greatest fear regarding his worsening Parkinson's was that he eventually might *not* being able to drive his beloved sports car. He completely recovered from every PD symptom except for one: when he reached for the gear-shift lever in his car, his hand, over the years, became increasingly rigid and immobile. All his other symptoms cleared up. His hand never *did* recover. His hand function grew steadily worse over time. This seemed very bizarre to me, until I was willing to consider a psychological component.

Also, *many* patients who resumed perfectly normal movement refused to believe that they were recovering from Parkinson's unless an MD said that they were recovering. Of course, no MD ever said that a patient of mine had recovered. Any patient who recovered had been "misdiagnosed." Many who were thrilled with their recovery suddenly doubted themselves if their MD didn't notice that they no longer had symptoms.

One patient, after all her PD symptoms were long gone, excitedly looked forward to seeing her neurologist. When she walked into his office, he didn't even look up. He stared at her chart and asked, "Are you ready for an increase in your medication?"

She replied, "I'm not taking any medication."

"Well then, do you want an increase in your medication?"

She repeated, "I'm not taking any medication. And my symptoms are gone."

He looked up, finally, and said, "So you *aren't* wanting an increase in your medication? Fine then, if you don't have any other questions, I'll see you in six months."

When she came to see me the next week, she was extremely upset. She thought she must be losing her mind. She asked me if she'd ever had symptoms, and if they were gone now. I assured her that she'd had symptoms, and that they were gone. She'd had recovery symptoms as well.

"Then why didn't my neurologist notice? I must be crazy! I probably never had Parkinson's disease! Or maybe I still have it! Why didn't the neurologist even *look* at me? What's the matter with me!" She was deeply upset and doubted everything that had happened over the previous six months.

I really got to resent the neurologists. Many patients were very invested in surprising their neurologists with their happy news. They dreamed of the day when the neurologist responded with amazement. Those days never came. I started warning patients that it might be a bad idea to see their old neurologist. If they were determined to get confirmation of recovery from a neurologist, they might be better off seeing a completely new doctor, explaining what their symptoms used to be, and then explaining that the symptoms went away following treatment. I also warned patients that, if they went this route, they might end up with "psychotic" or "neurotic" on their medical records. Many patients did end up with these notations on their charts. One even saw that the doctor at the prestigious Parkinson's Institute had added to her chart: "I don't know why this patient pretended to have Parkinson's disease for six years; probably to get high from the medications."

I was outraged by this. I got the patient's written permission to get a copy of her chart from the Institute and sent it off. In reply, the Institute sent me a letter saying that her chart had been lost.

About five years into the project, I began to understand why the doctor's approbation was so important. Many patients had been oblivious to how their bodies *felt* – they relied on visual analysis of their movements *or* the proclamations of their doctors to assess how their own bodies were doing. Even after recovering, they often did not trust the new *feelings* brought about by the changes that were occurring in their bodies during recovery. The new somatic sensations that confirmed that changes were afoot and that their symptoms of Parkinson's were decreasing were simply too strange and new to be trusted with regard to a syndrome that had been originally detected, or at least named, by the doctor. To be able to accept the idea that the Parkinson's symptoms were gone, they needed an MD's confirmation – a confirmation that was not going to happen. You will remember from chapter two, p. 22, the footnote about how doctors are trained to not accept the possibility of healing in the case of "incurable illnesses."

In summary, improved circulation and the gradual return of somatic, sensory awareness were often some of the first recovery symptoms. They might be unpleasant or a bit distracting, at the time. They were often the first steps on the road to healing the body. The next two chapters isn't about recovery symptoms, per se, but provides some help for people who have no idea how to deal with the new awareness of sensation in their bodies, the necessary pain of re-associating with an old, as-yet unhealed injury, and the sudden awareness of pain from old, significant injuries that have nothing to do with Parkinson's but which have been hiding dormant, not hurting, during the years on pause.

Chapter Twenty-three

Recovery Symptoms: Old Injuries

Many people have started to recover from Parkinson's only to find that some body part begins hurts in a way that it didn't hurt before. Very often, it's an old injury. In my experience, these old injuries are often in the neck, shoulder, or hip, but they could be in any part of the body. If the injury is *not* on the Stomach or Du channel, it was not directly contributing to symptoms of Parkinson's disease.

In my experience, most people assume that the new pain is a symptom of Parkinson's disease. It usually is not. When the body turns off pause mode, the pain of old, unhealed injuries might become feel-able. Even if they were barely felt, if at all, when pause was up and running, they might become quite painful when pause mode – a mode in which many types of pain are suppressed – turns off.

As the new pain makes itself known, and the body protectively stiffens up around it, or limps, or behaves as if favoring (protecting) the painful limb or joint, and maybe even tremors from the pain or muscle inhibition, the person often decides that the Parkinson's has come back or that the recovery has stalled out.

An example

One patient who'd never had tremor and was recovering nicely from Parkinson's found himself with a worsening left arm pain and weakness, and shaking in his left arm when he was stressed. He assumed that these were new symptoms of Parkinson's disease and that he wasn't recovering after all even though his other symptoms had cleared up and he was a new man, emotionally: able to cry and laugh for the first time in years.

However, based on all of his recovery symptoms, including increasing fluidity of movement and the emotional changes that accompany recovery, I suspected that he had a an old neck injury that was affecting his shoulder and left arm. He got a scan of his neck, and sure enough, he had a seriously displaced 5th vertebra.

A displaced 5th or 6th vertebra can cause shoulder pain, arm weakness and/or pain, and even shaking when trying to use the arm in a way that requires use of the inhibited muscles. This pathology pattern has nothing to do with Parkinson's. But because he'd had Parkinson's, the patient automatically assumed that his new arm and shoulder problems were a manifestation of PD.

He ended up working with physical therapists and an osteopathic doctor to resolve the old neck injury – an injury that was not in any way related to Parkinson's disease. Sure enough, the neck injury responded to treatment and the shoulder and arm pain slowly ebbed.

Sometimes the other, non-PD injuries appeared at the same time that an old, PD-causing foot or ankle injury started to show signs of bruising and swelling in response to Yin Tui Na treatment that re-associated the mind and the injry. Sometimes the other injuries appeared weeks, months, and even years after the foot injury healed.

Some people recalled the incident that caused the other, non-PD related injury. I was told things like: "I'll bet this hip pain goes back to when I fell two stories and landed on my hip; it sounded as if a bone had broken but my hip *never hurt*." And "Oh yeah! Eight years ago, when I moved the stove by myself, I thought I twisted something in my neck and I heard something pop, and my clothes have sat crooked at the neckline ever since, *but it never hurt*."

Other people have no idea how their bones articulations or soft tissue became so displaced. Either way, after turning off pause, these suppressed injuries really hurt, but they were *not* part of a PD problem. They were just injuries. However, in a person who has become accustomed to dealing with negativity and pain by invoking pause mode, the pain of the newly revealed injuries might cause him to re-institute pause mode. In which case, the Parkinson's *has* returned.

I have seen this sort of situation in many, maybe a majority of Type I patients.

As people begin to recover and their relative inability to fully feel pain begins to ebb, they become more aware of pain somewhere in the body. This pain might have nothing to do with a PD-causing injury. But the *response* to the pain is to assume that the Parkinson's has returned.

Making things even trickier, a person who has used self-induced pause in the past might, from habit, turn pause back on again to deal with the high level of pain from the long ignored injury, an injury that is finally being felt and is causing weakness and maybe even tremoring. A significant injury can cause all these symptoms, whether or not a person has Parkinson's.

Dystonia

The word dystonia often comes up in a discussion of Parkinson's. *Literally*, this word refers to incorrect muscle tone: too flaccid or too taut. In PD, the term usually means "too tight." Because of unaddressed injuries, including bone and soft tissue displacements, many people with Parkinson's have one or more muscle groups that are overly tight, causing a limb or the neck to pull to one side.

Dystonias are *not* directly related to being on pause mode. Instead, they are usually the result of an unhealed injury in the foot, leg, hip, hand, arm, shoulder, neck, or spine. The displaced tissues can cause the muscles in the vicinity of the injury to be imbalanced. This imbalance of muscle tone can cause the body parts to pull asymmetrically. The resulting muscle imbalance in various body parts can cause pain.

For example, an unhealed injury in the right hip might cause the right leg to pull to one side or the other. This might lead to a compensating pull on the left shoulder. In turn, this might cause tension in the neck and severe neck pain – even though the origin of the dsytonia is in the hip. A good body worker will be able to track these types of problems to their origin and resolve the problem. A mediocre one probably will not.

All people can develop a dystonic situation in some body part in response to unhealed injuries. Very often, the severity of a dystonia worsens over time. The pain of some dystonic situation might temporarily be more severe if the person is also experiencing fatigue or negative thoughts. This has nothing to do with whether or not a person has Parkinson's disease. Dystonias are *not* diagnostic for Parkinson's. However, because people with Parkinson's very often have significant, long-unhealed injuries, dystonias are somewhat common in people with Parkinson's.

When a person begins to recover from Parkinson's, his muscles get stronger and he becomes more aware of pain. This means that the asymmetrical muscle pull of the dystonia might worsen and the pain from the dystonia might become stronger. This doesn't mean the Parkinson's has returned. It means a person should get some professional help for the structural (bone articulation) and soft tissue displacements. The person should have done this at the time of injury, but if the person was on pause or dissociated from the injury, the injury might not have hurt much and could either have been intentionally ignored or maybe not even noticed.

Get help

If, after turning off pause, a new pain appears or a chronic pain becomes worse, and even brings some PD symptoms back due to your habitual way of dealing with pain and stress (going into pause mode), consider seeing an chiropractor, physical therapist, osteopath, craniosacral therapist, or whatever type of professional might be the best for addressing that pain.

You might be better off if you don't mention the words "Parkinson's disease." If you mention Parkinson's, the therapist will most likely presume that your pain is coming from Parkinson's and will try to explain to you why he can't help, or will suggest that you start taking L-dopa, CBD oil, or other inappropriate treatments.

If you mention the idea of *recovering* from Parkinson's, you will be considered a fool, in addition to the above.

If you are tremoring, you can look the therapist straight in the eye and lie to him: "I saw my MD and he says it's not Parkinson's. He says that I either have essential tremor or I have a tremor from a nerve impingement."

If you say this, the therapist will be more willing to do the radiology scans, if necessary, or at least start trying to figure out what the problem is and get to work on fixing it.

Chapter twenty-four

Recovery Symptoms: Processing Pain

Some people have never learned healthy ways for dealing with pain. As my patients with PD turned off pause or healed from injuries that caused pause-like channel qi flow, they often experienced the long-suppressed pains of dissociated injuries or the pains of suppressed emotional traumas. They were often baffled by the concept of *addressing* the pain instead of dissociating from it.

I was saddened to learn that many of my Parkinson's patients honestly had no idea how a person is supposed to deal with pain. Some of the pioneers even called my home phone in the middle night when they started feeling sensations they'd never felt before. One of them, at two in the morning, started off by saying, inaccurately, "I just *know* you'll want to hear about this right away. There's pain at the place where I broke my foot back in high school! What should I do?!!! " I soon unlisted my home phone number.

But I understood *why* they were reaching out. They were baffled or sometimes terrified because of a new sensation. That new sensation had been set in motion when pause or dissociation turned off. When these new sensations arose, patients knew they weren't supposed to dissociate from the pain or make themselves numb. But they'd *never* dealt with pain any other way. As patients experienced the pain of forgotten, unhealed injuries, including still-broken bones, they were often frantic, saying things like, "I'm feeling my foot! I'm *feeling* it. It *hurts*! What should I *do*?"

Many of my Parkinson's patients wrongly assumed that the healing of a dissociated injury and/or restoration of healthy Qi flow should be pleasant. The *end* result *is* pleasant enough. But many patients, after re-associating with an injured body part, experienced the long-suppressed pain of the injury. The sensations could be unpleasant, or even terrifying.

The book *Yin Tui Na: Hands-on Therapy for Traumatic Injury*, teaches the FSR (Forceless, Spontaneous-Release) technique. This is a specific type of Yin Tui Na that I recommend for patients with Parkinson's. "Yin Tui Na" is an umbrella term that covers any form of manual therapy that is subtle, slow, and supportive, as opposed to overt, physical manipulation (*Yang* Tui Na). The FSR technique *and* most other light-touch massage techniques all tend to work in the same way: they encourage a person's awareness and even subconscious to revisit a long-ignored injury and thus initiate healing. When the mind decides to acknowledge an ignored injury, the unexpressed, dormant symptoms of injury may appear. These symptoms might include bruises, tenderness, pain, swelling and heat. If a patient's injury had been only a dislocation or sprain, the reawakened pain wasn't necessarily severe. If the reawakened injury was a broken bone, the pain was sometimes considerable.

Many recovering patients who might have been capable of helping care for *other* people who were in pain often had no idea of how to care for *themselves* when they were hurt. I found myself teaching many of them the self-comforting and supportive physical and emotional skills that they should have learned as children. I also tried, not always successfully, to convince some of them that it was OK to reach out for help from others.

How to deal with pain

The appropriate thing to do, even if the actual injury occurred decades ago, is to treat the newly revealed injury the way that it should have been treated in the first place. Use common sense. If the foot or ankle or wherever finally starts to *hurt* a few hours, days, or weeks after receiving FSR treatments, then *favor* the injured area. If it's the foot, then limp a bit. If the area itches, scratch it. If it wants to be rubbed, rub it. Very often, an injured body part will appreciate support from a snug Ace (elastic) bandage. Have a good cry. Take an aspirin or some other mild, over-the-counter pain reliever. Listen to the body, and give it what it wants. Do *not* be stoic.

Treat your "recent" injury the way you would treat the new injury of a beloved child. Treat it as if *you* are the beloved child: ask for help. Or go to bed, call in sick to work, or take a hot soothing bath. Coddle yourself! Cancel your meeting and stay home and read a book. You might want to wrap it up in an elastic bandage.

In the rare case where it feels like a bone is broken, don't be stoic and force yourself to walk on the broken foot. Have it casted, or at least immobilized. Use crutches for as long as necessary or even stay home and lie on the couch for a few days. Leave the stoicism behind.

Chapter five in the book *Yin Tui Na* shares several methods for dealing with the pain from physical injury – methods that accelerate healing. This book is available for free download at PDrecovery.org.

Please do *not* take powerful prescription medication to help you sleep or deal with newly awakened pain. The rebound effect from many of these drugs can inhibit mid-brain function. Some can cause long-term or lasting brain damage.

Comfort the baby

In a healthy family, when a baby is crying, some adult picks up the baby and holds it to the left side of the adult's chest. The channel qi of the baby's pericardium is scattered, causing distress. The scattering might be due to hunger, pain, fear, or confusion. Whenever a person is upset, the channel qi flow in the pericardium becomes somewhat altered or scattered.

When the baby is held close to a relaxed adult's pericardium, on the left side of the chest, the baby's pericardial currents sync up with the currents in the adult's pericardium. The baby's *small* pericardial currents will begin to resonate with the much *larger* pericardial currents of the adult. If the adult is relaxed, there's a good chance that the baby relaxes – so long as there is no ongoing physical pain in the baby. The baby's brain interprets signals from its now-relaxed pericardium as a sign that everything's safe. The baby feels better.

As a baby grows older, he can still cry out for or run to an adult when distressed.

Between the ages of six and eleven, a child should learn how to calm *himself* when distressed or in pain.

Technically, when a person calms himself, he is reinstituting, intentionally, the pericardium signals that he associates with feeling safe and OK. He might take some deep breaths to help calm himself, as this helps restore parasympathetic mode function. He might do other physical or mental techniques to re-stabilize the pericardium.

Ideally, the child learns to restore destabilized pericardial signals prior to adolescence. The powerful mood swings of adolescence can overwhelm a person who has not already learned how his heart is supposed to feel when calm, and how to restore his heart back to that calm if it gets distressed.

Anyone who has *ever* felt calm has a memory in his brain of what "calm" feels like. "Calm" is a loving feeling that we can mentally call-up – unless we've mentally commanded ourselves not to. We can use this feeling to surround the heart and bring it back to stability. We can learn to install that feeling around the heart any time we need to – any time we are agitated or in pain. As we restore and then consciously sustain that feeling of calm, or what you might also call a feeling of "goodness," "soul," or "something within," the brain is then able to turn off its "Red Alert" signals: signals that are activated by pain or fear and that are quickly accompanied by pericardial distress. When the Red Alert signals turn off, the nerve impulses to the brain caused by pain then cease to register in the brain as "danger." They become indications of mere "sensation" instead of a potential danger. From here, the body or the thoughts can address the problem in a productive manner.

In some cases of physical pain, physical, supportive contact with the injured area *and* mental attention focused on the area also helps to restore the channel qi flow to a higher degree of parasympathetic mode. The restoration of channel qi to the parasympathetic mode flow pattern helps diminish the stress pattern in the pericardium, and allows the brain to move forward with processing the trauma.

Methods for self-calming

In *addition* to taking a few deep, calming breaths, physically holding the place that hurts and maybe consoling himself with a song or favorite adage, a person can quickly restore his pericardium to a condition of calm or peace and start to "process," start to heal from, the pain by using other, more focused methods.

The method he learns might be cultural. In China, a child might be taught to pay attention to the place that hurts and fill it with light and channel qi. In other cultures, a child might learn to ask for comfort from a totem animal or favorite saint. He might be taught a traditional song, chant, or hymn that helps with healing. H might be taught to offer prayers to a deceased elder, spirit guide, saint, or someone, anyone, who is listening. Hopefully, before the child is an adolescent, he has learned one or more ways of dealing with physical and emotional pain *besides* running to a parent.

Learning how to process pain should be a normal part of growing up. As the poet John Keats put it, "Do you not see how necessary a world of pain and troubles is to school an intelligence and make it a soul?"

Again, simply keeping one's focus on the area around the heart, paying attention to the feelings in that area, can sometimes calm the pericardium's electrical signals. If that doesn't help enough, mentally and/or physically holding the pericardium area or the injured area might help. Filling either area with light might calm the panic signals from the pericardium. Mentally asking for help from whomever comes to mind while continuing to mentally focus on the area around the heart or the injury can bring even greater solace. If the pain is large enough, a person might seek out hugs from another person. These hugs from a calmer person work just like they do in an infant. The close, chest-to-chest contact can help re-stabilize the chaotic signals in the pericardium of the injured party.

Whatever method is used to calm and comfort the pericardium or the injury, the pericardium signals should soon switch back to “All’s well” as soon as the chaotic channel qi in the vicinity of the injury stabilizes. The brain notes that the pericardium is OK now. Once the pericardium is OK, the brain can turn off the Red Alert signal in the area I sometimes call the brain’s “inbox,” the place for new, unprocessed information. “Processing the pain” involves moving information *out* of the brain’s “inbox,” *dealing* with the situation that created the pain, and moving the mental awareness of the pain to areas in the brain that direct healing or compile history.

In the USA, many children today are not taught *any* methods for dealing with physical or emotional pain. Some children are left to figure it out for themselves. Some do a good job. Some do not. If they learn to deal with pain by dissociating or turning on pause mode, they might not know what to do when finally re-associating with the pain, whether the pain is physical or emotional.

An example of a pain support technique

One method for dealing with one’s own pain requires paying attention to how one’s own heart (pericardium) feels when content or joyful. One can learn to consciously reinstate the calm, joy, or love feeling in the chest anytime the pericardium starts to feel distress. This basic human skill is not often known to people with Type I PD, so it must be learned, through practice.

Once a person has learned what the heart *feels* like when it is full of love or joy, then, if or when he feels pain, he can:

1) Pay close attention to the place where the pain is manifesting. Notice exactly what it *feels* like.

2) Summon up the feeling of a joyful heart.

3) Mentally imagine the *size* of the joyful heart feeling to be larger than the physical area that is being affected by the pain.

4) Mentally impose the heart feeling over and around the location of the physical pain. Leave the two sensations together. Try to feel *both* the sensations, the pain *and* the calm heart sensation, at the same time. Eventually, if you have made the heart feeling *larger* than the pain feeling, the area that was feeling pain will begin to resonate with the heart feeling. The pain signals will become mere sensations, and will cease to provoke fear.

As the great yogi Sri Daya Mata (1914-2010) often said, “In this world, your love must be greater than your pain.” Understand this phrase to be literal, not metaphorical. The frequencies generated by your pericardium when you are feeling joy can resonate with and alter your perceptions of pain, allowing the pain signals to be turned off, allowing the injury to be processed and healed. Once processed, the injury is only history: an event that you can learn from, but no longer suffer from.

Because this concept is *so* foreign to *so* many of my PD patients, I repeat: as the pain is assessed and assuaged, or begins to resonate with a calm pericardium, the brain’s interpretation of the pain signals will transition away from the part of the brain that perceives the signals as “Oh no! Pain and Fear!” and move the experience into brain areas that can help with healing.

After the healing work is underway, the injured area might still register as “highly sensitive” until the healing is complete. That’s good and healthy. It helps you be mindful and careful of the weakened area while it heals. Still, the event no longer has the ability to trigger the *distressing* type of pain response that unsettles the pericardium and causes fear. The pain has become neutral – the lingering pain, if any, becomes a mental reminder to be *careful* of the injured area until it is healed, but it no longer generates a pericardium-disturbing fear response.

Full healing does not occur while a person is in a high degree of fear. Most healing, and certainly deep, full healing, occurs while a person is in a high degree of parasympathetic mode: awake, curious, and content or, if the pain has been mentally processed, deep healing can also occur during sleep.

As adults, we have the legal right and the moral responsibility to re-install that remembered feeling of calm in our heart any time we don't feel good. We can re-install it with the help of friends, silent meditation, a calming physical exercise or even by just focusing the mind on past remembered sensations of calm and love. Failure to take care of pain, or worse, choosing to cultivate pain, dwell on it, dissociate from it, or use it as a self-pity device does *not* help heal the pain. Instead, these behaviors train the brain to focus on the terrifying or "un-healable" aspects of pain. Many of my patients with Parkinson's have had almost *no* idea of how to deal with pain and fear. They may not even know what "calm" feels like. Numb? Yes. Contented and calm? No.

Emotional immaturity

Once recovery from Parkinson's disease begins, a person's emotional maturity can be, briefly, very similar to the emotional maturity he had attained when he first started dissociating or using pause for the long term. For example, if a person first dissociated from pain or put himself on pause when he was five years old and never got to a safe place then, when as an adult, he finally does re-associate with the old pain, he might have the pain-processing skills of a five year old: yelling and sulking.

One patient, a middle-aged mother, when she began to re-associate with her foot injury, behaved like a three year old: throwing furniture, biting and doing wordless screaming. She had been three years old when her mother put her up for adoption.

Another recovering patient, after his birthday party, behaved "exactly like a nine-year old," according to his spouse. The patient had used the *exact* same sentences that their child had used twenty years earlier after his fabulous ninth birthday party was over: "Is that all I'm going to get to do for my birthday?" and "I never get to do what *I* want."

The spouse then realized that this particular patient's life-changing trauma had occurred when he was nine. At age nine, he'd come home from school and discovered his grandmother, dead of a heart attack, on the living room floor. He got out his Boy Scout book and gave her all the various treatments, including mouth-to-mouth resuscitation. He was still trying to revive her when his mother finally got home. The mother heaped praise on him for not having become emotional or given in to feelings at that time. For the *rest of his life*, his mother regularly praised him for not having had any *feelings* or *emotions* on the day that Grandma died.

Prior to starting to recover, this patient could not recall any negative events that might have led to emotional shut-down or going into pause. To his mind, his behavior with his grandmother had been heroic and a high point in his life, heroism for which he had received regular praise for decades. It was only when he started to recover and started acting exactly like a nine-year old that his wife recalled the dead grandmother incident.

This subject of patients' emotional-age reversions could fill a book. But this is enough to be getting on with. If a person can be circumspect, then if and when he starts to exhibit the emotional behaviors of a child, he can view his immature behaviors from the perspective of the most mature, adult parts of his mind. He can quickly "grow up" in his ways of dealing with pain. He *can* learn to apply adult *self*-comforting behavioral skills to any pain-causing events.

Fear of pain

Many patients were understandably terrified of pain. Some patients even expressed great fear in *anticipation* of feeling old injuries. Some were afraid to let me touch their feet. One person traveled hundreds of miles to Santa Cruz to be treated, knowing full well that the treatment, at that time, consisted of Yin Tui Na on the injured foot. When I asked her to remove her shoes, she balked.

She explained, "Not even my husband has ever seen or touched my feet." She went back and forth for about half an hour deciding whether or not she could allow me to even look at her feet. Then she made up her mind. No. She left. I never saw her again.

Others were terrified of what they might feel in *general* if they let their guard down. One PD patient, after refusing to even *consider* imagining looking inside her long-painful hip to see if it was dark inside and motionless or agitated, explained, "The whole point of life is to avoid pain." This same person, when asked if she could try mentally talking to some departed friend or higher power, told me, "I went to church once and *none* of the people there were perfect. So after that, I don't believe in church or God or a higher power or anything else." She reminded me, "Those other things don't matter: the whole point of life is to avoid pain."

Those patients whose stoicism level was *low* tended to recover from PD more quickly. They sometimes mentioned that they had been very stoic and guarded at the time of injury, or throughout childhood. But they had learned, in their *adult* life, that it *is* good to experience sensations and that it is not "bad" to feel and respectfully attend to the body's injuries and emotional traumas. These people responded more quickly to treatment. Some of these more emotionally mature patients had consciously worked, as adults, at learning that it's OK to ask for help. A few had even taught themselves how to cry.

The patients who were able to cry and mentally focus on the actual sensations of their own physical and emotional pain had fewer problems figuring out how to deal with any pain or bruising that arose when pause turned off and/or injuries began to heal.

Many patients, when starting treatment, were still proud of their ability to not feel pain. Some had stopped crying in early childhood and had not been able to cry since. Some truly believed that non-feeling or perpetual wariness was morally superior to acknowledgement of physical or emotional pain. In general, these people had Type I PD, and needed to first learn how to re-activate their striata and thalami. They were not even ready for Yin Tui Na treatments for their injuries. Often, these people were alarmed or anxious when the appearance and sensations of old injuries began to manifest. Although the pains were not necessarily severe, a few people veered into bouts of hysteria and paranoia when confronted with the pain of their old injuries.

Some patients had *no* ability to face pain and process it. One patient had full-blown bouts of hysteria every evening for months after he started feeling the injuries in his foot. We finally figured out that re-awakening awareness of his foot injury had also re-awakened awareness and an ability to feel the sensations of an excruciating childhood groin injury that was *still* in need of medical treatment, as well as awakening memories of heinous childhood abuse.

One (and only one) of my patients, within hours of being *diagnosed* with Parkinson's disease, had developed the same sort of daily hysteria, and it lasted for several months. He developed this hysteria a full month before he heard of our work and started being treated by us. His hysteria finally eased up after many months of foot treatment, psychiatric counseling, prescription-strength anti-insomnia drugs, and various homeopathic remedies prescribed by his homeopathic doctor. In his case, he was not even feeling long-suppressed pain, he was experiencing the *anticipation* of pain. In the face of being *diagnosed* with a terrible illness, he was unable to control himself any longer, after years of being stoic. In my limited experience, his case was unique.

In a few cases, patients decided that the appearance of pain in a previously numb foot was a sign of worsening Parkinson's disease. Some went to their neurologists in response to the sudden awareness of pain in a long-injured body part. And most of their *doctors*, confronted with the patients' new, bruised, throbbing, inflamed, injury-type foot or ankle pain, misdiagnosed the pain as...a symptom of Parkinson's disease! Parkinson's is a syndrome that is characterized by numbness in the face and feet. A neurologist should at least know that most of the pains that do occur in Parkinson's are due to steady worsening of stiffness and rigidity in the torso, biceps, and groin – or muscle spasms from overmedication – but *not* pains from inflammation due to an old injury finally being acknowledged.

The thoughtless prescribing of PD medication for treating non-PD pain

One patient who had thought she was recovering developed agonizing pain in both hips. The pain began when she finally became able to imagine herself having hips. Instead of seeing a pain specialist, she went to the neurologist who had diagnosed her with Parkinson's. This patient was *not* taking any antiparkinson's medications.

Her neurologist, thinking of her only as a Parkinson's patient instead of a patient in pain, prescribed a powerful anticonvulsant (anti-epilepsy drug). This drug is often used to sedate brain activity in people with Parkinson's *whose medications are at excessively high doses*. High doses of dopamine-enhancing antiparkinson's drugs can cause enormously powerful and painful muscle dyskinesias. To counter the excessive level of brain activity that triggers these spasms, anti-seizure drugs are sometimes prescribed for people *who are taking high, dyskinesia-inducing levels of antiparkinson's medications*.

This patient was not taking any medications. She was not having dyskinesia from drugs or dystonias (muscle spasms). She was not rigid: she was exceedingly limp, a recovery condition that you will read about in chapter twenty-six. Therefore, the anti-spasm medications prescribed by her neurologist for her pain were completely inappropriate. For over a year, she took the anti-convulsants that her neurologist gave her. The drugs made her even more limp, extremely groggy and confused. Because these drugs inhibit brain activity, they did reduce her pain a little: a *very* little. However, she was determined to keep as active as possible: she didn't want to "give in" to the pain.

After a *year* during which the almost paralyzing pain continued, she finally went to see a pain specialist. He took CAT scans of her hips, and discovered that both her psoas muscles were badly torn in the hip area – torn right through the middle of the muscle, from side-to-side – and inflamed. He prescribed medications to reduce the swelling and instructed her to minimize activity that used those muscles. As soon as she saw the scans, she suspected that this *extremely* unusual type of muscle tear had probably been received at age six during her father's "tickling games" in which he would have her lay down on the floor with her legs up in a fetal position. Then, he would force her knees apart to the sides. He would press her bent knees all the way to the floor and not let her get up until she cried. The "game" was to see how long she could go without crying.

This patient was a therapist in marriage and family counseling. She told me that she had no emotional feelings one way or the other when she realized that her father's "games" had probably caused the hip muscle tears. I asked her if those "games" might have been a little inappropriate. She replied firmly, with no apparent warmth, "I loved my father. *Everyone* admired him." Finally, after she started getting appropriate treatment and stopped being so stoic and driven, the muscle tears started to heal. It took more than a year for the lateral tears in her psoas muscles to heal completely.

The point is, she spent a full year in agony because she and her neurologist assumed that her pain from torn muscles was being caused by Parkinson's disease. Her error is understandable: she trusted her doctor. The neurologist's error was due to medical professionals' tendency to see every problem in terms of one's own specialty. The neurologist, assessing her in terms of overmedicated Parkinson's, assumed – incorrectly – that her hip pain was due to either dystonia (chronic muscle tension) or the violent dyskinetic spasms that Parkinson's patients often get from excessive levels of antiparkinson's medications, even though she had *no* muscle tension and she was *not* taking medications.

The three specialists

One patient in her early thirties, just starting to recover, had such horrible stomach and intestinal pains that she took herself to the emergency room at our nearby, top-level medical facilities at Stanford University. She called me first. I said that her sudden onset symptoms sounded like recovery from really horrible injuries. I also warned her that the doctors would be angry when they didn't find anything physiologically wrong. I also told her that she should go to the emergency room but she should not feel bad when the doctors got mad at her.

At the ER, she was in extreme pain but she had no fever and her blood work didn't show any signs of infection or elevated immune response. Her symptoms were baffling enough that three specialists were called in. Prior to the MRI scan, the OB-GYN told her it was endometriosis. The oncologist assured her that it was cancer. The internal medicine doctor told her that her intestines were "telescoping" and that immediate surgery was called for.

The MRI found nothing. She mentioned to them that the pains in her stomach and abdomen made her think of the times her father had attacked her with a hammer. In particular, there was one time when she was very young that he'd hammered her in her bath. To be fair, her father expected her to dodge the blows. She was not always successful.

All three of the specialists, never noticing her mild, remaining Parkinson's symptoms, turned in a diagnosis of psychosis. Not only this, they all were angry with her for having wasted their time for a mere "psychological event" that she was trying to pass off as a "suppressed memory." Obviously, any pain from such an attack would have healed decades earlier. She told me afterwards that she was *so* glad I had warned her that they would be angry. My words of warning helped her see the humor in their frustration instead of taking their insults personally.

This particular patient went through some pretty horrible pains during recovery, including many injuries from her professional work with horses. She was a high level horse trainer and her work was much in demand. Horses were her great love and passion even though her feet were a ghastly mess from having been stomped on so many times.

But all that was long forgotten on the day she came to visit my clinic after not seeing me for over a year. She was completely symptom free. She gave me a hug and asked, "Notice anything?"

I mentally scrambled to assess what might be different. "Your hair?"

"No!" Look at me!"

"You're even taller? She was a good six inches taller than me and always had been.

"No! It's so obvious! I'm wearing *sandals*! I just bought them. My very first pair. As soon I as got them I drove straight here. You're the first person in my whole life to ever see my toes out in public!"

We hugged. I might have cried a tear or two. People who have recovered from PD sometimes feel a special bond.

I've written up the above two, very abbreviated, case studies to demonstrate how doctors often assume that all syndromes are related to their own specialized field of study.

Very often, patients who had been given a diagnosis of Parkinson's *and* their doctors as well incorrectly assume that every problem and pain subsequent to the diagnosis must be due to Parkinson's.

For example, many recovering PD patients who developed flu symptoms when the flu was going around assumed that they felt worse than usual because the Parkinson's was getting worse. Sometimes, if they ran a fever with their flu, they insisted the *fever* was a sign that the Parkinson's was getting worse. And sometimes, their doctors incorrectly *agreed* that their flu symptoms and fever were symptoms of Parkinson's disease and suggested an increase in antiparkinson's medication to deal with the flu!

The same would occur when, due to recovery, the pain of an old injury, in the shoulder, hip, side of the neck, or some other area that was not related to pause mode suddenly made its appearance. The MD would say "That's from your Parkinson's getting worse!" and would automatically increase the antiparkinson's medications, or muscle relaxants, or anti-seizure medication (I'm not making this up) or some other drug that was completely inappropriate considering that the patient's pain was due to an injury. Some non-steroidal anti-inflammatory, or aspirin, or some other over-the-counter pain reliever would have been more appropriate, together with physical therapy.

Achy or stiff

I have *non*-PD patients who are middle-aged or older. Sometimes they come to see me because they are stiff or sore after a bout of unusual activity such as spending all day gardening or oppositely from an habitual lack of activity or exercise. They want relief from their pain, so they get a massage or come to me for an acupuncture treatment.

But some of my recovering Parkinson's patients, becoming mildly stiff or sore after doing an unaccustomed activity or after spending several days doing nothing, fell into a panic. They called me to announce that the Parkinson's was suddenly much, much worse.

I would ask them if they were doing regular stretching, swimming, yoga, or Tai Ji, or anything to keep the joints supple. They usually asked me in return why they should need to be doing such activities; prior to having Parkinson's, years or even decades earlier, they didn't have such pains and stiffness, even though they hadn't done regular stretches.

When I point out to them that, prior to recovering, they were pretty much numb, using a norepinephrine override, and only felt stiffness if the joint was so locked up that they couldn't move it, *and* they are getting older, they struggle to understand my point. I tell them that any person who is middle-aged or beyond, who fails to work at staying loose, might start to tighten up, even if they are recovering from Parkinson's. This idea is usually met with disbelief, or the statement that, "I'll start doing stretching exercises if the Parkinson's goes away completely."

Many of my patients with Parkinson's struggled to accept the idea that bodies can have pain for reasons *other* than Parkinson's disease. As mentioned in the previous chapter, many patients discovered, during recovery, that their neck stiffness was due to old neck and shoulder injuries, *not* advancing or returning Parkinson's disease. These injuries often responded very well to gentle styles of chiropractic or osteopathic treatment, or light-touch therapeutic treatment such as craniosacral therapy. Recovering from Parkinson's might have *exposed* the pain from these injury-based problems because recovering means you're no longer numb. But Parkinson's didn't *cause* the injuries, nor did the sudden appearance of pain from these old injuries mean that the *Parkinson's* was getting worse.

Many patients have said things such as, "That neck injury occurred decades ago and it never hurt, even at the time. The Parkinson's is what's making the neck injury become a problem. Therefore, since my neck hurts worse than ever [since the foot injury healed and I've become more sensitive], it's proof that I'm *not* recovering from Parkinson's disease. "

The *fact* that the injury hadn't hurt at the time might have been related to Parkinson's or pre-Parkinson's: blocking out pain so that injuries couldn't heal was the problem. So many patients are not able to even *consider* this possibility.

Increased awareness of body pains can become a real problem for some recovering patients: after first recovering from Parkinson's, some people temporarily develop fibromyalgia or hypochondria, two conditions in which a person is hyper-sensitive to pain. In all but one of the patients that *did* develop fibromyalgia or hypochondria, these syndromes went away within a few to six months. One person who never exercised, ever, had fibromyalgia symptoms for years after recovering.

Getting back to the main point, many people with Parkinson's literally do not know how to deal with pain or fear. They may have *never* learned the usual pain assuaging mechanisms that young children slowly master during the years from around age three to age eleven (approximately). For many of my PD patients, the only fear- or pain-treatment mechanism they'd ever known was mentally blocking out the pain or fear: either dissociating or commanding themselves to feel no pain. The concept of *addressing* fear or *feeling* pain, maybe having a good cry, taking an aspirin and then consciously soothing the pain, or asking for help to soothe it, thus neutralizing the pain and allowing healing to move forward was *absolutely* new to them. Many thought that *processing* pain was impossible, or a very bad idea. So many felt that the whole point of life itself is not so much experiencing joy but avoiding pain.

A lengthy aside: pain from other injuries

Sometimes, at the same time that healing took place in an injury along the Stomach channel area that was causing pause-type circuitry, some *non*-Stomach-channel area spontaneously manifested a bruise or soreness. Sometimes, the patient then recalled having injured both areas at the same time.

It does *not* matter whether or not the patient is able to remember the painful incident(s). Some patients (especially those that have raced bikes and motorcycles) have had so many injuries that there is no way they will ever sort out which incident caused which injury. That's fine; this lack of memory will not impede recovery.

Some of the injuries that surfaced only appeared as faint bruises with no pain. Some were full Technicolor bruises, featuring blues, yellows, and greens, with streaks of fresh red under the skin. Sometimes there was pain with no bruise. Sometimes there was bruising *and* pain.

Although unhealed broken leg bones from decades earlier were relatively rare, the people who had them experienced a tremendous amount of pain and bruising at the site of the break. As the pain arose, all of my patients with an unhealed leg bone (femur, tibia, or fibula) break recalled *vividly* the event during which the bone had been broken, oh so many years earlier.

Many of my patients had these bone breaks confirmed by x-ray. The x-ray technicians all insisted that the breaks were very new, within the last few days or weeks, based on the amount of healing that was visibly occurring at the broken ends. When the patients described the injury event as having taken place years or even decades earlier, the x-ray techs told them that they were wrong. Every technician insisted that there was no way a broken bone could remain painless and unhealed over a long period of time. These x-ray technicians were wrong, but there was nothing to be done about it.

Many patients were relieved to see in an x-ray that the area of intense pain was in fact an area with an obviously broken bone – not cancer, gout, carpenter's nails, or broken glass. Sometimes, in cases of very severe pain from a broken leg, a new type of rigidity or a desire to hunker down and/or a new type of either local *or* intermittent body-wide tremor accompanied the pain and shock of the broken bone for a short time, maybe a few days – as it *should*, when the body is badly injured and maybe at risk of imminent death. These new, pause-like symptoms went away as the healing progressed – as they should, when a person turns off pause and starts to heal.

Staggered recoveries

Although some patients had arm, leg, neck or head injuries that appeared at the same time as the foot injuries came to the surface, it was more common for the various injuries to show up in a staggered fashion.

Research has proven that a person who receives severe multiple injuries cannot feel the pain of *all* injuries *simultaneously*. In these cases, the body seems to "decide" which injury is the worst at any given moment, and addresses that one. When appropriate attention has been given to that worst injury and/or healing has begun in that most problematic area, a different injury is then able to receive the brain's foremost attention.

A person whose bicycle accident has bruised his ribs, sprained his knee, scraped skin from many places and thrown his back and neck out will know what I am talking about. Even though he may have a general sense that he hurts all over, only one injury at a time will *truly* stand out as being the thing that needs to be addressed immediately in any given moment. And as soon as that particular problem starts to feel better, a few seconds or minutes, or a few days, or a few weeks later, another injury will move to the fore. Sometimes the immediate pain cycles quickly from one area to the next, every few seconds, over and over, as if checking in with the injuries in rapid rotation.

It is not uncommon for a person with or without Parkinson's disease, who has injuries in multiple areas from a really bad accident, to spend *months* healing. As soon as the neck pain starts to heal a little, the hip pain might demand attention. As soon as the hip pain starts to resolve, the neck pain might resume where it left off *or* the knee pain might arise. Once some amount of healing of the knee is underway, the knee pain might be temporarily silenced and the shoulder injury might start to squawk.

In some of my PD patients, once they started being able to tune in with their bodies and feel long-forgotten pain, one or two "new" injuries showed up every few months, or once a year. In some cases, this delayed type of healing continued for several years even after completely recovering from Parkinson's. The recovery from Parkinson's does *not* require healing of all suppressed injuries. The recovery from Parkinson's, including the person's ability to experience dopamine release as demonstrated by a return of automatic motor function, often started up as soon as pause or pseudo pause turned off. The presence of other injuries – injuries that didn't necessarily cause the channel qi to flow in the pause pattern – did *not* necessarily inhibit the recovery from Parkinson's.

Then again, *many* people went back into pause in response to the new appearance of pain from an old injury.

Others, those still in partial recovery, whose injuries had healed but who were still using self-induced pause, often insisted that they couldn't recover yet because they might not have found "all the injuries" yet. Watch out for this attitude: it's a ploy by the Blocker.

It's never too late to learn how to respond to pain in a way that moves you forward into healing and forgiveness. When a person learns how to deal with pain, he finds to his surprise that pain, or even the mere *idea* of pain, is no longer able to scare him or drive him into, or drive him *back* into, pause mode.

Chapter Twenty-four

Recovery Symptoms: Fungus and the Red Rash

Only about twenty-five percent of people recovering from PD get the red rash. However, the rash is a very important recovery symptom: it can provide a *visible* sign that the blood circulation is improving *and* gives still more proof of the new hypotheses in this book regarding PD. Dead dopamine cells do *not* cause toenail fungus, nor does "misdiagnosis" explain the red rash during recovery. The channel qi patterns during pause *do* explain why fungus is able to penetrate into the Stomach channel areas in the feet, legs and face (facial seborrhea) in people with Parkinson's disease.

Many people with Parkinson's have foot and/or toenail fungus. The toenail fungus causes the nails to be thick and gray, or even misshapen and chalky white. In some patients, this fungus has moved into the tissues of the feet, as well. The fungus might "blossom" or "fruit" (present an itchy, red rash, or itchy or mildly painful sores) during the summer months or anytime that the feet are hot. The fungus might become dormant when the weather is cold.

In areas of the body where channel qi does not flow and therefore blood circulation is poor, fungus can thrive, unmolested and invisible. When circulation improves, the body's immune system becomes able to *notice* the presence of the fungus. Once the body *notices* the fungus, it will take steps to kill it. The ensuing battle can lead to the appearance of the little red blisters or a red rash.

Microscopic fungus is everywhere. Our bodies are constantly being exposed to fungal spores. It's normal. It's *healthy*. The white tip of a healthy fingernail is white from fungus: fungus is chewing away at the underside of the nail, making the underside of the nail microscopically rough and opaque (white), instead of clear. Healthy blood circulation keeps the fungus from establishing itself in the pink, attached-to-the-nailbed section of the nail. The faint, very thin line of deeper red where the nail goes from pink (attached to the nail bed) to white (free standing) is the inflamed red of a tiny biological battle line. These red lines show where a healthy body's immune system is keeping the ever-present fungus at bay.

In body areas with poor circulation, the immune system cannot not fight the fungus very well, if at all. Fungus can thrive in these areas.

Because most people with Parkinson's have poor circulation in their toes and feet, they often have fungus invading and becoming established in the nail-bed (under the pink part of the nail) and just under the skin of the feet.

The numbness, poor circulation and poor body awareness that allows the fungus to slowly move deeper into the body may start decades before a person is diagnosed with Parkinson's.

For example, at age seven, about two years after having my foot smashed in a car door, I noticed that I couldn't tell *exactly* where my *finger*tips ended and the air started. In my twenties and thirties, I arrogantly assumed this vagueness as to the borders of my own body was a sign of advanced spirituality – my body consciousness was contiguous with the universe! I never even realized that I had *no* idea where my *toes* ended. I developed toenail fungus in my second and third toes (the termini of the Stomach channel) in my mid-forties, just two years before I was diagnosed with Parkinson's. I only had fungus on my toenails, not my fingernails. I knew my fingertips were hard to feel, somatically, but evidently, my toes were even more numb than my fingers – so numb I didn't even know how numb they were. After turning off pause, the toenail fungus in my feet cleared up on its own over about six months.

In addition to often having obvious fungus in their toenails, people with Parkinson's often have thriving fungus in the skin of their toes, tops and sides of the feet, and sometimes even on the soles of the feet.

If the *leg* is somewhat numb and there is poor circulation in the skin of the leg along the path of the Stomach channel, the fungus sometimes spreads farther up the skin of the leg. In areas where the blood circulation *is* sufficient to keep it at bay, the fungus is *not* able to thrive. Thus, its presence in the *legs* is generally limited to an asymptomatic sub-dermal invasion, usually only along the path of the Stomach channel.

As noted above, these areas *might* break out into an itchy, red, and sometimes painful rash when the weather is hot. But in most of my patients, the fungus was always lying low, invisible and undetected, except for the toenails, until the person started to recover from Parkinson's.

During recovery, circulation almost always improves quickly in patients' feet. As circulation improves, it seems as if the patients' immune system becomes able to detect the fungus, if there is any, and initiates battle against it. This often causes a reaction on the part of the fungus. The fungus, coming under attack, reproduces and "blooms" aggressively. Possibly this helps produce spores before being killed. The "blossoms" of the fungus are itchy, red bumps, sometimes a quarter inch across, sometimes very tiny. If there are a lot of the very little bumps, they look like a red rash. Sometimes, if they are scratched enough, the bumps open up, releasing a tiny bit of fluid.

As the fungus comes under attack from the body's newly improved circulatory system, itching red sores might break out wherever the fungus had been living quietly, invisibly under the skin.

In some patients, the fungal infection has pervaded the skin of more than just the foot. The single red blisters or the mass of tiny blisters making up a red rash might extend up the lower part of the leg(s) and, in a few cases, I've seen it extend up even to the thighs. Again, the presence of fungus is usually limited to the path of the Stomach channel, and is worse on the side where PD symptoms first appeared.

No treatment is necessary.

The red rash can be hot and itchy, but in all cases that I have seen, the red rash has gone away by itself. Once circulation is restored, the body is able to recognize and destroy the fungus that, over the years, had snuck into numb areas with poor circulation.

Some patients found that an athlete's foot salve was somewhat helpful during this time, but others said that it was not. Others found that aloe vera lotion was useful in soothing the heat and itch until the battle is over. Others disagreed. One patient had good luck temporarily numbing the painful itch by rubbing raw garlic on the rash.

The red skin rash always ceased eventually. Even the fungus in the toenails often decreases or disappears, although this usually takes much longer. Watching the healthy new nails slowly grow in, pushing the diseased toenails out, can be a cause for gentle celebration. In some cases, the toenails return to complete health.

I find it interesting to note that toenail fungus is an illness that some doctors consider to be superficially treatable but ultimately incurable – just like Parkinson's.

Pills to treat the fungus

Some patients have asked about the internal (pill form) antifungal medications. Fungus in the toes and feet is not a dangerous condition. Internal antifungal medications, however, are extremely toxic and hard on the liver. In fact, the internal antifungal medications (as opposed to the external-use ointments and salves) are far more dangerous than the fungus itself.

Most of the doctors I know personally will not let their own family and loved ones use the FDA-approved *internal* antifungal medications. Besides, when a person uses internal antifungal medication, the *dormant* portion of the fungus doesn't die from the medication. The fungus will resume growth and thrive again within a few weeks after a person stops using the medication. In other words, the anti-fungal medications do not *eradicate* the fungus. The fungus can remain in the body, dormant, as long as a person is taking the medication. Therefore, the medication doesn't actually "cure" the fungus; it just *temporarily* prevents it from thriving or "blooming": it just masks the symptoms.

Duration of the red rash

The red blisters or the red rash sometimes last for a few short weeks. Sometimes it goes on for over a month.

One patient who had the red rash go all the way to the top of his thigh was a neurologist. It was exciting for him to observe this utterly unexpected manifestation of submerged illness. It was clear to him that there had been something wrong with him that was not related to "dead brain cells," and that his body was healing from some previously unrecognized numbness. I asked him if he would tell his colleagues at one of our top east coast medical schools about our theories and his treatment. He said that he would not. "They would think I was crazy if they knew I was seeing an acupuncturist."

If you get the red rash, celebrate. Your body is waking back up. It's taking notice of pathogens that have been silently munching on you, maybe for years, and your body's now noticing them and killing them. Congratulations!

Chapter Twenty-six

Recovery symptoms: Rigidity and Limpness

While recovering from Parkinson's, muscles that *had* been rigid lose their rigidity and instead became limp and unresponsive.

Unresponsive is different from "weak." When you first begin to wake after a deep sleep, you become aware that you are conscious *but* your muscles might still be limp and unresponsive. Even if you are in perfect health, even if you are a powerful weight lifter, your muscles will be limp as you feel the first stirrings of consciousness. After a few moments or a few minutes, as the mid-brain resumes running awake-time electrical currents with steadily increasing amperage, the brain's automatic motor function, which has been disconnected during sleep, reconnects. You begin to *imagine* moving a muscle or two, and suddenly, you can move.

Effortless, "automatic" movement: not the same as emergency movement

Then again, if you are awakened by some calamity in the night, you will be able to move instantly, using the brain's norepinephrine emergency motor activation system. If you hear a crashing noise that wakes you out of a deep sleep you can jump out of bed, heart pounding, and run down the stairs to confront the crisis. When you go back to bed after realizing it was just the raccoons getting into the garbage again, your legs might feel wobbly and strange. You were using emergency movement, using your body mechanically. You *weren't* using what's called "automatic movement," meaning *effortless*, parasympathetic mode movement.

Even people with advanced Parkinson's can move easily in a genuine emergency. Even if they can *no longer* sustain a *contrived*, purely mind-created sense of emergency that's convincing enough to override their use of pause mode, even if they can *barely* move at all due to *advanced* PD, they *can* move in a way that appears perfectly normal during a real emergency, when the full-strength norepinephrine surge kicks in.

When the parasympathetic, *automatic* motor area (as opposed to the emergency system) is *not* turned on in a healthy person, such as occurs during sleep, during periods of insufficient dopamine, or due to an inability to consciously imagine movement, the muscles feel unresponsive and limp. Not *weak*. Disconnected. Therefore limp. Turned off. This chapter discusses the unresponsive and limp behavior in previously rigid muscles that can occur while recovering. This limpness can occur when pause turns off *but* the automatic motor function doesn't turn back on right away. Automatic motor function uses a sequence of steps, including *imagining* oneself moving. After long years of dormancy, this sequence for movement initializing might not start up again right away even after pause turns off.

People with Parkinson's tend to speak of this phase of recovery as "weak muscles." If they think of the muscles as non-responsive, mentally inaccessible, or disconnected, rather than weak, they are more likely to remember to do the exercises that can hasten re-activation of the brain's motor imagining area – a crucial step in the process of generating automatic movement.

Recovery from rigidity

Rigidity is a correct physiological response to backwards-flowing channel qi. Following a severe injury, such as a leg-break, the subsequent backwards-flowing channel qi helps the injured body part or most of the body stay rigid, thus inhibiting movement and preventing further damage until the injury is able to heal. As soon as the channel qi flows the right way again, in a healthy blend of the parasympathetic and sympathetic pathways, these rigid areas are once again able to use dopamine-based movement. Dopamine-based movement uses a very different pathway in the brain than the norepinephrine pathway. The dopamine motor pathway flows through the motor-imagining route in the brain. This helps ensure that automatic movements can only occur when a person is safe and is able to imagine himself making the movements – in other words, the person has to be conscious and *not* at risk of imminent death.

An hypothesis: when a person has been on pause and the channel qi has been flowing backwards for *years*, various sectors in the motor imagining area in the brain becomes dormant. People with Parkinson's, for the most part, cannot *imagine* themselves moving. When people begin to recover from Parkinson's, the motor-imagining area might *not* resume function right away. Or it might be able to imagine *some* movements, but not others, in the beginning. The dormancy in this imagining area might recover function fairly quickly. But until it does, people recovering from Parkinson's might go through a period in which their muscles feel limp and unresponsive.

The above hypothesis, supported by the brain research mentioned in chapter fifteen, is backed up by the peculiar events that occur during recovery.

Again, during recovery, the ability to *imagine* certain movements might still be dormant for areas where the body has been rigid, as opposed to numb. The muscles for these areas, muscles that had been rigid while on pause, become *limp* and unresponsive when pause turns off. It seems as if, when pause turns off after decades of inhibiting the brain's motor-imagining area, the use and coordination of some of these muscles *cannot* be accessed right away. If they can't be accessed, the muscles behave as if they are *asleep* – still *disconnected* from the mind's motor imagining area.

Becoming limp

Prior to recovery, many of my PD patients imagined their rigid, even rock-hard muscles, and the anterior-lateral thigh muscles in particular, to be proof of healthy, well-toned muscle. However, these muscles were *not* "toned." They were perpetually somewhat contracted and wooden. They could *not* relax. They were *not* vigorous.

During recovery, the tissue in these muscles softens. When the backwards-flowing channel qi ceased to flow through these muscles, they lose their rigidity. They often become limp or even mushy, for a while. It's not that they are *weak*: they can't even tighten or loosen a *tiny* bit in response to the brain commands to move. They behave as if they aren't receiving brain commands, as if those muscles are sleeping. Although the problem *seems* to be one of weakness, it is more likely a problem of certain brain-to-body instructions not getting through. Based on what happened when patients *worked* at *imagining* the desired movement, the problem was one of dormancy in the motor-imagining area of the brain. This area of the brain has been suspected of contributing to the symptoms of Parkinson's as far back as the year 2000. [1]

These body parts hadn't responded to brain commands during the years on pause, either, but because these body parts were rigid, they could be used as supports. The other, still-functional muscles in other parts of the arms, legs, back, and buttocks, areas that had channel qi flowing in the right direction, *could* push off against the rigid muscles or compensate for them. Many patients had actually thought that their lifeless, rigid muscles, especially those in the thigh, were *extremely* healthy: *super*-toned. As proof of their superb muscle tone, many of my patients pointed to their ability to climb stairs two at a time. The mechanisms enabling this fairly typical PD behavior were discussed earlier, in chapter fifteen.

Although the muscle limpness and unresponsiveness during recovery was most noticeable and problematic when it occurred in the thighs, it sometimes was noticeable in other muscle groups that had been rigid. Then again, some patients experienced an effortless return to healthy muscle tone in some or all of the previously rigid muscles, with *no* noticeable period of limp, unresponsive muscles.

Not a question of atrophy

Some patients wondered if the sudden flaccidity was *atrophy* (weakened muscle). It was *not*. Based on what I saw during recoveries, it seemed as if the flaccidity was due to a disconnect between the mind and that body part – and it happened when pause turned off and the person was once again predominantly in parasympathetic mode.

I can venture this hypothesis for two reasons: first, in cases of true emergency, people were still able to use these otherwise limp muscles. Second, these areas did not *slowly* regain strength. Instead, it seemed as if the problem was utter: all or nothing. When the muscles suddenly did make the connection, the previously limp body parts suddenly moved perfectly normally.

For example, recall the situation described in chapter twenty-one when, five years after recovering, my right leg suddenly, spontaneously, lifted up off the floor and rested over my left knee so that I could put my shoe on more easily. The muscles in my right leg had been strong and healthy for nearly five years. Since recovering, I had long been able to physically do everything I wanted to do, including hiking, swimming and going to the gym. But when it came to the very specific, coordinated movement of lifting the right leg up and putting it across my left knee so I could put on my shoe, I still needed to use my hands to do it. I never even questioned it. I'd always needed to do that. I just assumed it was normal, for me. When it came to performing that particular movement, my leg was essentially limp and powerless – not responsive to my mental suggestion that it lift up.

And then, one day, out of the blue, my leg spontaneously did that movement on its own. I wasn't *trying* to do that move. I was just sitting down, putting on my shoes without thinking, mentally reviewing the dozen things I needed to do that day. This sudden, smooth movement had *nothing* to do with muscle strength. It was as if my brain suddenly re-established the connection with that specific, long-dormant leg-movement sequence.

---

[1] "Motor imagery in normal subject and in asymmetrical Parkinson's disease"; Thoois, Dominey, Decety, et al; *Neurology*; Oct 10, 2000; 996-1002. For more information about this and other footnotes related to the motor imaging area, please see p. 82.

(When it comes to complex motor sequences such as lifting one leg and resting it on the opposite knee, and based on what we know about the different brain areas, it's likely that the motor imagining area is also having to link up with the cerebellum. The cerebellum is considered to store information about complex motor sequences. But this is more detail than we really need in this book.)

Ever since that moment, that particular motion now occurs whenever I start to put my shoes on. It's become, once again, an "automatic movement."

This mind-to-body disconnect only seemed to apply to those body parts over which channel qi had been running backwards. I had to wonder, in my patients with Parkinson's, had this mind-to-body disconnect been in place for decades? Did this mind connection start breaking down when the person first started using pause mode? If so, that might explain why some people who started using pause in early childhood had severe limpness and unresponsiveness during recovery. Others, those who hadn't started using pause until they were in their teens or later, had fewer muscles that seemed limp and unresponsive during recovery, and the limpness was of shorter duration.

During patients' recoveries, it did seem as if the absence of a mind-to-body-part connection, and not atrophy, was the primary cause of the limpness: as *soon* as the mind-to-body connection was restored in these areas, the muscles instantly resumed some degree of tone, or at least experienced the tingling and spasms that suggested a return of muscle function. As soon as healthy *awareness* of the limbs *and* their repertoire of movements resumed, it was as if the brain connections abruptly ended their dormancy. The muscles functioned again – spontaneously.

No workouts at the gym were necessary to get these muscles functional. In fact, until these muscles resumed responsiveness, trying to use these muscles at the gym didn't help at all. Going to the gym was an exercise in futility. A person could keep mentally *commanding* a certain limp muscle to move in some manner, the way he used to command himself to move when he was stuck on pause, but with pause and the norepinephrine override both turned off, no movement ensued. If any movement was produced, it was produced by the splinting muscles, the *alongside* muscles that "help out" when another muscle isn't functional.

Reactivating automatic movements

The best way to rebuild the brain connection to limp, unresponsive body parts turned out to be pretty simple: imagining the desired movements. If, after turning off pause, a person could no longer get up from the toilet, he could spend as much time as possible every day *imagining* himself getting up from the toilet. He could be lying on his back on the sofa or resting in a rocking chair while doing this. If he *mentally* imagined getting up from the toilet over and over, for as many minutes or hours a day as possible, it seemed to *greatly* accelerate the mental reconnection for the imagined automatic movement.

While a person is using pause mode, he can't *do* this type of imagining. But when pause turns off, a person can once again imagine anything he wants to.

Many top athletes these days do regular *mental* exercises, *imagining* their performance in order to improve their performance. It turns out, athletes attain *faster* improvement if they repeatedly *imagine* themselves doing the high jump or doing their gymnastic routines than if they only do the *actual* jumps or routines. This counterintuitive approach started being used by top coaches and their athletes around the beginning of the twenty-first century. [1]

"Conscious strength"

Usually, after turning off pause, within a few days, many *numb* (*not* rigid) muscles resumed normal tone and responsiveness, especially the muscles of the face. However, the muscles that had been *rigid* might not resume function for days, weeks, or months. In a few cases, it took *several* months.

I started referring to this resumption of normal tone and responsiveness in previously *rigid* muscle as "return of *conscious* strength." It was a resumption of strength similar to that which a person gets when he returns to a fully awake state after having been deeply asleep or in a coma.

At first, when a person wakens from a deep sleep, he feels limp. Then, a surge of body consciousness and strength surges through the muscles. In some people recovering from Parkinson's, after turning off pause, the surge didn't happen right away, or it only occurred for some muscle behaviors, but not others.

This was *not* a dopamine-related problem. *Some* of the muscles might work just fine. I am certain the root of the problem was a brain disconnection at the motor imagining level. I repeat, for many patients, their learned, coordinated movements that had been turned off while using pause mode for a long, long time seemed to be dormant. Muscles over which the channel qi had been running backwards had essentially been put on hold at some spot, some location, in the brain's movement-initiating sequence that controls automatic movement. The location in that sequence, based on recovery behaviors, seemed to be the movement imagining area.

A most difficult phase

The limp muscle stage was the most *emotionally* difficult phase of recovery for some people. It was also *physically* difficult because, during this time, certain muscles might behave as if they were made of limp rags when attempting some particular movement.

Making it even more stressful, a patient might still have rigidity in some areas while having limpness in others. For example, if his foot injury was healing, he might

---

[1] A book that touches on this and other brain change subjects is *The Brain that Changes Itself*, by Norman Doidge, MD, Penguin Books, New York 2007. While I do recommend *this* book, I do *not* recommend Doidge's later works in which he hypothesizes that Parkinson's disease is caused by people being mentally lazy. He created a whole theory of Parkinson's disease based on one man's ability to keep moving in spite of PD by forcing himself into physically challenging, even dangerous situations: bolstering his faltering norepinephrine override. The patient still had severe symptoms of Parkinson's, especially when his daily exercise challenges were over for the day. Dr. Doidge clearly knew very little about the Parkinson's personality, the mental intensity of purpose – *not* laziness! – of most people with PD and the fact that *most* people with Parkinson's keep themselves moving by creating mental threats. His example patient was more *typical* for PD than unique. He thought that this one man's highly self-promoted story was singular and that it pointed the way for everyone with Parkinson's to keep moving despite the steady worsening of symptoms. Still, I enjoyed his previous book, the one about how the brain changes itself in response to mental behaviors and exercises.

develop limp muscles in his legs. But if he still had an unhealed neck and shoulder injury, maybe even one completely unrelated to causing the circuitry of pause mode, he might still have painful *rigidity* or dystonia in his neck and arm while having such extraordinary *limpness* in his leg muscles that his legs could barely support him. When combinations of limp and rigid occurred, it was sometimes extremely difficult for patients. They had no idea what was going on.

Those who were content to enjoy or be amused by the process had fewer problems with these changes. Those who were still predominantly fear-based became highly distressed when conflicting muscle behaviors presented at the same time. Some reverted to the familiarity of using pause mode to deal with their confusion and fear.

Limpness in the body, part by part

In the following examples, the patients were not doing mental exercises. They were *not* practicing imagining that their limp muscles were moving. These examples are from the early days of my research, and the behaviors described in the sections that follow were spontaneous and not influenced by actively imagining.

As an aside, asymmetry often occurs during recovery from rigidity. Many patients have noticed muscles pulling to the left or the right as the opposing muscle group became limp. The *less* damaged muscle group was usually the one that started recovering first: it became limp first and it started working correctly first, sometimes before the same muscle group on the opposite side of the body even started showing signs of going limp.

Neck limpness

Examples: a patient experienced softening in the rigid muscles in her neck. Within two days of her neck starting to go limp, she couldn't hold her head up. To hold up her head at work, she placed a stack of law books under her chin so that she could read her legal paperwork. Several days passed before she had enough conscious strength in her neck to use her muscles normally.

Another patient, a graduate student, asked me to write a doctor's note explaining she could not take an oral exam because she literally couldn't hold her head up. She didn't want to tell the professor that she was recovering from Parkinson's. I think she just told her prof that she'd "hurt" her neck. A week later, she was able to hold her head up perfectly normally.

Another recovering patient went through several days during which her head pulled to the right. This occurred when the rigid muscles on the left side of her neck began to melt while her right-side neck muscles were still rigid. Her Parkinson's symptoms had first occurred on her right side. Her right side symptoms were more severe, and they were also slower to heal. Several months later, after the two *sides* of her neck had resumed healthy balance, the front and back of her neck went limp and her head flopped gently forward for several days. After that, she experienced no more neck weakness.

I personally *never* noticed a time when my neck muscles became weak. I only realized that my neck muscles were no longer rigid one day when I tried to look to my left side while slowly steering the car out of its parking place. In recent years, I'd gradually grown accustomed to looking to the side by turning my head *slightly* to the left – as far as I could – and putting all my strength into twisting as hard as I could all along the spine. This allowed me to look to the side.

When my neck muscles loosened unbeknownst to me and I applied the usual amount of extreme strength, I found myself looking *behind* me when I intended to merely look to the side. With almost no effort, my neck had pivoted nearly 120 degrees, as far as any healthy person might be able to turn his head. Together with my powerful, well-practiced spinal twist, my head ended up 180 degrees from where it has started. I had to learn how to moderate my head-turning strength to accommodate my new neck flexibility. But the point is, my neck muscles never became problematically, or even noticeably, weak or limp.

Ankle limpness

Sudden limpness in the area just above and below the ankles sometimes caused swelling in the ankles. This condition did not seem to be related to poor kidney function or any of the usual problems that might cause water build-up in the ankle. The root problem was *not* water build-up, per se. It seemed more as if the muscles above and below the ankle had become so limp that they did not present enough tension to force fluids back up the legs. Consequently, fluids built up in the saggy areas of the ankles. No exercise of this area was necessary, or able, to reduce the swelling: as soon as the muscles of this area resumed healthy mind-to-ankle awareness, the ankles soon resumed their slimmer, pre-recovery lines.

If your ankle swelling scares you, gently wrap the ankle in an Ace (elastic) bandage until the muscle tone wakes up. And/or elevate your legs as often as possible.

Leg limpness

The legs often become *very* limp. Many patients experienced a period during which their legs were so unresponsive and limp that they could not get up from a chair or from the toilet. This inability to stand up due to limp or "mushy" muscles *felt* different from the patients' previous inability to initiate movement. For one thing, the patient was able to *feel* his legs, as opposed to objectively observing the poor functionality of the legs.

The upper legs in particular often felt profoundly weak, even like "custard pudding." Patients who were in partial recovery, so that the Stomach channel qi was running somewhat correctly *sometimes* but the mind was still highly wary and usually unable to release dopamine for motor function, nearly always felt that this new utter inability to stand up from a sitting position was much more of a problem than their previous inability to initiate movement.

This was an especially challenging time for people who were stuck in partial recovery. Prior to recovering from the injury that caused Type II PD, the patient might have had difficulty in figuring out *how* to make his legs move. When the legs turned to mush, he still couldn't move them *and* they were limp, to boot. Many patients decided, at this point, that they had rapidly gone from bad to worse. If they plunged into fear and amped up their use of pause mode in response, they often found the rigidity rapidly returned. Which meant that they were no longer limp. They were often emotionally relieved by this resumption of pause mode, even though all their other PD symptoms then got much, much worse, sometimes very quickly. The tremor often become far more severe than it ever had been because of their now-heightened use of pause mode.

I know that I've already discussed the treacheries of partial recovery. But I keep bringing it up because it was such a large part of my experience in working with people who were trying to recover, and also, I really want this point to be heard, no matter on what page a person picks up this book: a person wants to recover from Type I PD *before* he works on healing any injuries that might be contributing to Type II PD.

Whether the condition lasted only a few days or a few months, the leg non-responsiveness while trying to stand up was sometimes the most challenging phase of recovery from Parkinson's disease. Many patients found themselves humiliatingly inconvenienced: needing help with bathing and toilet. This phase was exhausting for some caregivers, especially elderly ones. This phase was the one in which many recovering patients began to doubt the wisdom of trying to recover.

I eventually came to see that those patients who could feel and *imagine* movement in their legs rapidly overcame this phase: mushy legs started to firm up in a few days or a few weeks. Those who were in partial recovery, who were still using self-induced pause and were therefore unable to *imagine* their legs moving sometimes found themselves stuck in this phase indefinitely – until they decided they could *not* recover, after which, they fearfully *increased* the use of pause mode, stiffened back up, and could use their legs again in a PD-like manner.

Feet sticking to the floor with rigid or limp legs

The inability to lift the legs due to limpness in the anteriolateral muscles of the upper leg during recovery was *different* from the Parkinson's symptom of "feet sticking to the floor." Patients' feet might stick to the floor whether the legs are rigid *or* limp.

The foot stuck-ness of Parkinson's can be caused either by aberrant channel qi flow set in motion by an injury on the foot, *or* by a particular electrical pattern in the feet that is *supposed* to kick in during pause – an electrical pattern that, when severe, can cause a person to feel *magnetically* stuck to the floor. It can even feel as if the foot is being "sucked into" the floor. These sensations are due to electrical currents on the sole of the foot that "ground out" into the floor instead of flowing up towards the medial ankle.

Limpness in the legs can also make it difficult to pick up the feet. This situation does *not* feel as if the feet are glued, magnetically attached, or being sucked into the floor. This latter type of stuck feet just feels as if the legs are too limp to raise the foot.

While recovering from Parkinson's, a person who *used* to feel his feet being magnetically attached to the floor due to being on pause might find that his feet are now merely stuck on the floor because he can't *imagine* how he moved his legs in the days *before* he developed PD.

Torso limpness

Many patients, often well before they were diagnosed, noticed an increased difficulty in rolling over in bed. A recovery landmark that was often disturbing was the *change* in how the patient couldn't roll over in bed.

Typically, as Parkinson's worsens, a patient lying on his back may need to turn over in bed in the following manner: he brings the knees closer to the chest and pulls the head forward, as if in a fetal position. Then, in one strong movement he jerks his whole body, as a single rigid unit, over onto his side. As the Parkinson's progresses, he may need help to do the heaving bit: a strong shove by the spouse will usually shift him.

In recovering patients, the rigid muscles of the torso become limp. Patients become *unable* to pull themselves into a fetal position. Instead, they can only lie floppy or limp on the bed.

It might not be too difficult for a healthy spouse to shove a rigid, fetal position person with PD from one side to the other. It is *much* harder for the spouse to shift a person who is limp, whose body behaves like deadweight.

This limpness while trying to turn over in bed was clearly *not* characteristic of Parkinson's – a disease that features rigidity in the torso. However, the new utter inability to turn over in bed often convinced patients that they were far worse off than before.

Those with a curious and positive attitude and an ability to feel their muscles appreciated that having the muscle tone of mayonnaise was a shift in the right direction. Some patients reported feeling genuine pleasure from the new awareness of sensation in the muscles of the torso and limbs, whether limp *or* strong. In the past, they had been accustomed to jerk themselves over quickly and efficiently without *noticing* any somatic sensations created by these movements. They began to appreciate a new way of moving: noticing the internal sensations that languid movement conveyed to the heart and mind.

Eventually, these patients were able to turn over in bed.

I remember how I managed to turn over in bed after my torso muscles became limp. Starting at the shoulder, I very slowly managed to drag one limp arm in the direction that I wanted to turn over in bed. Then I slowly oozed one leg over in the direction in which I wanted to turn. I slowly moved my head to the side. Slowly, moving one body part at a time, I was able to get enough body weight turned to the side so that my hips then followed my arm, legs, and limbs, slowly pouring myself over onto my other side.

Even doing this "slow motion" style of turning over, some patients needed help rolling the hips over until they regained conscious strength in those torso muscles that are used to turn the hips. But in time, these people learned how to turn over *languorously*, a movement style that many of them had *never* used since childhood.

Oppositely, as you've already guessed, those who were in partial recovery were usually *terrified* if the body became limp in response to their injury becoming healed while the mind was still on pause. When the body become limp and they had even less ability to turn over in bed, they sooner or later enhanced the degree of self-induced pause mode that they'd been using. Their minds increasingly raced, day and night, through worst-case scenarios, their tremors sometimes became more violent, their slowness became glacial, and their rigidity became painfully tight – which at least caused the limpness to go away.

It seemed as if their bodies were going through the motions of healing from the foot injury, causing them to experience *some* recovery symptoms. Because they were still using self-induced pause and its highly wary mindset, they were terrified beyond reasonable logic by their recovery symptoms. Therefore, they soon increased the *degree* to which they used self-induced pause. I'm aware that I'm being redundant. I *really* want to drive home that partial recovery is worse than mere Parkinson's disease.

Back limpness

Many recovering patients had a spate of back limpness, causing their torsos to bend forward, so that the head hung down in front, sometimes almost to the knees. This condition usually healed up fairly quickly, in response to repeatedly straightening up.

Early on in my Parkinson's research, two recovering patients did *not* recover quickly from this. They were utterly unable to stand up straight. They might pull themselves to a standing position for a few moments, but within less than a minute they were once again bent over from the waist, head facing the knees. In addition to this, they seemed to lose all of their drive and focus. They had both been taking antiparkinson's medications.

In these two cases, I did not figure out how to effectively treat this situation. Both of these patients lived far away – one on the opposite coast and the other in Europe. I only saw them a few times. I wish that I'd had more opportunity to work with both of them.

As I learned more about the other channels, not just the Stomach channel, that are involved in pause mode, I hypothesized a cause for this very rare pathology. I now guess that there might have been an inhibition of the adrenal glands *and* the small of the back muscles due to the Urinary Bladder (UB) channel leaving the body just above UB-11, thus failing to provide energy to the back muscles *and* to the adrenal glands. I have since done a research project showing that people with minimal adrenal function very often have a glitch somewhere along the UB channel, causing failure of UB channel qi to make it far enough down the body to activate adrenaline release and muscle function in the small of the back.

My patients' sudden postural collapses were so impossibly bizarre that I found myself grateful for Oliver Sacks' photos and descriptions of this exact same postural problem in one of his patients, in his book *Awakenings*. (See footnote on p. 33.)

In Dr. Sacks' patient, the bent-double posture occurred, practically overnight, in one of his sleeping sickness patients after she was dosed with high levels of L-dopa (dopamine). I suspect that her extremely high doses of L-dopa (thousands of milligrams per day) may have caused a shift from chronic sleep mode into parasympathetic mode.

I'm purely guessing here, but this re-awakening of parasympathetic mode via L-dopa might have exposed a lurking UB channel qi aberration that was preventing activation of the muscles in the small of the back – an aberration that wasn't significant so long as the person was "sleeping" from sleeping sickness.

Had it not been for Dr. Sacks' photographic documentation of this patient, I might not have believed my eyes when, in response to turning off pause, two of my patients became bent double from small-of-the-back limpness and stayed that way.

Urinary Bladder channel not flowing correctly

At any given time, the amount of channel qi in the UB channel reflects the degree of sympathetic mode a person is using at that moment. Even a healthy, contented, and happy person, while awake, uses *some* amount of sympathetic mode channel function in order to be lively. Use of almost pure parasympathetic mode occurs when one is highly consciousness, in perfect health, and with *motionless* body and mind, as one is in single-focus meditation. While in sleep mode, the UB channel is very nearly shut down, running with a minimal amount of channel qi.

If this situation of no energy in the low back does arise, the patient might either mentally examine the flow patterns of the UB and Kidney channel qi or get someone else to feel the channel qi of his UB and Kidney channels. There will likely be a spot somewhere along one of these two channels where the channel qi flow seems to stop or else flows outside of the body.

If the problem is one of channel qi flowing out of the body just above UB-11, the patient needs to mentally imagine the flow of that channel flowing down his neck and *staying under the skin* all the way down to the back torso. This sometimes brings immediate results. Sometimes, the person has to repeat this mental exercise several times a day, over several days, or for weeks, until the fix becomes permanent.

If the UB channel is stopping or running sideways from some location other than UB-11, Yin Tui Na treatment (in the case of injury) or mental reconstruction of the channel at that location (in the case of mental habits) might be needed. This mental reconstruction can be done by the patient imagining the correct flow pattern over and over, until the healthy flow pattern is stable. A map of the correct path of the UB channel is in Appendix II.

In a few cases, the back of the knee shunt from UB-40 to Ki-10 is not working. More on this subject is presented in *Tracking the Dragon*, in the chapter on sympathetic mode.

If a friend learns to feel channel qi or a local acupuncturist is familiar with channel theory (unlikely), he/she can help track the patient's UB channel, find where it is flowing outside of the body or flowing sideways into another channel, and then show the patient just where that is happening. The patient then will need to imagine the UB channel going back on course.

Working with the doctor when the limpness appeared

Sometimes, people who were in the midst of limpness went to a doctor to ask, "What the heck is going on?" They were sometimes told, during this mid-recovery visit, that they evidently never had Parkinson's disease in the first place: what they *actually* had was Multiple System Atrophy. Although MSA is an *extremely* rare condition, I recall a one-month period in which three of my recovering Parkinson's patients were re-diagnosed with MSA.

Or, if the doctor was less well-informed, he incorrectly decided that, in some people, leg and/or torso *limpness*, not rigidity, were the main symptoms of Parkinson's disease. Or the doctor simply changed the diagnosis to "parkinson*ism*" (a catch-all term), or even "*atypical* parkinsonism" (an *extremely* vague catch-all term), and left it at that.

Multiple system atrophy is an *extremely* rare syndrome in which a person becomes steadily more limp and weak. Multiple system atrophy (MSA) is not in any way related to Parkinson's disease. But if the patient reminded his MD that, prior to entering a recovery program, he'd had problems of *rigidity*, not problems of limpness, the doctor might ignore these statements. Other MDs explained, patronizingly, to the recovering patient that it is always hard to get a firm diagnosis in the beginning. No MDs, in my patients' experiences, changed their minds about the MSA when informed that the patient had been *rigid* prior to becoming limp. And when the recovery limpness went away the diagnosis was changed to either neurosis or psychosis.

It was hard for patients to stand firm in their knowledge of what their own symptoms had been when their doctors told them that they'd never had Parkinson's after all. One of the first patients who received the altered diagnosis of Multiple System Atrophy was the neurologist mentioned in the previous chapter (the one whose red rash extended up to his thigh). When he started to be as limp as a blob of jelly, he asked his doctor for an assessment. His neurologist told him that he'd never had Parkinson's: he'd had Multiple System Atrophy right along. My patient was also a neurologist. He knew darned well that his previous symptoms had *not* been characteristic of Multiple System Atrophy. His symptoms *had* been those of Parkinson's.

Even so, when his colleague told him that he had Multiple System Atrophy, he decided he could not trust his own judgment any more. (This was probably accurate: his mental clarity had become heavily fogged by his antiparkinson's medications.) He was willing to accept that his PD diagnosis *had* been incorrect even though, as a neurologist, he had originally concurred in every way with his diagnosis of PD.

The first time this happened, I was surprised. PD and MSA are *very* different illnesses. After this happened several times, I realized anew the difficulty that doctors have in accepting the idea that a person can have Parkinson's disease and recover from it.

Now, I tell patients that if they *used* to have rigidity and the usual symptoms of Parkinson's, but when recovering they become limp and their doctors tell them that they were misdiagnosed and that what they've had right along is Multiple System Atrophy, it is time to celebrate: they no longer have Parkinson's disease. And in all likelihood, *despite* what the doctor says, they don't have Multiple System Atrophy, either. Sometimes, instead of MSA, a patient in recovery was re-diagnosed with parasupranuclear palsy (PSP). The above observations for being re-diagnosed with MSA also apply to being re-diagnosed with PSP.

Medical reports are not detailed enough

I was seeing most of my patients every week, for an hour. I kept extremely detailed notes on their symptoms. They usually expected the same level of interest and detail from their MDs. I frequently had to point out to my patients that it was *not* reasonable to expect a neurologist or any other doctor, who might not have seen the PD patient for six months, to quickly examine him and decide if his symptoms had changed away from their original condition: most MDs do not make thorough enough notes to be able to tell if a person's symptoms have changed significantly, and memory of a fifteen minute visit, six months prior, is rarely precise. The doctor usually made a diagnosis of Parkinson's based on an overall picture of what seemed to be going on after having ruled out, via a brain scan, brain tumor and stroke. He may *not* have even noted in his records the exact symptoms or the exact location of symptoms that the patient presented. His notes might merely say something along the general lines of "tremor, rigidity, cogwheeling, lack of facial expression." His notes may not even mention the *exact* locations or the severity of the symptoms.

Therefore, if a patient has a 75% return of facial expression, but one corner of the mouth still turns down a bit, the MD may look at that corner of the mouth and say, "Continuing lack of facial expression." The MD will have no way of remembering that the condition used to be far worse.

I had patients who'd lost their voice to PD but who subsequently regained the ability to talk, who'd been expressionless but had regained the ability to smile, and who had lost the use of their hands but had regained it again. They eagerly awaited a surprised look on the doctor's face, only to be told by their MDs during their next bi-annual visits that "nothing had changed."

If they pointed out these obvious changes to their doctors, the doctors might reply with something along the lines of: "So you're having a good day today." In the case of one patient who had never taken antiparkinson's medications in the three years since his diagnosis, the doctor said, "It's nice to see that your medications are finally starting to work."

I also reminded my patients that the MDs are probably accustomed to seeing *medicated* patients. In these cases, the doctor will *expect* the patient to be moving better in subsequent visits for the first year or two – thanks to the medication. Therefore, he may not be surprised to see the patient moving somewhat better than before: it's what he's used to. Even if he is reminded that the patient *isn't* taking the prescribed antiparkinson's medications, the significance of this might not sink in.

One recovering patient who pointed out to old Doctor Dorosin, his doctor for twenty years, that he was once again making his own meals after *years* of not being able to use his gnarled hands at all *and* that he no longer used a walker, which he'd needed for several years, was told, "Your symptoms aren't declining as quickly as before: your wife certainly is taking good care of you!"

An admission of recovery

Except for one delightful exception, no doctor in my experience was willing to say that a patient was recovering from Parkinson's. In the one exception, a *group* of doctors officially stated, for political reasons, that a person "might have recovered from Parkinson's disease."

The case involved a high level French magistrate (a federal judge). The reason behind the statement was this: because her Parkinson's symptoms were waning, she was facing a new diagnosis – a diagnosis of psychosis. From her doctors' point of view, the only possible reason that she could have previously exhibited "false" symptoms of Parkinson's disease for several years would be that she'd been having a psychotic episode that whole time. However, *if* her diagnosis was changed to "psychotic episode," or psychogenic parkinsonism, she obviously could not remain in her position as magistrate. Psychotics cannot be judges.

The patient asked me for advice. She was working with the top neurologists in Paris at the time. I suggested that she tell the doctors, in all honesty, that I had some patients in Germany who were recovering, and that the German patients would be more than happy if the first European recoveries from Parkinson's occurred in Germany, not France. When the patient presented this information to her team of doctors, her diagnosis was changed to "possible recovery from Parkinson's." She was allowed to continue working.

A few curious doctors

To be fair, I must say that a few doctors have said things like, "Your case is baffling," and, "I would have expected you to be much worse by now," and even, "Your other symptoms are gone. If it wasn't for that one arm still not swinging [or whatever symptoms was remaining, and these were often dystonia-related problems and not actual symptoms of Parkinson's], it would seem as if you didn't actually have Parkinson's disease." But these comments, though observant of change and improvement, are not statements as to the reversibility of Parkinson's. Rather, they suggest that the doctor was considering a change in his original diagnosis: the patient had been misdiagnosed.

A patient should not expect his neurologist to pick up on *recovery* symptoms and to notice that they are the opposite of PD symptoms. If muscles go limp, the doctor only notices that the person's problems are worse off than before. Doctors are trained to focus on what is *wrong*. If a patient became limp in certain muscles, the MD focused on that. The doctor often said, accurately, that in terms of movement, a patient going through the limpness phase of recovery was obviously much worse off than before.

Trusting only the doctor

Many people, even while clearly recovering, trusted their doctors' diagnoses more than their own personal observations. Oppositely, some of my patients who had successfully turned off pause tended to dismiss the whole subject of doctors. Their new attitude was expressed in statements such as: "Who the hell are they [doctors] to tell me that I've got an incurable illness? What an idiot I was to have been so emotionally influenced by them! Why did I fall for their stories? They don't know everything!"

These people had become able to *feel* the burgeoning changes within themselves, and had no reason to rely on any outsider's opinion as to whether or not they were doing better. I was actually a bit surprised at the level of anger, even disgust, that many recovered patients felt towards their doctors when they realized that doctors were fallible. Doctors are only human. Their attitudes and expectations reflect their training.

Duration of limp muscles

The amount of time necessary to recover function in limp muscles varied from one person to another and from one muscle group to another. You knew I was going to say that. When working on the 2012 edition of this book, one of my many proofreaders was annoyed by the redundancies that I inserted into these chapters about recovery symptoms, redundancies such as "time needed for recovery will vary."

However, another one of the proofreaders who had been on the Parkinson's Treatment Team (which ended in 2013, for reasons noted earlier) said, "I'm so glad you're starting to be redundant about the most important bits. So many of our patients have been *so* resistant to the key ideas that they need to hear them over and over. So many don't even understand principles such as 'each recovery is different' until they've heard it twenty times."

Summary

Some patients had limp and unresponsive muscles for a few hours or days, or a week or even a few months. When they were able to easily *imagine* themselves moving the limp body part, that body part usually recovered full function fairly quickly. The muscles in which this occurred were usually those that had previously been rigid: along the Stomach channel between the jaw and the top of the foot, or along the Large Intestine channel between the neck and the wrist. The muscles of the small of the back, along the UB channel, also were susceptible to a period of inaccessibility and severe limpness.

This was not weakness, per se: the muscles did not need to grow *strong*. The nerves that connected the imagination to the muscles needed to be hooked back up.

Chapter Twenty-seven

Recovery symptoms: Dyskinesia

Dyskinesia literally means "incorrect" movement. Dyskinesia can refer to movement that occurs spontaneously, that has not been *consciously* initiated.

In the field of Parkinson's, the term "dyskinesia" almost always refers to the uncontrolled movements that occur in response to excessively high levels of antiparkinson's medications. When dopamine levels are excessively high in the brain, the body might erupt in violent arm flailing, head jerking, and even wild swinging movements of the torso and head that might throw a person onto the wall or to the floor. Smaller movements such as tics and twitches might also occur, such as facial grimacing and hand and/or foot twitching. Other dyskinetic movements from overmedication might not be fleeting: excruciating muscle cramps might last for minutes at a time. *Tremor* is not considered to be dyskinesia.

Dyskinesia is *not* a part of classic, idiopathic, *un-medicated* Parkinson's disease. If you are not taking antiparkinson's medications, you do *not* have Parkinson's-type dyskinesias.

Dystonia, as was already discussed, is more of a "locked" muscle problem, such as constant rigidity in a muscle that pulls to one side all the time, or pulls during specific situations such as while walking or lying in bed. Technically, because "dystonia" means "wrong *amount* of muscle tone," this term could theoretically be applied to a muscle with *insufficient* tone. However, in Parkinson's, customary usage of this word is a reference to an *excess* level of muscle tone in some muscle or group of muscles: a muscle pulling too *hard*, so as to prevent normal relaxation in that muscle.

During recovery, when long-dormant motor imagining starts to wake up, muscles along the Stomach and Large Intestine channels and sometimes along the UB channel might behave dyskinetically for a short period. Unlike the violent and painful dykinsesias set in motion by overmedication, recovery dyskinesia is gentle, only occurs when a person is relaxing and feels safe, and can even be mildly amusing. Muscles might start to perform spontaneous, effortless, often graceful, repetitive movements or muscle contractions with *no conscious instruction*. These movements might last for up to twenty minutes per episode, one or more times a day, and might occur in a single muscle or in muscle groups until full brain-to-muscle function is restored in the muscle or muscle groups.

Spontaneous movement

The dyskinetic moments during recovery can be delightful, inasmuch as they are the very opposite of the forced, difficult movements of Parkinson's. They occur when previously rigid *or* numb muscle begins to receive dopamine-driven, "automatic" motor nerve signals once again. When this first occurs, the muscle coordination is often poor, even gently spastic, at first.

When the brain begins to connect to these muscles, so that the recovering patient can somatically *feel* their existence and imagine them moving, they often move imperfectly, even immaturely: these muscle movements are sometimes like those of a baby. A baby happily grimaces asymmetrically while learning to use his facial muscles. He joyfully, repeatedly, helplessly, bangs a spoon on the highchair tray while learning to use his arm. These exact same movements might occur in an adult after turning off the circuitry of long-term pause or pseudo pause.

I named this spontaneous, usually gentle, non-intentional movement "recovery dyskinesia."

Some recovery dyskinesia events are spontaneous, *one-time* muscle spasms or contractions in a previously unresponsive muscle, followed by perfect conscious control. For example, after the one time my right leg spontaneously lifted itself up and placed itself over my left knee, it never happened again spontaneously, meaning *on its own*, without conscious initiation. After that, I could perform that particular move automatically, whereas before, I had to lift that leg with my hands.

Sometimes the recovery dyskinesia events were repetitive: gentle flexions and extensions of a single muscle or muscle group, repeated a few times, or a hundred times or more, every day for a few days or months.

Do not confuse recovery dyskinesia with the rhythmic movement of Parkinson's *tremor*. Parkinson's tremor, whether it is the resting tremor of the fingers, shaking of the arms, legs, or chin, or the "amplified tremor" that shakes the whole body, is always at its worst when the person with Parkinson's is stressed or thinking of something worrisome, and it ebbs when he relaxes or dozes off.

Recovery dyskinesia, on the other hand, occurs when a person is relaxed and feeling safe. In my patients, it occurred most often when the person was watching TV in the evening or lying down before falling asleep.

Another distinction is that Parkinson's tremor is generally somewhat vexing to the person experiencing it, while recovery dyskinesia is generally described as an enjoyable experience, even amusing.

Finally, the movements themselves are different: Parkinson's tremor is usually a predictable, rhythmic vibrating or shaking, whereas recovery dyskinesia, as you will read in the coming sections, is more like muscles gently exercising themselves. In some patients, recovery dyskinesia is only a fleeting event that happens once or a few times. Some recovering patients have *no* episodes of recovery dyskinesia.

Examples of recovery dyskinesia

I will describe only a few examples of recovery dyskinesia. I cannot possibly describe *all* the instances and styles of recovery dyskinesia that I saw or were described to me by astonished patients.

Toe wiggling

Recovery dyskinesia might appear in the toes, shortly after the return of sensation. After the circulation in the toes improves and the tingling is over, some people have gone through a very short phase in which their toes spontaneously wanted to move and stretch. It was as if the toes moved or "wanted" to move without conscious instruction: moving "on their own."

Patients said that they *could* inhibit the toe movement if they wanted to. But they found it more pleasant *not* to get consciously involved, for a change, and to allow the toes to simply express themselves. Even if the toes went into a mild cramp, they usually wiggled themselves free pretty quickly.

Movement in facial muscles

When patients' long-dormant facial muscles began to function, the resultant facial expressions were much more obvious than the spontaneous toe movements. The fleeting facial contortions often resembled those of an infant who cannot yet control his face.

Anyone who has spent time with an infant knows that babies can make some pretty funny facial expressions. Their facial muscles don't work in a coordinated manner for the first several weeks of life. These same immature types of irregular, spontaneous, or even spastic movements of the facial muscles might occur when recovering PD patients' facial nerves awaken from their dormancy.

From an advice column on babies: www.thebump.com: "You should only worry if your baby *isn't* exhibiting jerkiness or spastic movements…"

Some patients, trying to decide whether or not to attempt recovery, are afraid that they will spontaneously make a goofy face while out in public and wonder if recovery is worth the risk. Again, most episodes of recovery dyskinesia take place at home, while relaxing in front of the TV, or while falling asleep. No one has experienced facial spasms while giving a presentation at work. It seems that the body only enjoys the liberty of exploring new muscle function while a person is in a relatively high degree of parasympathetic mode: whenever or wherever he is safe and relaxed.

Recovering facial muscles: an example of "safe"

During my own recovery, after experiencing all manner of fleeting, small facial tics and spasms over a period of two months, I found myself having a major "face recovery" moment while enjoying a rare lunch at a classy restaurant with my daughter. We were seated on the rooftop patio, the warm sun was shining down, we were both laughing.

I was at peace with the world. Suddenly, the entire right side of my face went into a powerful spasm. My right eye was squeezed shut, the right cheek muscles were bulging outward, and the right side of my mouth was pulled up towards my eye. On the right side of my face, *all* the muscles that should be used during a heartfelt smile kicked in at once – at full strength. These muscles were still a bit clumsy, and hadn't worked together as a unit in at least ten years.

As the muscles locked into a powerful spasm for over a minute, screwing up and immobilizing the right side of my face, I finished my sentence by speaking out of the left side of my mouth.

My daughter replied, and we continued chatting. After the facial spasm had been in place for what seemed like a full minute, my daughter said, "Mom, I'm not sure that 'look' really *works* for you," and we both exploded into laughter.

After a few more moments, the spasm melted away. A new sensation of warmth and power pervaded the muscles in my cheeks and the skin of my face. From then on, my face was far more expressive and I was better able to feel a breeze or the sun gently kissing the skin of my face. After that, I had no more episodes of facial dyskinesia.

I chose the above anecdote as an example because many patients have been terrified of having an obvious recovery symptom at a "wrong" time or place, such as when out in public, or in front of some judgmental person. The point I am making here is that, if the person feels safe, it won't matter to him if a facial spasm appears in public. But if the person is in a situation that renders him self-conscious, that situation will *not* be safe. Therefore, he is unlikely to experience a recovery spasm in that setting.

Patients only experienced recovery symptoms when they felt safe. Location, per se, did not make a place safe or not. What made a place "safe" was the attitude of the patient.

A sudden arm stretch

One recovering patient was practicing piano when suddenly her right arm gracefully straightened itself sideways and extended to the keys at the high end of the keyboard. After a moment, the arm returned to its previous position. This happened several times that evening, and then never happened again. It was *not* a muscle cramp. The movement had been graceful, powerful, and completely unexpected.

The neck pivot

Another patient – one who had not gotten an MD's diagnosis and who therefore did *not* know she was actually recovering from early-stage Parkinson's (I never told her) and hence had *no* knowledge of recovery symptoms – was standing up singing in the choir when her neck muscles painlessly but powerfully pulled her head to the left. She found herself staring at the person next to her. The person next to her stared back.

"Cramp in my neck," she explained. After a split second, the neck muscle relaxed and she found herself facing forward again. It had not actually been a cramp. Cramps are overly tight and painful. This neck movement wasn't painful. It had been an involuntary, gentle contraction in a neck muscle that she hadn't used in years. Moments later, it happened again.

"More of a twitch, really," she whispered to the person next to her.

After half a dozen episodes over the course of an hour, it never happened again. Prior to this event, she had not been able to turn her head easily to the side. After this event, she could effortlessly move her head to the side.

Her favorite activity was singing in the choir. She was not embarrassed by the "twitches." She thought they were funny. She was relaxed and didn't care that it happened.

The waving lady on a pancake house

Another recovering patient described recovery dyskinesia in her upper arm. "Last night while I was watching TV, my right arm lifted up and started waving back and forth, back and forth. It wasn't fast. It was like that plywood woman on the roof of the pancake house who mechanically waves back and forth. It kept up for about ten minutes. Never went slower or faster. It didn't hurt. I probably could have stopped it, but I didn't want to. It was bizarre. My adult daughter was kinda worried about it, but I thought it was kinda funny. It felt nice. It wasn't *anything* like tremor."

Marching in bed

Sometimes, when sitting on the sofa or lying in bed, a recovering patient's leg (or legs) starts rhythmically "marching." Sometimes the arms join in, moving in time with the legs. This is *not* restless leg syndrome. This is recovery dyskinesia.

Fixing the foot

One recovering patient felt an urge to bang the top of his foot against the bottom of the coffee table. Every evening, relaxing after dinner, sitting on the sofa in front of the TV, his leg "wanted" to bang the top of his foot against the coffee table. So he let it. He would let his leg gently rise up a few inches, causing the top of the foot to get a gentle whack. The movement was steady and rhythmic. Each evening, the foot was whacked at least a hundred times or so. The whacking ceased on its own one day when his leg no longer "wanted" to do it anymore.

He said it felt really good, as if his leg knew that something in his foot wasn't quite right, and needed to be gently knocked back into place. The foot had received many Yin Tui Na treatments. The foot already felt completely healed, in terms of a return to suppleness and all the other things I look for when treating an old injury. The foot's channel qi was all running the right way. And the patient had no *conscious* understanding of something in particular that needed to be done to the foot. His leg just "wanted" to gently whack the top of the foot, that was all.

After doing this gentle whacking every evening for a few weeks, the patient noticed that his toes seemed "happier" and more flexible. He also realized that his leg was no longer wanting to bang his foot on the bottom of the coffee table in the evening.

Technically, this might not be considered a form of recovery dyskinesia. But the movement felt almost spontaneous, it was repetitive and rhythmic, and so I'm including it in this section.

King Kong

One patient, relaxing at home in the evening, beheld her alternating fists beating on her chest as if she were doing the "proud gorilla" move in slow motion. Alternating, left, right, left right, her fists pounded her chest for nearly ten minutes. She was a very delicate, petite woman: the next morning she had bruises on her chest. She only had this experience once, and afterwards, her arm movements felt more fluid.

Hand positions

In some recovering patients, the muscles in the hand tighten for a while – never for longer than twenty minutes at a time. This sometimes creates weird hand positions: dancer-like, stylistic hand positions. In my case, I experienced them for about three weeks. They usually occurred about forty minutes into my hour-long early morning walks in the woods as I slid into the day-dream phase of my walk. Other recovering patients noticed them most often while sitting around in the evening watching TV.

The voice

Patients' voices suddenly reappeared after months or years of being reduced to a whisper. The return of voice is not always a straight line. The muscles that opened up in the larynx sometimes open very wide, without warning, and an embarrassingly big booming voice issued forth for several minutes – or on and off over a day or two. And then, sometimes a few days later, the voice might temporarily disappear altogether. The full, consciously controllable "normal" voice soon becomes consistent, usually within a few weeks.

One patient called his sister when his voice returned after nearly ten years of almost inaudible speech. His sister accused him of being a prankster. "You're not my brother; my brother only speaks in a whisper." She hung up on him.

Chest muscle spasms

Several patients have grown mildly concerned while experiencing recovery dyskinesia in the chest. In Parkinson's disease, the muscles that run down the mammary line of the torso become rigid. During recovery, these muscles sometimes experience recovery dyskinesia: either they tense up for about twenty minutes and then relax, or they tighten and relax over and over again, somewhat quickly. Either way, the event usually lasts no more than twenty minutes at a time.

During the tightening up phase, recovering patients sometimes felt they could not take a deep breath. A few then wondered if they were having a heart attack. Some went to the hospital. By the time they arrived at the hospital, the tightness had ceased. One patient stuck around at the emergency room for a full heart work up, to reassure himself that nothing untoward had occurred. The next evening when it happened again while he was watching TV, he stayed home.

An aside: I always tell patients to see a doctor immediately if they think they might be having a heart attack. Do not ignore symptoms that give cause for concern. If it turns out that the chest spasm was only recovery dyskinesia and not a heart attack, no harm will have been done.

None of my unmedicated patients had heart attacks during their recovery from Parkinson's disease. Many did have chest muscle dyskinesia. My own occurred while I was enjoying my morning shower, for several days in a row.

During the *relaxation* phase of chest-muscle recovery dyskinesia, the opposite occurs. Patients who experience this feel as if the chest is so wide open that there is no need to inhale. In my case, I was in the shower when I suddenly realized that I hadn't inhaled in a *really* long time. I was a little concerned, but I just didn't feel any need to inhale. My chest felt very wide open and relaxed. Finally, I did inhale and exhale, and *again*, a long time passed before I felt the need to take another breath. This glorious sensation of chest hyper-*expansion* started several days after I'd had the chest *tension* episodes.

Recovery dyskinesia in the tongue

Many patients experience a bout of clumsy speech: the tongue feels as if it is moving on its own or not moving the way it used to. It may seem, for a short while, as if one needs to relearn how to use the tongue. However, the speaking skills usually come back *very* quickly. In some cases, after recovery, the tongue seems to be positioned differently. This may be caused by a change in sensory awareness of the tongue or a change in the position of the palate. In my case, it seemed to be some of both.

Many people bite their tongues and/or the inside of their cheeks during this phase.

I personally had a curious tongue situation develop during recovery: when concentrating deeply on anything, I would stick my tongue out on the right side of my mouth, ever so slightly. Just the tip of the tongue was visible. I had been doing this for several weeks when I remembered an old photograph of myself playing the violin when I was age twenty. In that photo, my eyes were closed and I wore a look of deep concentration – and the tip of my tongue was sticking out the right side of my mouth. I knew that I had not put my tongue out to the side for *decades* but evidently I was now reverting back to a specific time in my youth.

After a few months, after my palate lifted and my teeth spread apart, I no longer stuck my tongue out to the side. I was certain that my age twenty tongue-to-the-side had not occurred when I was healthy, and only begin after initiating self-induced pause at age seventeen. I suspect that I started doing it shortly after my weird brain spin event that occurred shortly after inducing pause mode.

In other words, the age twenty tongue asymmetry and protrusion had been a very early symptom of left-right imbalance and internal tension – a very early symptom of pre-Parkinson's disease – and not a healthy idiosyncrasy. Since fully recovering, my tongue now stays centered in my mouth even when I'm concentrating.

Recovery dyskinesia in the palate

A person's upper palate (top of the mouth) is held in position by muscles. These muscles sometimes change their degree of tension during recovery. If the muscles above the upper palate gently tighten, lifting the lateral (outer) sides of the upper palate, a gap may appear between the two front teeth, as if the teeth have suddenly moved apart. This sudden, very visible movement of the teeth is painless. The teeth have not actually moved in their sockets: the two sides of the upper palate have lifted up, and the teeth came along for the ride.

While recovering, the roof of the mouth sometimes feels as if it has assumed a new position. Again, this movement in the upper mouth is not painful. Just the opposite: it feels pleasant, if it feels like anything at all. It seems to be caused by a return of vigor in previously weak palate-support muscles. Sometimes, the lift in upper palate position can bring about a welcome reduction in snoring or sleep apnea.

Many patients, including me, *prior* to recovering, experienced an increasingly frequent sensation as if the upper palate was falling down into the mouth now and then, partially blocking the airways and the sinuses. The resumption of healthy muscle tone in the muscles of the upper palate cure or greatly improve this problem.

Recovery dyskinesia in the eyes

During recovery, changes sometimes occur in visual acuity. Many patients noticed a sudden, extreme improvement in vision that lasted for a few minutes or a few days, which was followed by a return to normal vision or a temporary worsening of vision.

For example, one patient said, "I swear, yesterday, I could see a bird sitting in a tree a quarter mile away!" A few days later, the same person was hardly able to focus her eyes. Over a period of a month, this occurred several times. After that, her vision settled back down to exactly what it had been.

Based on patients' reports, I hypothesize that patients' eye focusing muscles can go through tightening and relaxing exercises. The muscle tensions and relaxings cause the temporary changes in vision.

After this occurred several times in several recovering patients, I told patients not to rush off to the optometrist for an eye exam or a new pair of glasses if the vision suddenly alters. In my limited experience, once the recovery dyskinesia in the eye-focusing muscles was over, the vision always settled back down to something very close to what it had been prior to recovery.

Speeding up

A few patients had the strange experience of the body briefly moving faster than they could control. While doing an ordinary, mundane and repetitive chore, such as chopping vegetables, it felt as if the *correct* arm muscles for the chore suddenly kicked in. The muscles then moved very quickly, effortlessly, in an exaggeratedly rapid manner. The *effect* is that the knife seems to be suddenly chopping the vegetables *much* faster than before: hyper-fast. The *feeling* is effortless, as if the arm is "moving by itself."

This "speeded up" movement might happen during all sorts of activities, ranging from practicing piano scales to chopping celery. The commonality is that it only happens while a person is relaxed or enjoying himself. This was a fairly unusual recovery symptom.

Not uncontrollable

Patients nearly always wanted to explain to me that they probably *could* have stopped the dyskinetic movements in the arms or legs or hands if they'd wanted to, but they didn't *want* to. It's as if some muscle wanted to work out or stay in a new position for a while, and it felt good when allowed to do so. The patient *enjoyed* feeling the sensation of the moving limb or vigorous muscle contraction *and* enjoyed the general good feeling of expansion in the chest (heart feeling) that came from *paying attention* to how the sensation *felt*.

These repetitive types of recovery dyskinesia usually last somewhere between a few moments and twenty minutes. Even the most relentless recovery dyskinesia usually peters out after about twenty minutes.

In most cases, recovery dyskinesia is amusing. If it ceases to be pleasant or amusing, it might soon stop. If a person stops being relaxed or becomes stressed during an episode of recovery dyskinesia, the movements soon cease.

Enjoying the body

Recovery dyskinesia is wonderful. Several patients have said that they felt as if they were coming back to life when the body starting relearning, on its own initiative, how to feel and use muscles that had been rigid and somewhat numb. The feeling that one is starting afresh, growing a whole new body, is so very delightful that a few people have even said that they feel as if they have lived two lives in one lifetime: they had their first life, and they were dying from it; then they were given a second chance and they got to start again from the beginning – learning what it's like to *enjoy* having a body, and learning how to *enjoy* using it.

Using a body versus enjoying a body

Some patients have protested my phrase "learn to enjoy having a body." They declared that they *do* enjoy having a body, or always *used* to before they had Parkinson's. Now they just want to get their old bodies back.

I recall one patient who was adamant that he loved his body. After we'd been working together for several months, he finally healed from his foot injury. He had *not* yet turned off his self-induced pause. He was in partial recovery. He related the following experience.

The previous weekend, he'd spent an hour floating in his daughter's swimming pool, lying on one of those floating rafts with arm rests and a holder for a beverage. His mind was blank and the sun was shining down. He felt a wave of peace flood over him, and he realized that he was *feeling good.* He realized that he could feel the sensation of the sun on his skin, and the sensation of floating. It was a rare moment. He marveled at the sensations that he was experiencing.

Then, his wary, partial-recovery mind kicked in. He immediately wondered to himself if this was the type of "enjoyment from the sensations of the body" that I was always "badgering" him about. His next thought was, "Heck, I can't be expected to *feel* this much *all* the time. That's ridiculous." As soon as he thought this, he realized that he could no longer perceive the *somatic* sensations of being in his body, enjoying the sun and the floating somatically rather than intellectually. Instead, his self-awareness was back in his word-based, racing mind.

The moment of pleasure from body awareness had snuck into his consciousness when he'd somatically felt his body, but he'd quickly brushed it away with his negative thoughts. As soon as he thought to himself, "Heck, I can't do this…," and re-immersed in negative thinking, he realized that he was unable to feel his body in the same way. He was unable to recapture the sensation of sun, the feeling of floating, and the good feeling inside his own body. He certainly was no longer *enjoying* it in the manner that he'd done a few moments earlier.

As noted earlier, he was in partial recovery. He did *not* fully recover. His fleeting experience in the sun, instead of being encouraging, awoke a powerful Blocker. His experience in the pool served to convince him that he would never be able to recover. So he stopped working on turning off pause.

I have had *many* patients who have insisted that they always enjoyed their body, who realized, during recovery, that they actually hadn't. They may have enjoyed *using* the body like a tool, they may have enjoyed having the body obey their instructions when they worked it hard during sports, but they hadn't actually noticed or enjoyed the *somatic* and sensory experiences produced by the body, or hadn't in a long time.

For some patients, the heart-felt relaxation that occurred when pause turned off and the spontaneous, gentle movements of recovery dyskinesia began were like beginner's lessons in how to *feel* being in a body and *enjoy* having a body.

The spiritual question

More than a few patients, prior to recovering, have been certain that sensory awareness of the body and/or enjoyment of the body was self-indulgent, or even "not spiritual." They disagreed with my suggestions that the sensations generated with a healthy body are, like flowers and beautiful music, something that can and should be enjoyed. Spiritual injunctions in *many* faiths warn against excessive body attachments. The concern is the problems that arise from wrong identification: when a person imagines himself to *be* the body instead of being the soul. Also, *excessive* fascination with the inherently restless body, which occurs when the mind is undisciplined, can be a distraction when trying to stay focused on uplifting activities or on the inner stillness that can occur during communion with one's soul or with the Divine.

However, the sensations that arise from having a body, which include vision, hearing, taste, smell, feeling, and movement are *not* inherently bad. If you have spiritual inclinations, you might want to consider that these sensations can be enjoyed as perceptions of the Divine, of God's vibratory energy that that underlies and permeates the universe and all objects, even bodies. So long as a person does not *identify* himself as his ever-changing body or become overly attached to it, he risks no "sin" in enjoying the sensory experience of being able to proprioceptively feel the energy inside his own arms and legs, torso and head. Then again, many people with Parkinson's cannot even fathom what is meant by the phrase, "Feel the energy *inside* your own arms and legs" until after they recover.

An infantile demonstration of repetitive, dyskinetic movement

Once, in the early days of this project, I was on the road, breakfasting in a diner. I was musing about the unexpected bouts of recovery dyskinesia that had recently occurred in a few of my pioneer patients. At the table next to me, a baby was sitting in a high chair. I watched as he was handed a spoon. He had little control over his movements. As he focused on keeping the haft of the spoon clutched in his fist, his bicep began to contract and relax.

The result was that his arm, and the spoon, started moving up and down, up and down. The rhythmic movement continued for several minutes. The proud parents said that he was banging the spoon on the tray. But I could see that he was *not* banging the spoon intentionally: he clearly did not have the coordination necessary to bang the spoon so rhythmically on his tray. His non-controlled muscles were firing off on their own. His biceps were flexing and extending, flexing and extending. The infant was not doing it consciously. He looked happy and surprised at the movements occurring in his arm.

As he continued helplessly banging the spoon on the tray, the proud parents beamed as his movements became more vigorous. His other arm started moving up and down in time with the first. He was obviously enjoying himself. Within moments, his legs started moving in time with his arms. His Stomach channel muscles along the torso started tightening and relaxing. Soon, all the muscles along the baby's Stomach channel and Large Intestine channel were tightening and relaxing, tightening and relaxing. After several minutes, he stopped moving. His parents kissed him and fussed over him.

He had not been making these moves consciously. His brain was just starting to form awareness of motor imagery. The muscles were starting to learn how to integrate with signals from the brain. It would be many years before the child would be able to exhibit supremely elegant motor control over his fingers and arm muscles. But the process had to start somewhere.

His spontaneous, repetitive movements, set in motion, perhaps, by the curious sensation of the spoon in his hand or maybe by his desire to imitate the hand-to-mouth movements he had seen performed by his parents, looked exactly like the several instances of arm or leg recovery dyskinesia that I had witnessed.

This vignette makes two points: the repetitive, spontaneous movements that occur in specific muscle groups during recovery from Parkinson's are not pathological: they are perfectly natural; they occur as the brain is becoming re-familiarized with imagining specific motor functions. Second, with the right attitude, this re-learning can be fun.

Infant dyskinesia occurs on the Stomach and Large Intestine channels

The infant described in the above section was learning to control the muscles that underlie the Stomach and Large Intestine channel: the two channels that are not functional until the moment of birth. The muscles regulated by these channels are the last muscles to become active in a developing child. These channels do not even *start* to be activated until birth, when the baby takes his first breath.

These two channels drive the peristalsis of the gut. An infant in utero should have no gut movement whatsoever: any activity in the large intestine might eject sticky meconium (fetal fecal matter) into the amniotic fluid. If meconium gets into the fluid, and thence into the lungs of the unborn baby, it can be fatal. The baby has no need for activity in the gut: all his nutrition comes in through the umbilical cord and goes directly into his bloodstream.

All the other channels, the other ten primary channels and the eight extra channels, are functional in utero. Only the Stomach and Large Intestine channels are dormant until the first breath. All of the functions that are nearly impossible for an newborn (control of thumb and index fingers, facial muscles, neck muscles, arm bending, standing, walking, holding the head up, bowel control, and so on, are regulated by these two channels. In contrast, the muscles that move the diaphragm, heart, bladder sphincter, that arch the back, and even the muscles under the skin that regulate the pores, are all smoothly operational at birth. These muscles are active no matter which neurological mode we are in and are driven by brain systems that are *not* consciousness- or breathing-related.

It was no coincidence that recovering patients with long-dormant Stomach and Large Intestine channels found themselves performing movements that brought to mind the spontaneous muscle activities of infancy. Even after being born, these two channels are only supposed to be *fully* activated when a person is awake and healthy. It is also no coincidence that a severe trauma can trigger a chain of electrical events that cause these two channels to shut down until such time as it is safe to heal and safe to come fully "back to life." While on the verge of imminent death, a person does *not* want to squander energy on the smaller details of healing, nor does he want to be distracted by non-essentials such as eating and digestion: activities supported primarily by the Stomach and Large Intestine channels.

Fear of recovery dyskinesia

Although I always make the point that recovery dyskinesia feels good, many potential patients are afraid of it. Some potential patients have been far more worried about momentarily "looking like a fool" than they have been about having Parkinson's disease. Some potential patients, having read through the earlier editions of "Recovery Symptoms" concluded that they didn't want to risk experiencing a recovery symptom while out in public. They told me, in all seriousness, that they were afraid that, in a moment of weakness, recovery symptoms might occur that would make them look "stupid," "wrong," or "sick." Several people have admitted that they would rather believe that Parkinson's *is* incurable than risk recovery incidents in which they might lose face. After all, Parkinson's is a respectable illness.

The reader who does not have PD might think that I am joking. Surely, no intelligent adult would rather be rigid and shaking for the rest of his life than possibly have a few moments of perfectly understandable loss of motor control. But be assured, reader, that many people with Parkinson's are reading these same words and thinking, "Yeah. I'd hate to lose facial control or have my arms jerk around while someone was watching. I'm not sure this program is for me." Being on pause can make a person wary of changes and extremely, even illogically, fearful of being judged.

A wild, but gentle and even amusing ride

Recovery symptoms such as dyskinetic movements might happen at the same time as other recovery symptoms, and in the same body part. A person might be feeling pins and needles in his face, be suddenly aware of how horribly numb his face has been, and be having powerful spasms or gentle rhythmic dyskinetic movements in his face muscles, all at the same time.

Do not hope for any sort of linearity or regularity. The body wants to heal as quickly as possible, and all sorts of recovery symptoms might overlap in the race back to health. Or recovery symptoms might ease off for a month or longer and then start back up. Please don't worry.

Some patients have thought they noticed a pattern of more or fewer recovery symptoms in sync with the full moon, the days of the week, or whether or not they ate noodles for breakfast. So many patients were looking for a system against which they could measure and anticipate their recovery, but every person's recovery was unique.

Summary

Recovery dyskinesia events occur over a relatively short time: weeks, not years. The rewards are thrilling and sweet. The recovery dyskinesia period was usually one of the more glorious phases of recovery from Parkinson's. People could somatically *feel* themselves. Their own brains were exploring and *imagining* new connections with the body. It was usually a delightful time.

I recall, at the same time I was going through various types of recovery dyskinesia, I was clipping my fingernails one day and suddenly experienced a wildly new sensation: my fingers were each feeling the mutual presence of my other fingers as they touched each other. I had never lost the ability to mechanically use my fingers and I still had awareness of superficial, skin-deep sensitivity. But suddenly, for the first time, it felt as if my awareness in each finger, in the *depths* of the finger, was checking in with each other, "saying hello" to each other. At first, I was amazed that such a high degree of proprioceptivity and awareness could even exist. Next, I was giddy with gratitude that I was discovering it.

The gratitude felt as sweet as the new awareness of mutual finger communication.

Chapter Twenty-eight

Recovery Symptoms: Muscle Soreness

Arm swing: bicep soreness

Prior to recovering, many patients with arm-swing inhibition can generate a short-term, mentally forced arm swing, a swing that *doesn't* use the biceps, but uses the muscles on either side of the biceps. After resumption of normal channel qi flow through the arms, the biceps start to function after what may have been decades of dormancy and, in most cases, atrophy. When, during recovery, a patient's arms resume true, automatic, bicep-based arm swing, the biceps may become very achy and sore, at first.

This arm swing pain is *not* recovery dyskinesia. Dyskinesia means "abnormal movement." Recovery dyskinesia occurs when a muscle resumes connectivity in the dormant brain pathways that allow for automatic movement motor. When dusting off these dormant pathways, the body *clumsily* starts relearning how to integrate the brain instructions and the associated motor behaviors.

Achiness, tenderness, or soreness occurs in the biceps after they become *correctly* operational. The biceps, after not having been used in years, begin to tighten and relax automatically a few *thousand* times a day without your even thinking about it.

Prior to recovery, most of my PD patients no longer had the synchronized electrical pattern that automatically swings the arms – using the correct muscles. During recovery, the biceps, muscles that contribute to a *correctly* performed arm swing, may start to automatically contract in synchrony with the opposite-side leg stride. Once the arm-leg connection is working correctly, biceps muscle contraction automatically occurs with *every single step*. After walking more than a dozen steps, the arm muscles may soon feel a bit sore, even a bit painful.

In the beginning, even if the new *automatic* arm swing is very tiny, almost invisible, that tiny movement is the result of contraction in the feeble biceps. Again, this muscle might not have been used for years. During recovery, the biceps automatically make a healthy contraction followed by relaxation a split second prior to *every* opposite-side footfall.

If a recovering patient walks fifty steps, the convalescing biceps contract and relax fifty times. If he walks at a good clip for half an hour or so, the biceps might contract and relax more than a thousand times.

When the biceps begin to work, their usage rate might be going from zero contractions per day to many thousands. Over the next few weeks, walking often becomes difficult because of the accompanying arm soreness. Even if a recovering patient *tries* to inhibit the arm swing while walking, the reconnected biceps will do their healthy contraction in sync with the footfalls.

Many recovering patients who previously mourned the loss of arm swing noted the irony of trying to *prevent* their arms from swinging. "My arms are *so* sore. When I go for my morning walk, I cross my arms over my chest and try to press my upper arms to my chest so they can't move. Sometimes that helps, a little. But it's getting so that the arm soreness is limiting the distance that I can walk. I used to go three miles a day. I've cut back to half a mile a day because of how sore my arms get. It's a good pain. It's like the soreness I used to get when I was in high school sports, after doing those conditioning exercises. And my arms *are* getting a lot stronger. But this last week, after just half an hour of steady walking, I was so sore in the arms that I just wanted to go home and lie down the rest of the day so that my arms wouldn't swing."

This soreness and pain eases up as soon as the muscles in the arm become accustomed to the thousands of daily repetitions that a healthy person automatically makes while walking. But for a short period, maybe a few weeks or a month, the new arm swing and the resultant workout for the budding biceps can be a bit painful.

Prior to recovery, many patients assured us that they were still swinging their arms, or *could* if they thought about it. They were surprised when the arm soreness began. Truth was, even if they'd been swinging their arms or doing biceps building reps at the gym, they had *not* been using their biceps.

When other muscles take over the job of an injured muscle or help stabilize an injured area, it is referred to as muscle splinting. Muscle splinting is a common, normal occurrence following an injury or loss of some muscle function.

For example, some patients had generated an arm swing by *throwing* the arms forward using other, nearby muscles. Others had an arm "swing" in which the hands and forearms stayed in front of the torso, elbows out to the sides, sashaying widely from left to right instead of front to back, in time with the footfall.

Although I wrote in a previous chapter that previously rigid muscles were not atrophied, the biceps *was* atrophied: an exception to the rule. The chronic tension in the upper arms that causes the arms to stay bent at the elbow and the accompanying mental disconnect to the biceps did lead, over the years, to some amount of atrophy.

Prior to recovery, no amount of gym work on the part of patients ever helped the biceps get strong. If a patient worked out in the gym, doing exercises that are *supposed* to develop the biceps, the only muscles that got stronger were the ones that splinted for the biceps. As long as the biceps remained out of reach of the mind's movement imagining area, no number of weight lifts did anything for them. The biceps do *not* work if the Large Intestine channel qi is flowing backwards over them.

Ever since I was about twenty-five, I had not worn a sleeveless shirt. My arms didn't look right. I was very fit (or so I thought), and my arms were *very* strong: I'd competed in rowing in my high school years. I hadn't been able to explain exactly what was wrong with the look of my arms. After I recovered and my biceps returned, I suddenly realized what had been wrong with my arms all those years: they'd been missing the bulge of the biceps. My biceps returned after I recovered. I started wearing sleeveless shirts again – *not* because my arms finally looked normal, but because I no longer *cared* whether or not they looked "right."

But the main point of this section is this: the biceps hurt when a patient starts automatically using them again. The pain eventually eases up as the biceps build up.

Back soreness: universal symptom of recovery

Up until now I have frequently stated that any given recovery symptom might or *might not* occur in any given patient. My constant cry has been: "Each person's recovery is as unique as his symptoms!"

However, when it comes to *back* soreness, this recovery symptom is almost universal. In my limited experience, all but two recovering patients had back soreness.

The small-of-the-back soreness was usually referred to as back "pain," but it was not back pain in the classic sense. It was soreness, like a gentle ache or pulling in the small of the back. The instant cure for turning off this particular pain was simple: stand up straight.

The back soreness occurs when the muscles in the small of the back, the lumbar quadratic muscles, begin to resume strength. During Parkinson's, these muscles are over-relaxed, overly loose. The lumbar quads, when contracted, serve to straighten the low back for when you are standing or sitting up straight. If they are *highly* contracted, they allow a person to perform a gymnastics move called a "backbend" in which the lower back is curved anteriorly: towards the front of the body.

For a good visual of the lumbar quads at work, look at any video of the gymnast Simone Biles doing a full floor routine and see how tightly arched is the small of her back. This tightness is *very* healthy, and is the opposite of the limp lumbar quad muscles in people with Parkinson's.

The psoas muscles are the paired, oppositional muscles for the lumbar quads. They work to pull the chest forward and bring the front of the thighs towards the abdomen, making the front of the torso into a concave curve while the low back spine is pushed posteriorly: towards the back of the body. The psoas muscles go all the way from the mid-thoracic spine down to the tops of the upper leg bones and pull the knees closer together as well as bringing the front of the thighs closer to the abdomen. Again the lumbar quads and the psoas work as a team: a pair of opposites.

During pause, the psoas muscles are highly tensed and rigid. This means that the strength of the lumbar quads is correspondingly reduced. The torso and legs are constantly being pulled towards a fetalesque position. The lumbar quad muscles, the small of the back muscles so beautifully demonstrated by gymnasts, are turned *off*.

During recovery, when the rigid psoas muscles along the front of the torso begin to loosen up and *relax*, the back-straightening lumbar quads in the small of the back are once again able to tighten up and *contract*. These small-of-the-back muscles might not have functioned correctly for years. When they begin to contract, the lower back will feel sore.

Sometimes these back muscles tighten up only briefly, then relax, then tighten again and relax again: the back "pain" comes and goes as the muscles play at finding their correct tension level. The soreness is felt when the muscles are trying to tighten – *if* the patient happens to be standing in his habitual, forward-leaning posture. When the lumbar quads tighten up *while the body is bending forward* at the waist, in the habitual PD posture, they feel sore. Only one maneuver will stop the mild soreness in the low back: standing up straight.

This soreness is *not* true back pain. Back pain that is due to injury, nerve damage, or pathological spasm usually causes a person to stand crooked, in such a way as to "favor" the pain or minimize the pain. The small-of-the-back muscle tightness that occurs during recovery from Parkinson's disease does *not* feel better if the patient stands crookedly to favor the pain.

Chiropractic treatment, hot or cold packs, and other back treatments do nothing to reduce the new health and vigor in the lumbar quad muscles that are causing the soreness.

The only thing that makes these healthy back muscles feel good is standing up straight, allowing the tightening back muscles to assume their correct positioning relative to the spinal bones.

This back soreness might last for weeks or even months. During this time, leaning forward aggravates the sore feeling in the back. By leaning forward, I mean the type of gentle leaning forward that occurs while washing the dishes or reaching across the bed to straighten the covers. These gentle, forward-leaning movements may cause a mildly unpleasant pulling sensation in the newly functional muscles. However, this problem is not severe, and can be easily remedied at any time by throwing the shoulders back and standing up as straight and tall as possible.

I ask concerned patients to keep in mind that this is not a physical problem: this is your body teaching you to stand up straight once again after having been increasingly hunched forward for years. This is a *recovery* symptom. It's a good thing.

Cases of no back soreness

As mentioned in an earlier chapter, two patients did not experience the back muscles pulling tight. Healthy tension in the back failed to automatically kick in. These recovering patients found themselves bent far forward, with their faces nearly touching their knees.

In these two cases, I did try many acupuncture and moxa (locally applied heat) techniques to strengthen the low back. These techniques did not work, even temporarily. Both of these cases occurred in the early days of my research, prior to my discovery of the UB channel qi's tendency to stop flowing past UB-11, on the neck, when a person is on pause. I now suspect that fixing the UB channel at this point would have allowed the back muscles to resume function.

Frequent urination: oversensitivity of the bladder nerves

At about the same time that a recovering patient experiences small-of-the-back soreness, he may feel drastic changes in his sensitivity to bladder signals.

In his youth, the pre-Parkinson's patient may have had powerful bladder control. He may have been able to go *all day* without feeling a need to urinate. This was not because he had a "strong" bladder. In these patients, this lack of "need" to urinate occurred because the bladder nerves were somewhat numb. Only the very strongest signals from a *very* overstretched bladder could generate a strong enough signal to get through the relatively numb area in the low-ish back, near where the bladder nerves enter the spine. The feeble bit of signal that got through to the spine and then traveled to the brain was all the person might have gotten, even if the bladder was actually saying "I'm really overstretched down here."

Oppositely, some people, in the decades prior to manifesting Parkinson's, have extremely "weak" bladders: they must urinate every hour or so. The problem is one and the same: the signals to and from the bladder – signals that travel through the area of the low back, and which should be regulated by the parasympathetic and sympathetic nervous systems – are not running at full capacity.

When an animal is highly dissociated or on pause from a high degree of trauma, when he is behaving as if dead, the animal might not register signals from the bladder. He might find himself *unable* to *hold* his urine or, oppositely, he may find that most of a day goes by before he *feels* the need to urinate.

One elderly patient told me how, during World War II, his buddies highly resented his ability to stay in a trench all day. He never *felt* any urgency to urinate more than twice a day. The other soldiers had to leave the safety of the trenches every few hours in order to use the latrine trenches, thus exposing themselves to risk.

I heard many fascinating bladder stories, and other health stories, that all helped me put together a very full and three-dimensional picture of Parkinson's disease. Our modern system of medicine, in which a neurologist sees a patient for a quick fifteen minutes, twice a year, almost guarantees that doctors will not be able to make the connections between seemingly unrelated symptoms: connections that, in my research, led to a much deeper understanding of the physiological changes that can accompany Parkinson's disease.

The combination of pause and/or the lack of flow in UB channel qi in the small of the back may have been the cause or at least contributed to the somewhat common, liftime bladder irregularities of people with Parkinson's disease.

As the spinal nerves of the low back begin to be invigorated, at about the same time that the back soreness begins, the adjacent nerves from the bladder also begin to resume healthy sensitivity.

During the decades that the Parkinson's was silently worsening, the patient's brain had, in many cases, become accustomed to a *very* low signal from the bladder nerves. Because the "fullness" nerves from the bladder (the stretch receptor nerves) had barely gotten any signal through to the brain, the brain had slowly trained itself to respond to the least little signal, if any, from the bladder. The brain learned that even the smallest signal from these nerves indicated a very full bladder.

Some patients, prior to recovery, got few or no bladder signals during the day, until the bladder was horribly full. The only time they felt genuine bladder fullness might be at the first urination of the morning. A few had trained themselves to urinate at regular intervals – every three or four hours – regardless of whether or not they *felt* any urgency. But even so, sometimes, they got home from work at the end of a long day and, as they noticed how much urine was passing, said to themselves, "Huh. Looks like I forgot to use the toilet when I was at work today. Again."

In my research, I only thought to ask my PD patients about this because "forgetting to urinate" was one of the symptoms on my personal long list of "things that are unique about me." Turns out, I wasn't so unique.

In recovering patients, as the bladder-signal nerves begin to revive from their partial dormancy, they began sending healthier, more vigorous signals. The brain, accustomed to a *tiny* nerve signal, misinterprets these healthy, larger signals: it assumes that *extreme* bladder stretching must be occurring. When the recovering patient's brain starts receiving what seems like massive, steady surges of bladder information, the brain's response is to assume that the bladder is constantly, *painfully* full.

There is actually no fullness pain in the *bladder*. The sensation of bladder fullness is a purely mental response. It occurs in the brain. During recovery, the feeling of urgency is a brain response to the new, healthy intensity of the bladder's stretch receptor nerves. They send a *mild*, healthy, normal, signal up to the brain when the bladder is *empty*, as they should. They send a *really* strong, vigorous signal when the bladder is full.

Eventually, recovering patients' brains recalibrate their responses to the healthy bladder signals. But until then, while the brain is still overwhelmed by the new, mild, healthy nerve signals from the bladder, some recovering patients felt the "urgency to urinate" signal getting triggered every few *minutes*. This was very frustrating, because the amount of urine passed each time in response to the panic call could be measured in teaspoons, or even droplets. Nevertheless, the brain signals were adamant.

The recalibration of the bladder-urgency signals occurs over a few days, a few weeks, or a few months. Just as the increased sensitivity and awareness of a previously numb foot tapers off when the brain accommodates to it, the increased sensitivity to the bladder signals tapers off over time.

Going through hell

If the bladder urgency phase occurs at the same time as the extreme limpness in the legs phase, the recovering patient might find himself in a difficult situation. Some patients have been so unresponsive and limp in the thigh muscles that they've needed help to stand up and get to the toilet *plus* help to get up off the toilet. During the night, they have quickly exhausted their spouses with their need to use the toilet every half hour or more. Some patients – and their spouses – have referred to this phase of recovery as "hell stage."

Some patients merely went through a *mildly* annoying period of increased bladder sensitivity. Others found the frequent bladder urgency/ limp legs combo to be the most soul testing, hellish part of the recovery process.

If the bladder urgency was severe and preventing the person from getting sleep, I suggested wearing adult diapers at nighttime, or even in the daytime, for as long as is needed.

Bladder infection

I warn patients that a bladder infection can often cause symptoms of bladder urgency. It is reasonable to ask the doctor for a urine test (urinalysis) if one develops symptoms of bladder urgency. Many people develop bladder infections during times of stress. Recovery from Parkinson's can be stressful, especially during the limp muscles and frequent urination stages.

Bladder infections are a serious illness, and must be treated. Bladder infections in younger people are usually associated with frequent urination, burning pain when urinating, darker urine and sometimes fever.

However, in older people a bladder infection may be nearly symptom-free, in terms of bladder-specific problems. In older people a bladder infection can be present with no fever, no pain, or not even noticeably frequent urination, though the urine might be "cloudy" instead of clear. But even if no fever is present, a bladder infection is still a serious health problem. In older people, a bladder infection can cause extreme weakness and mental instability, even if there are no obvious bladder symptoms whatsoever. If there is any possibility that a recovering patient might have a bladder infection, he should seek diagnosis and treatment.

Please know, many people with Parkinson's, after having read about recovery symptoms, have wondered whether or not they should risk entering into a program that offers such opportunities for humiliation and inconvenience. Is recovery from Parkinson's disease worth it? Everyone who has fully recovered has felt so grateful for the return of a healthy body that the short-term recovery symptoms, in retrospect, were nothing to complain of.

"You look terrible!"

Very often, patients look haggard during the phase of frequent urination and its corollary of poor sleep.

This might be due to the fatigue, but in some cases, the haggard look was due, in part, to the greatly increased expressiveness of the face. If, prior to recovery, the person had a fairly inexpressive face, and his face was now projecting "I feel exhausted and discouraged, I can't get up out of chairs, I pee all the time, my feet hurt and I'm crying a lot," his best friends may tell him how bad he is looking.

This new development – frank concern from friends – can be a completely new experience for some previously stoic people with Parkinson's.

When such comments arise, recovering patients might feel deeply concerned. They are going through so many changes and they can't be certain these changes are for the better. When someone says, "You look terrible," the patient usually understands this to mean, "Your symptoms of Parkinson's are getting worse." Very often, this *is* exactly what the well-meaning friend *does* mean.

Also, some people with PD do not have the intuitive social skills to know how much information should be shared with concerned friends; in many cases, people with Parkinson's are not accustomed to being on the receiving end of sympathy.

Prior to recovery, most of the patients I've worked with didn't mind *giving* sympathy – but they didn't like to receive it. They didn't like appearing vulnerable. The instinct of an animal that is on pause or is dissociated from an injury is to lie low and be invisible – the opposite of crying out and saying, "Comfort me! Care for me!"

I also have to wonder if one reason for the outpouring of compassion from friends and co-workers is that the patient had finally ceased projecting supreme competence. Many people with Parkinson's from self-induced pause project an air of inapproachability, especially with regard to personal matters. Spouses of several patients have assured me that the patient had, for decades, projected the signal "I don't need your help."

Prior to recovery, the patient's facial immobility might have conveyed internal strength and/or lack of compassion. After recovering tone in the facial muscles, that immobility is gone. The person no longer has a poker face or an "intentional" smile. As the face becomes more expressive, emotions such as sadness, fatigue, boredom or resentment became apparent.

During recovery, as the face becomes expressive and protective walls crumble, the patient may start to come across as a person who *could* conceivably be comforted. His wounded body and fatigue send signals to his family and friends: "I'm tired and I'm sick and I need help." Any sensitive human can pick up on these electrical, chemical, and body language signals. But many recovering PD patients have little or no experience at being on the receiving end of compassion.

Some family members have been grateful that the loved one was becoming more "humanized." Oppositely, sometimes, when a patient starts coming across as more vulnerable, family and friends are horrified by the patient's changes. The patient, in many cases, is "The Rock" or "The Capable One" of the family or social group. When he or she becomes less heroic, less stoic, and more "human," maybe even more emotionally needy, family members sometimes resent the changes in family dynamic and their new need to step up to the plate.

Children of people with Parkinson's disease

I've had some long heart-to-heart talks with adult children of people with Parkinson's. Very often, the adult child has long harbored mixed feelings towards the parent who didn't go in for hugs and/or easy, self-deprecating laughter. Not knowing why the parent was so darned stoic, the child often assumed that he, the child, was unloved. The parent might have been deeply attached, loving, responsible, hard-working, and logical to the point of exasperation, but the child was often hoping for something different: playful love, cuddling, even silliness and joy.

As mentioned earlier, it can be physically painful to be in proximity with a person whose electrical systems are running differently from one's own, let alone cuddling or hugging with that person. As for providing unconditional love, a person on the verge of imminent death might not be very good about paying attention to the "childish" needs of the youngster.

I mention it here because this might come up when the adult child is asked to provide physical and emotional support to an aging parent who is working on recovering from Parkinson's. Very possibly, in the child's eyes, the parent never came across as very physically and/or emotionally supportive to others. Just a head's up. [1]

The change in facial expression

There may be some *very* temporary, very mild soreness in the muscles of the face as strength returns to the cheeks. This brings up a completely different subject: the change in expressiveness.

Many a person with Parkinson's who assumed that his friendship was shown through his actions, who imagined that he was projecting sincerity and friendliness, and who prided himself on his never-changing look of stern intelligence, was stunned when a "friend" or co-worker told him, during recovery, "I always assumed you didn't really like me because you always frowned at me" or "...because you never smiled at me."

One relatively young patient, after fully recovering, was told by senior management, "We're impressed at how much you've matured in your social skills in the last few months." His supervisors never knew he'd had Parkinson's disease, and they suspected nothing while he was going through recovery. But after his full recovery, they noticed with pleasure that he'd somehow changed: "matured." He confided in me that "all" he was doing differently was smiling more, joking more easily, being more genuinely empathetic and not over-thinking everything.

Some patients were outraged over these types of remarks. Others loved them.

I suggest to patients that they should celebrate if family and friends start to express concern that the patient looks exhausted, worried, or suddenly "looks his age" (instead of looking sort of frozen).

---

[1] See: *The Distinguished Guest*; Sue Miller; Harper-Collins; 1995. This acclaimed work of fiction details the relationship between an aging, powerful personality with Parkinson's disease as she becomes physically dependent on her son.

Then again, many patients, even while recovering, have found themselves under attack by loved ones because the loved ones do not believe that a person can recover, they *wrongly* think that the medication will prevent or slow the progression of the illness or, for whatever reason, they want the person with Parkinson's to "just stop being an idiot and do what your doctor tells you (take drugs and be normal again)!"

One person was only able to turn off self-induced pause when he decided "To hell with my brothers!" and stopped listening to their well-intended insistence that he take medication, and lots of it.

Warning

This chapter is a good place to repeat that not everyone is a suitable candidate for turning off pause after using it for nearly a lifetime.

Very elderly people who are no longer mentally driven enough to practice imagining motor function and thus restore motor connections in the brain might never be able to fully recover their muscle function. A person who is no longer able to learn the new mental habits that can turn off pause might not be able to terminate pause, and might find the work to be an exercise in futility. Even if the person *is* able to turn off pause, he might still need to work for hours every day on imagining the motions of limp muscles – more brain retraining. While recovering, he might find himself recovering from Parkinson's but going through a hellish period of life with very weak muscles, extreme urinary frequency, and an inability to get up from a chair, roll over in bed, or stand up straight. In this case, his problems will be due to severe limpness, rather than the rigidity of Parkinson's disease. If he is living alone, this might be a trial the person would rather not undergo.

Even short term, the severe limpness can be a very debilitating condition, exhausting to both the patient and the caregiver. If it lingers for many months, the patient and his loved ones will have to wonder whether the person might not have been better off with Parkinson's, particularly if the symptoms were mild and the person was already quite elderly and/or losing mental acuity.

It is impossible for me to state "How old is too old." It is impossible for me to guess whether or not a given person is a good candidate for full recovery. Please do not ask me. In general, if a person is over eighty years old and only recently diagnosed, that suggests that his Parkinson's is developing very, very slowly. He may be uninterested in or incapable of making the mental changes required for recovery. He may be better off if he just continues with his gradually increasing symptoms. Maybe, when he's genuinely unable to move, he can use the medications at the lowest, safest doses, and live out his life slightly stoned from the drugs, but safe and somewhat independent.

Please do not contact me to ask if your loved one should try to recover. I often receive inquiries saying an elderly loved one has Parkinson's disease and is not capable of or interested in reading the material about Parkinson's, but the concerned writer wants my help in "fixing him."

A difficult message

I respond with something like:

"Your loved one might not be a good candidate for recovery. Recovery can require the conscious re-making of a personality. If your loved one is not keen to do this, or does not understand the need for this, it may be *impossible* for him to fully recover. He may be better off just waiting for as long as possible before starting the medication. They only work for a few years, regardless of the PD stage at which they are started. But if he keeps his doses as low as possible, just strong enough to make him stoned enough to override pause, but *not* strong enough to make him feel genuinely happy or giddy, he may be able to get acceptable results from the medication for many, many years.

"Please read *Medications of Parkinson's or Once Upon a Pill*, available for free download at www.pdrecovery org.

"Please do not ask for *my* help in making this decision. If your loved one has Type I PD and is no longer *capable* of reading and/or understanding this book about recovery from Parkinson's, or is not *interested* in reading it, that is a large tip-off that he is probably not a good candidate for recovery."

Chapter Twenty-nine

Recovery symptoms: Changes in Sleep Patterns

One of the more pleasant or, for a few people, more aggravating, symptoms of recovery is the change in sleep patterns. During recovery, even people who had been plagued by insomnia often find that they are suddenly sleeping very well.

"Too much" sleep

Many recovering patients find themselves wanting to go to bed early, wake up late, and take naps. They often worry that they are sleeping too much: "I'm sleeping my life away." A person recovering from a serious injury or ravaging illness needs to sleep a lot. A person who is growing new nerve cells, muscle cells, and brain cells needs sleep: lots of it. Some people accept this. Some are unable to accept it and feel chagrined, even ashamed, about how much sleep they now need.

Concerned about sleeping too much

Many people with Parkinson's, by the time they are diagnosed, are starting to have a hard time sleeping through the night. In the beginning of recovery, this new ability to sleep well and long seems like an answer to prayer. However, many people have to pit their glorious new ability to sleep against their lifetime conviction that people who sleep a lot are lazy and bad. While this may not seem like a big problem to the reader who does not have PD, the extra hours of deep sleep can be a true emotional challenge for many recovering patients. *Many* of my patients have trained themselves to be judgmental towards anyone, including themselves, who isn't accomplishing a lot.

Prior to their diagnosis with Parkinson's, many patients, unable to feel their own bodies and, in some cases, their own emotions, had valued themselves because they "get a lot done." During recovery, many of these same people avoided doing anything that wasn't a stark necessity. One patient reported, "I plan my days around being able to get as much sleep as possible. If an activity isn't absolutely necessary, I won't do it."

When the ability and *desire* to be a workaholic drops away, some patients feel ashamed and even depressed. Depression is a condition in which the release of movement neurotransmitters is minimized. Depression can put the brakes on recovery. If you start feeling depressed by the changes in your body and the seeming loss of qualities on which you used to pride yourself, please go through the steps in the book *Feeling Good*, by Dr. David Burns, MD, referenced in the footnote on p. 126.

A case study in "laziness"

One patient recovering from Type II PD had, like many people with Parkinson's, often worked three jobs at a time. She was a math professor by day, a software designer in the evening, and a regularly performing professional musician on weekends. During the "increased need for sleep" phase of recovery, she found herself turning down music jobs, unable to stay up at night to work on the software, and even parking as close as possible to her classroom to minimize her walking distance. She didn't *need* the extra money from her side jobs. She was a successful single woman with no dependants, so her "problem" with working less was purely a self-worth issue.

While she was in the thick of this phase, she came into my office and exploded into tears. When she was finally able to talk, she told me about the above changes in her lifestyle. I asked why this was a problem. She replied, "I'm turning into the people I hate! *But that's not the problem*. The problem is that I never knew I hated *anyone*!"

She was very loving, kind, and generous. She had always assumed that she loved everyone. But when she found herself minimizing her daily activities so that she could sleep more, her inner thoughts screamed at her, "You're turning into a lazy person, a *bad* person!" This realization, that she had been subconsciously judging – and finding lacking – those people who did *not* work three jobs and constantly exert themselves, made her deeply ashamed of herself.

The reader may think that patients like this are making a big deal out of nothing. But the increased need for sleep and the decrease in "getting things done," or "making things happen," was sometimes a devastating emotional experience for those people who had only valued themselves on the basis of what they were able to accomplish. Some also worried about becoming a burden or an increasing burden to their spouse or other family members.

How long did the need for extra sleep last?

The need for extra sleep is not a straight line. Some people have needed a few extra hours a day, or a nap on weekend afternoons. Sometimes, this increased need lasts for months. In some cases, it lasted for years. Very often, the "new" amount of sleep is actually a far healthier amount of sleep. Many of my PD patients have chronically shorted themselves on sleep. In some recovery cases, the patients never got back to their old patterns of getting by with less sleep than most people. As people recover, they no longer feel the pause-based internal agitation that might have forced them to sleep as little as possible. The new, "lazy person" sleep pattern is usually a *healthier* sleep pattern.

Some patients happily accept the new amount of sleep that their bodies need. Others slide into despair because they honestly feel that they are sleeping their lives away, with no end in sight.

In general, younger people needed much less "extra" sleep during recovery than older people. For example, one patient in her thirties, who started the recovery program immediately upon diagnosis, only needed several days of staying home and sleeping all day. A retired patient in his late sixties who had an advanced case of Parkinson's found that, during recovery, he slept long and hard at night and then needed two naps in the daytime. However, there are no hard and fast rules, and there are variations and exceptions. To say nothing of the fact that some people in their thirties have an advanced case at the time of diagnosis and some people in their eighties have a mild case at the time of diagnosis.

Shifting sleep patterns

Some people's sleep patterns go through *several* changes. A recovering patient might fall asleep at nine at night and awaken at seven in the morning – much more sleep than he used to get. And a few months later, he consistently might not be able to fall asleep until three in the morning and then would sleep until noon. And then, a few weeks or months later, the pattern might change again: going to bed at seven, waking at five.

Anyone who has raised a child will recall that children go through periods when they need an enormous amount of sleep, and other periods when they don't even need to nap. These periods of increased sleep and altered sleep patterns correspond to periods during which the child does an enormous amount of mental, emotional, and/or physical growth. In a person recovering from Parkinson's these periods of increased sleep very likely correspond to enormous amounts of healing *and* re-growth.

Two-hour intervals of deep stillness

A few recovering patients have noticed that, even if they didn't feel tired, their bodies fell into heavy, drugged-like physical immobility for about two hours a day. These two hours of stillness sometimes occurred at the same time every day, and went on for several days or even for months. This very weird type of sleep feels similar to the motor stillness induced by strong pain medications such as Demerol, a drug that allows the patient to remain absolutely conscious but not able to move or talk.

The recovering patient might be perfectly conscious, deeply relaxed, and yet unable to move any part of his body – even *appearing* to be asleep.

This type of "sleep," or utter immobility while alert, usually only occurred, if it occurred at all, for about two hours at a stretch. After the two hours of feeling drugged was over, the recovering patient quickly resumed whatever his normal movement ability happened to be. But the next day, at about the same time, he might, once again, have two hours of gentle, but utter, immobility. And again the next day. And the next.

Only a small percentage of patients had the two-hour, same time every day, limp paralysis. Of those that did, most of them only had it for a few days. Some had it for a week. A few had it for several months. The people who had it for several months also seemed to me to recover more quickly, in general, though of course meaningful research comparisons have been impossible.

More channel theory

The two-hour periods of extreme limpness and immobility correspond to healing activity in specific electrical channels. Every primary channel has a specific two-hour period during the day when that channel runs at its highest amperage.

For example, the Lung channel runs at its strongest (its highest amplitude) from 3:00 to 5:00 a.m. People with lung problems are often awakened during this two-hour span as their lungs do healing work, which can include coughing and expectorating. The Large Intestine channel revs up from 5:00 to 7:00 a.m., as the gut is starting to wake up for the day. The Stomach channel carries the most current from 7:00 to 9:00 a.m., and so on. This ancient circadian Chinese medical theory is known as "The Law of Midnight-Midday." This theory has many applications for medicine. Even western doctors have noticed that surgeries for particular organs go better at particular times of the day. You can read more about this topic in *Tracking the Dragon*. This theory is far more sophisticated than the relatively new guesses about circadian theory that are being proposed in allopathic medicine.

The times of day with heightened amplitude in a given channel's qi flow are also the times of day when healing is most likely to occur in body parts that are influenced by that particular channel.

These times are approximate and are based on the sun. For example, "6:00 a.m." actually refers to sunrise, *whenever* that might occur. 6:00 p.m. means sunset. The hours are *not* based on Greenwich Mean Time.

If a body area primarily serviced by the Stomach channel needs intensive repair, the body is most likely to do this repair work between 7 and 9 in the morning. During these two hours, if the body is doing *enormous* amounts of healing work on any damaged places that are served by the Stomach channel, a person who is emotionally relaxed may not be able to move any part of his body. He might feel limply, gently paralyzed, or very, very sleepy, from 7 to 9 in the morning – Stomach channel's "prime" time. He will snap out of it and spring back to life when the Qi starts flowing more heavily in the next channel in the sequence, the Spleen channel, from around 9 to 11.

When this type of two-hour limpness does occur, the person – who might have nearly normal physical function during the rest of the day – has a bit of warning time: he can feel himself slowly relaxing, over a period of about ten minutes, into the deeply calm stillness. Once he is comfortably ensconced in it, nothing short of an emergency can pull him out of it. And at the end of the two or so hours of gentle, "soft" paralysis, he finds himself able to move perfectly normally again – until the same time the next day.

If the patient can take them in stride, these bouts of non-moving are pleasant, even amusing. They might or might not occur on a daily basis until the area being worked on is healed. Also, after a person no longer has 7 to 9 in the morning (or whenever) soothing paralysis, he might develop a different two-hour stint of calm stillness at some other time of day.

For example, one person who needed a lot of repair work around his shoulder blades found himself unable to move from 1 to 3 in the afternoon for a few days while the shoulder blade area recovered more movement and feeling. The previous week, he'd been limp from 7:00 to 9:00.

Again, it was *not* the rigid type of paralysis that a person might have following a stroke or polio. It is a time of softness, a deeply calm period during which a person might be awake or asleep, during which his ability to move is turned off. It is somewhat similar to the deep, relaxing rest that can come after a high fever has broken and a person slides into a deep, healing stillness during which he is awake but feels absolutely no interest in moving a single muscle.

This stillness will not occur if stress or any sort of emergency is ongoing. It happens in people who are free to surrender to their bodies' inclinations to whatever extent is reasonable.

An example

I was one of those who had morning "zone outs" for nearly two months. I could get up any time in the morning so long as it was before 7:00 a.m.. I could rise early and get my day started: have breakfast, exercise, read the morning paper. At around 7:00 a.m., I would slowly become limp, unable to move or talk. At around 9:00 a.m., I would snap out of it. Within fifteen minutes, I was back on my feet, functioning normally. I rescheduled my work, changing my start time from 9 a.m. to 11 a.m. No one I was working with ever suspected that I spent two hours every morning awake yet utterly unable to move.

During this phase, I desperately wanted to attend a rare, traveling exhibit of works by Leonardo DaVinci. The only venue hosting this show on the west coast of North America was a museum in Victoria, BC, Canada.

I arranged to stay with a friend up in nearby Seattle but even with her taking care of me, our attending the exhibit was going to be a challenge: we had to leave the house at 5:30 a.m. to take the 7:00 a.m. ferry from Seattle to Victoria. I warned her about my little bouts of "limpness" between 7 and 9. Now, I always have loved being on the water. I never feel safer than when out in a boat. I've since learned that many people with PD feel this way. Maybe it's because no one can "get you" when you're far enough off shore. At any rate, I had no emergency thinking going on. Just the opposite: I felt great, and was anticipating much joy from the DaVinci exhibit.

I went limp at around 7 a.m., just as we were boarding the ferry. My friend helped me, almost dragging me for the last few yards, to a seat in the ferry café. Maybe it was because we were on a boat, which meant I was feeling extra safe, but I went into one of the deeper of my "immobilizations." I sat, slumped, eyes opened, body unmoving, unable to talk, for nearly two hours, while Sandy chatted to me about what her kids were doing at school. Then, about twenty minutes before docking in Victoria, I sat up. I started conversing with Sandy, ending her monologue. Within a few minutes, I was gesturing and joking effortlessly.

Sandy was mildly alarmed. "You're normal again! You told me about these two-hour 'quiet times,' but I didn't believe you. That's the weirdest thing I've ever seen. I've been sitting here wondering how the heck I was going to drag you all over Victoria. I thought you were sick or something. I was getting ready to call for a doctor, and now you're perfectly normal! Absolutely normal! This is the weirdest thing I've ever seen. And you've been doing this every morning for how long?"

Shortly after that, I was finished with the two-hour "zone out" interludes. During the time I was having them, I helped plan, and then hosted, a huge family wedding at my house. I was also working full time. So you can see I was *not* incapacitated during this period. I just couldn't move between 7 and 9 in the morning.

Afraid of needing sleep

I've heard from a few people with Parkinson's who have decided not to try to recover because they were frightened by the idea of needing lots of sleep. They've explained that they cannot afford to miss any days of work. Some have even asked if I know of a way they can recover without going through the recovery symptoms(!).

Some have also feared that, in order to explain to the boss or co-workers that they need more sleep, they might also have to confess the horrible fact of having been diagnosed with Parkinson's disease. They fear that either the increased need for sleep *or* the admission of having a physical illness will cost them their jobs.

Being afraid to miss work, or being afraid of appearing lazy (another popular reason for not wanting to attempt recovery) during the period of increased need for sleep, is a fear-based attitude that slams right up against what many people with Parkinson's think they need: accomplishments. As noted before, many value themselves only in terms of what they accomplish each day.

Seen in this light, it is understandable that many people are *afraid* of anything that might rock the I Get Things Done boat – including recovery.

But, as noted above, in an emergency, people recovering from Parkinson's *are* able to move. We've observed that, if showing up for work was crucial for a recovering person, he was able to attend work. However, if this was the case, he might spend his days *off* sleeping around the clock. Recovering patients seem to be able to work around employment or other "emergency" needs while still doing whatever recovery work has to be done – within reason.

Periods of insufficient dopamine

In addition to becoming limp during the time of day when a significant amount of healing was happening along the path of a given channel, a person who is recovering might become limp for a short while if/when the brain's dopamine supply temporarily runs out. During these fairly short periods, which occur when there is no emergency on the horizon, the person feels limp and relaxed – which is *how* a person feels when dopamine is sufficient for consciousness but insufficient for motor function. Over weeks or months, as the recovering brain steadily increases the amount of dopamine in response to need, these short-term, temporary events become further spaced apart and last for shorter durations until, at some point, they never occur again. This subject was discussed in depth in chapter four, pages 40-41, in the section on the substantia nigra.

I should mention that even after a person no longer has these episodes on a regular basis he still might have another episode months or even a year later, following a severe chill or some other dopamine-depleting event such as a severe illness. Two years after I had completely recovered, I spent a whole winter's day on a boat in the northern Pacific, exposed to the winds and spray. It was exhilarating even though I was wet through and freezing cold the entire day. It took me hours to really thaw out after I got home. The following morning, during a mild hike, I fell into a twenty-minute "low dopamine" event in which I gently collapsed and sat on a log in the brittle winter sun, utterly limp and calm, unable to move. I think the severe chill was a helpful dopamine-increasing brain challenge. In the nearly twenty years since that day, I have never experienced another "motionless event" from dopamine insufficiency.

"Cure me fast so no one will suspect I've had Parkinson's"

One patient came to visit our (now ended) program in Santa Cruz, and opened his first appointment by asking, "Can you cure me really quickly so that no one will ever know I had Parkinson's disease?"

I said that I couldn't promise anything, and asked why it mattered if people knew he'd had PD. He replied that he was a physical fitness coach. "I make a good living because my clients think that I'm healthier than they are. If they knew I had a physical problem, they would reject me."

I told him that he might be wrong, and that if he was able to show his clients how he could confront and recover from a difficult illness, they might respect him even more. He was adamant that I did not understand, and that everyone would despise him and accuse him of being a liar if he promoted fitness when, in fact, he had Parkinson's.

I said that it seemed to me that if he truly felt that he was sick, and was pretending to be well so that he could continue to mislead his clients, then he *was* lying. He replied that he had to lie to be able to make a living. So I asked if maybe his problem wasn't so much that people might *think* he was a liar, but that they might find out that he actually *was* a liar. He agreed, and didn't seem to understand that the *latter* situation reflected the more poorly on him.

He replied that people would *hate* him if they knew that he was being a fitness coach while having Parkinson's disease. We went back and forth on this for some time. When I refused to guarantee that he could recovery quickly and in such a way that no one would ever suspect he'd been "unfit," he decided to not to attempt recovery. He went for the medication.

He was not the only one. Many people with Parkinson's have shared their fear that, by divulging the fact of physical imperfection, they would make themselves vulnerable to scorn or even place themselves in some sort of unnamed danger. It was years before I figured out that avoiding the appearance of vulnerability is a biologically normal part of pause mode and the Parkinson's personality. A severely injured animal, one that is in pause mode, dare not show any signs of weakness to a nearby predator *or* competitor.

Many patients, neurologically behaving like injured animals, or "walking wounded," feel that they are not yet in a place that is safe enough to allow them to let their guard down. Sadly, some have cultivated such a powerful attitude of wariness for so many decades that they cannot easily change even when tempted with the possibility of recovery from PD. Some people felt that any *change* in attitude would be a sign of weakness, a sign of surrender. As mentioned earlier, if I had to pick one word that my PD patients dread more than any other, it would be "surrender."

Quitting the job

Oppositely, faced with the idea of *possibly* needing to miss a few days of work because of needing more sleep, many patients decide to quit working altogether. They always told me they would recover faster if they had time off to focus on their recovery. They were wrong every time. Those who quit work to "focus on recovery" never recovered and their symptoms worsened more rapidly. I discourage this very common type of thinking.

I've seen that patients who *continue* on at their regular jobs while they also work on turning off pause fare much better. Isolation does not encourage learning a new mindset – it allows a person to wallow in his habitual ruts. The regular presence of others, including work colleagues, was usually a boon to patients who had never known that "other" people can actually be extremely helpful – even if "other" people were usually thought to be slower, stupider, and lazier by the person with Parkinson's. Learning to *accept* help from others is a part of learning to feel safe. And feeling safe releases dopamine. Dopamine release does *not* occur when a person is hiding and in fear.

What dopamine release is not

Many a person trying to recover simply cannot understand that parasympathetic mode and its concomitant dopamine release is *not* the result of getting what he *wants*, often phrased as "being happy." Dopamine release is *not* the result of retreating or hiding in the benumbed calm that borders on falling asleep. Dopamine release is *not* the result of suppressing or stifling emotions in order to present a calm face to the world. Dopamine release is *not* the result of achieving "safety" by acting on fear-based impulses for self-protection and self-preservation. Dopamine release is *not* the result of receiving praise from others. It is *not* the result of attaining lauded victory or material success.

What dopamine release is

Dopamine release occurs when a person feels safe enough to be unguardedly alive – which includes being alive to risks, frustrations and failures: in other words, safe enough to be alive no matter what happens. Dopamine release occurs when a person *expects* to experience the joy of being alive *whether or not* he gets to do what he wants – whether he wins or loses, whether he's calm or dynamic. Staying home from work in order to micromanage one's time so that one can practice "being happy" *and* avoid confrontation or risks is the exact *opposite* of expecting to feel the joy of being alive *no matter* what the circumstances. Reveling in life, risks and all, is the *opposite* of playing dead.

Life is fraught with risk. Commanding oneself to play dead, automatically, except during those times when one gets exactly what he *thinks* he wants, is one way to avoid risks, but at the cost of eventually developing Parkinson's, a syndrome in which one becomes a living corpse. [1]

Help in unexpected places

Those people who continued working, who even shared with co-workers the fact that they had Parkinson's and that they were trying to recover often found an enormous weight lifted from their shoulders when they learned – often to their shock and amazement – that their co-workers were able to take their "failure to be perfect" in stride. Some even received unexpected support and strength from co-workers.

One recovering patient who had always stared at herself in the mirror when needing to summon up extra numbness had a messy accident at work: a friend bumped her. She stumbled and fell to the floor. Her drink spilled all over the front of her blouse. She pulled herself up and headed to the lady's room to stare into the mirror where her mirror image, known as Mirror Lady, would command her to make herself extra numb so that she wouldn't feel the shame. But a co-worker who knew what she was going through stopped her. "No. You don't do the Mirror Lady any more. Let me go with you and clean you up. I've got a clean tee shirt you can put on." My patient told me the next week that this was the moment that she started to embrace her relationship with her invisible friend and reject the lifelong power of the pause-inducing tool that she had named Mirror Lady.

I recommend that a person continue working or performing his normal activities of daily living to the best of his abilities, while allowing recovery symptoms, including his increased need for sleep, to freely manifest, whenever doing so is reasonable.

---

[1] When I was a girl, the phrase "living corpse" was actually used to describe the eventual, utter paralysis of Parkinson's.

As for the issue of celebrating life whether or not you get what you *like* or *want*, read Kipling's "If". Sometimes misinterpreted as a paean to stoicism, it is actually a tribute to "not being attached to outcomes": an underlying principle of Hinduism. Kipling wrote this after his experiences in India, where he marveled at the utter trust in the Divine and the non-attachment to outcome that he saw in the Hindu population. India, until the recent rise of the middle-class and its severe pressure to "succeed," was historically one of the countries with the lowest per capita rate of Parkinson's disease. Today, urban India has the same per capita rate of PD as other developed nations.

Chapter Thirty

Recovery symptoms: Brain Shifts

Some of the most bizarre symptoms of recovery, a symptom that could not possibly have been expected by anyone, were the intra-cranial brain reorientation movements.

These movements, which I named "brain shifts," were fleeting events that felt as if different brain sectors were shifting position relative to each other.

There were three types of brain shift: front-to-back, top-to-bottom, and side-to-side.

Front-to-back brain shift

In what I call a "front-to-back" brain shift, a person feels as if the front and back parts of the brain have moved further apart.

The shift often starts with a feeling that the frontal bone (forehead) was gently pulling away from the rest of the cranium, moving forward a fraction of an inch. Just after this, the head feels very relaxed and light as if there's been a decrease in internal pressure in the cranium. Next, a sensation occurs as if the front lobe of the brain was gently floating upwards and forward. The back of the brain moves slightly down and back at the same time or a moment later.

The sensations pass very quickly, in the time that it takes a muscle to relax. The sensations are non-dramatic, and are followed by a faint awareness of decreased tension in the head.

Top-to-bottom brain shift

The top-to-bottom shift can feels as if an enormous internal pressure was compressing the brain down onto the brain stem. This brain shift was described as feeling as if a "too-tight hat" or "swim cap" was compressing the head. During this brain shift, people sometimes feel a strong urge to stomp the feet, almost as if they are trying to tamp their spines down into a better position while the head pushed down onto the top of the spine. There were variations that didn't include the "too tight hat" sensation but which seemed overall to fit the idea of a top-to-bottom brain shift.

For example, one person gave this description of the event: "I was sitting in the concert hall listening to a piano recital, and all of a sudden I turned my head and there was this deep piercing pain in the very center of my head. It went from the very top of my head down to the neck part of my spinal column. How can I describe it? I could say it's like I pulled a muscle or something, but that wasn't really the feeling. It was like a big train running through the center of my head down to my spine. Was it painful? Well, it didn't really *hurt*. The big shock went away in a few minutes, but the aftershock stayed for about twenty minutes more."

In my own case, it felt as if a massive weight was bearing down on my head, and it made me want to stomp the floor. My husband just stared with raised eyebrows as I vigorously raised alternating legs and brought them down hard on the floor. It felt *so* good to stomp. It seemed as if I stomped for ten minutes, but it might have been a much shorter time than I thought, probably less than a minute. When the pressure and tightness around my head stopped, I stopped stomping. And then I felt *really* relaxed inside my head.

Side-to-side brain shift

The side-to-side adjustment was the most strange and glorious. It usually begins on the healthier (less PD-affected) side of the brain. For example, if one's symptoms are worse on the *right* side or started on the *right* side, this phenomenon will usually begin on the *left* side of the head, and vice versa. It usually begins behind the ear, just above the mastoid process.

It may start off as a low rumble, so slow as to be barely audible. In this stage, it is almost more of a vibratory sensation than a sound. As the vibration picks up speed and rises in frequency to an ever-higher pitch, it vibrates through the very center of the head.

At this point, the patient may find himself thinking with awe and acceptance, "Wow. I'm about to die." The vibration continues to increase in speed and rise higher in pitch until it vibrates its way out through the opposite side of the brain, in the area near the temple. After this, a deep stillness is felt in the head.

After the vibration exits out the side of the head, the *internal* tremor, if any, might stop or become greatly diminished. Some people's tremor stops long before the brain shift. In my case, the brain shift occurred several months after the tremor stopped. Some people's tremor stopped long *after* the brain shift. And yet, for some, the brain shift seemed to turn off or greatly reduce the tremor.

The sensation of internal stillness that follows the side-to-side shift is so profound, so peaceful, that some patients assume, for a moment, that they have died.

After experiencing a side-to-side brain shift, a person sometimes needs a few moments to ascertain that, *despite* the interior stillness, he is still alive. Sometimes, only after noticing that he is breathing does the patient realize that he hasn't died.

Years before any symptoms of Parkinson's disease had appeared, many people with Parkinson's have felt the presence of a constant internal tremor, a tremor that *eventually* drove the physical tremor. Others had always thought that the vibrations in the head were normal, and only realized that they'd had a pathological level of agitation in the brain when it stopped. Either way, it feels *unbelievably* good when the internal tremor stops for good.

The side-to-side brain shift is usually a deeply significant moment in recovery, mainly because it can solidify the feeling that Parkinson's is not coming back. Some people told me that they must have had a brain shift in the night but slept right through it because they wake in the morning with a sense that something unspeakable is gone from their life.

Most of my patients who have been awake during the brain shift say that they assumed that they were dying. And when they decided that this death was going to be OK, even wonderful, that's when the vibrating rose in pitch and finished its work. The word surrender comes to mind…

One patient who experienced the head shift but who continued to tremor slightly told me that, even though she was still tremoring, it was now only a physical tremor not connected to anything in her brain, and not nearly so annoying.

She explained further, "There's no tremor in my head any more. I have a shake in my arm when I'm standing, but it feels as if it's because my arm is weak. And it's in my hip when I'm lying down, but it's more like just a weak-muscle shaking, not a tremor. It's not nearly as annoying. Before, *I* was shaking; something inside of me was shaking. Now just my arm or my hip is shaking. It feels more like a muscle habit; I can laugh at it, now." (As we were to discover, she still had yet another unhealed injury that was affecting her hip.)

In my own case, my internal tremor stopped after the epiphany. Even so, I experienced a side-to-side brain shift about two months later, after which I felt even more calmness inside.

In my office

I was fortunate enough to observe one person experience a side-to-side brain shift while she was in my office, while I was holding her shoulder, doing Yin Tui Na.

Her eyes got huge. She brought her hands up to the sides of her head. Her mouth opened in a silent scream. The whole thing lasted less than a minute. [1]

After several minutes of trying to describe for her husband and me what had just happened, she laughed and exclaimed, "I feel so *good*! I feel so *good*!" She still had a few recovery symptoms to go through, but she felt at her core that she had suddenly, unmistakably, become "all better." [2]

One patient's description

The following is a partial transcript of a tape recording made in my office of a patient who had experienced the side-to-side head shift a mere four hours before coming to my office. "You'll want to get this down," he said, when he arrived for his weekly session. He was my first patient to experience the side-to-side head shift. Since then, others have shared similar stories. This person was a psychotherapist, and was accustomed to writing up case studies and analyzing mental experiences. I turned on my audio recording device. As he spoke, he also made a few arm gestures. This is transcribed from the recording:

"I had an awesome experience, just awesome…the upshot of it is that some life form, or some piece of me, some part of me, died during the night. And it may have been the Parkinson's part…I had the feeling that something was coming to an end, it was as though I were dying, but I was aware that I didn't think I was really dying…I wasn't getting ready for my own real death, but as though some part of me or something in me was dying. And it was a totally unique experience.

---

[1] When another patient emailed to me that he had experienced the side-to-side brain shift, he described it as being "a Silent Scream, like in the famous painting" by that name. The term fits so perfectly that I have used it since then to describe the fleeting moment when it feels as if the brain hemispheres are vibrating themselves back into their correct position.

[2] I write this in 2020. I saw her just a few months ago for a chest cold. She has had no Parkinson's symptoms since her brain shift occurred in 1999. She'd been diagnosed by two neurologists. When she saw the second one again *after* recovering, that neurologist told her she was psychotic and had obviously had psychogenic parkinsonism.

"I went with it, breathing was fine, and whatever it was then moved to the point of dying, letting go…(long pause). And I still am not sure what are the best words to use. (His eyes filled with tears.) Time will get some perspective on that too. But it's as though something was lifted. And I gave it plenty of time to go, and respectfully said goodbye to it. And then when I was sure it was gone, realizing that would be the end of whatever that was, I got up on the side of the bed. (Long pause.) At that point, I was aware, more keenly than before, that I was actually alive, that it was not a death experience, that I wasn't getting ready to have a heart attack or die, but something was dead, something was gone, something was lifted and I had a strange experience of…lightness and …smoothness (tears)…those two words were real clear. And I knew at that point that I was not dying, that I was not dead, that I was continuing to live…

"I was clear that this was an experience about me, and the interesting part was that I felt free of tremor, and it was unbelievable. But I've made a career out of being open to believing the unbelievable, so wait and see, time will tell, but clearly this was some kind of important experience.

"It was clear that I was tremor-free. I had a sense of balance and solidness that was new, that I didn't really want to test, for fear that it wouldn't really test out. So I started gently testing it. Oh. There was also a sense of symmetry that hadn't been there before. So I kept testing it putting my arms above my head, by putting them out in front [He gestured, with hands straight up, then out to the sides, then out in front and demonstrated the wrist movements.], looking for tremor, turning 'em, looking for cogwheel, not seeing anything, doing a bunch of touching, testing, touching the back of my head…and in the middle of this, I got up, twice, and tested my stability and balance, and ease of movement, and it was there!

"It was easy movement, it was as though I was without Parkinson's…oh, then at one point, I said to myself, 'I wonder what my writing is like?' So I have a pen, and a notepaper right by the bed, right by where I was sitting, to the left of where I was sitting, so I got that, held the little telephone note pad in my hand. So it's not the steadiest thing, so I wrote something. What I wrote, interestingly enough, was 'I am a renewing person. I am a renewing being' and I (long pause) looked at it and it was (tears again, choking a few times) luh… luh… large (choking) handwriting. (Crying.) Not micrographia! And it was a little scrawly, but then I reminded myself that my handwriting had always been scrawly, but it was just naturally as big as it used to be!" [He made a hand gesture for me, using thumb and forefinger to show an inch in height.]

Other patients, after the side-to-side brain shift, also have a similar sense that Something Had Changed. Each person explains it differently.

Some fully recovered patients have experienced none or just one of the brain shift patterns. A few, including myself, experienced all three.

Fleeting dizziness

Not everyone who recovers feels a distinct pattern of brain shift. Sometimes, the patient just has a moment of dizziness, as if the room is spinning, after which, they feel calmer inside and the internal and external tremor is gone.

One patient reported during her weekly visit that she'd been sitting on her living room couch between her husband and her grandson, watching TV just prior to going to bed. When the earthquake hit, she dove to the floor and threw her arms over her head to protect herself from falling objects. When the shaking stopped, several seconds later, she looked up at her husband and grandson who were staring in amazement. "Didn't you feel the earthquake? It was huge! The whole room was spinning around." They slowly shook their heads. There had been no earthquake.

Another reported that he'd had a brain shift while he was relaxing, with eyes closed, during a plane flight. He felt the airplane dip one wing deeply to one side until the plane was almost sideways. Then the plane dipped deeply to the other side.

"*Violent* turbulence!" he said to himself. He grabbed onto his armrests, braced for anything, and opened his eyes. That's when he saw that no one else was reacting. The flight attendant was calmly pouring a beverage. He looked at his own beverage. The liquid was not sloshing. The fleeting turbulence had been inside his head.

His tremor had been small and intermittent. After the "turbulence," he never tremored again.

Various terms such as "room spinning," "loop-de-loop" and "earthquake" have been offered to describe the fleeting perceptions that occurred while it seemed as if the brain was repositioning itself. These were painless, fascinating shifts that sometimes resulted in a decrease in or cessation of internal tremor. In my limited experience, no one ever had repeats of the any of the three types of brain spinning events.

Again, many people did *not* experience these events, at least not while awake. But many suspected that some distinct event, possibly one of the brain shifts, *had* happened to them in their sleep because they woke up and felt unaccountably different: taller, calmer, and in some cases, permanently free from tremor.

A possible explanation

I have to wonder if the brain spin mentioned in chapter fifteen, p. 184, that might occur when the pause pattern is first becoming established, is related to the brain shifts that occur when Parkinson's turns off.

My memory of my age-seventeen brain spin, after which, in retrospect, I always felt a bit agitated, felt somehow related to the side-to-side brain shift that occurred while I was recovering, after which a very profound level of constant inner tension turned off. The corrective recovery event that seemed to realign the hemispheres sometimes felt something akin to the vibrating and roaring inside the head that originally *mis*aligned them.

If the brain spin *was* caused by an actual physical shift in the hemispheres set in motion by an asymmetrical current flow (Stomach channel shunting into the Gallbladder channel on the right side of my head *only*), we're probably talking about distances of microns here, not millimeters, so it won't show up on a brain scan.

Fear of the brain shift

As you have no doubt already guessed, some patients have told me that they dare not enter into a recovery program because they might experience a brain shift while driving. And by now you can probably provide the same reply that I gave them: brain shifts have only occurred when the person feels deeply peaceful. These events have never occurred during times when alertness or mental intensity was called for.

Recovering patients have experienced their brain shifting events while resting, daydreaming, or while half-awake. Others concluded that a head shift must have occurred during sleep because, upon awakening, the head felt different: larger and/or more relaxed. Or else the internal tremor was gone or they felt a new sensation inside: profound stillness.

No one, in my experience, underwent a head shift while driving, while bustling about, or while generally combatting the everyday crises of life.

Chapter Thirty-one

Recovery symptoms: Changes in Attitude and Personality

Introduction

The previous chapters focused on those recovery changes that are related to muscles, nerves, sinews, and even brain hemispheres. Those were physiological changes, changes that had a physical basis.

This chapter describes a few of the recovery symptoms that were more mental and emotional than physical: mood and personality changes.

Crying

At some point after turning off pause and/or pseudo pause, recovering patients often found themselves bursting into tears at the least little thing. Various patients told me, prior to recovery, that they rarely cried, or that they *never* cried, or even that they *couldn't* cry. During recovery, for a few weeks or months, they often found themselves crying at almost anything.

Typical reports included "I'm turning into a sap! I saw a little child walking a puppy on a leash, and it was so cute, I burst into tears…"; "I read the headlines on the newspaper and I was so touched, I started crying!"; and "I caught myself crying at *Oprah*, for God's sake."

Usually, the onset of easy tears was a wonderful feeling, accompanied by a feeling of openness in the heart and the end of a long-time fear that tears would lead to being condemned as a sap, a weakling, or stupid. Then again, the onset of tears could be very painful.

One patient who did not recall ever crying since she was six years old started crying one day after a session in which we'd worked on the blockage at UB-11, helping her to feel as if she was back inside her physical body. As her UB (Urinary Bladder) channels started flowing in her neck and back instead of floating out into space, her "imaginary body," her sense of the body that contained her heart bridged the several-foot gap that usually separated it from her physical body, and the two merged.

She started crying in my office, after blurting out, "Why are people so mean to one another?! Gee…I'm crying." And then she started crying harder. Soon, she was so violently wracked with sobs that I suggested she not return to work, that she go straight home and call in sick for the rest of the day.

She assured me that she wouldn't have any problem at work: she had always been able to stay in control of her emotions.

She called me the next day, from home. Following our session, she had returned to work, started sobbing hysterically at her desk, and actually fell on the floor and was unable to stand up. A co-worker drove her home. She stayed home from work the next day and cried. She was unable to staunch the tears, but more importantly, she was unable to stop the flood of emotions that surged in her breast. She was feeling emotions for the first time since she was six years old. She felt emotionally drained by all the feelings and the crying, but she optimistically figured that it was all to the good.

Three days later, a horrible tragedy occurred.

Her best friends, a couple that she had introduced to each other, died in a car crash just three days after she'd called me from home. Her friends had been on their way back from Disneyland. Their infant daughter also died. Their eight-year old child was injured, but survived.

This patient, now in her mid-fifties, had not cried *or felt any emotion* since she was six years old. She was slammed with the full force of real-time emotional loss. She told me, the next week, that when she got the news of her friends' deaths, she cried so hard that her chest hurt, her eyes hurt, her face hurt. Her arms hurt, her skin hurt. At some point, she was in so much pain that she couldn't tell if she was crying because she was in such physical pain or if she was in such physical pain because she was crying. She feared that she might go crazy from the emotional pain, the physical pain, and the crying.

She truly did not have the emotional skill set to deal with this tragedy. She had the emotional strength and savvy of a six-year old.

A week later, she told me that, for several days, she questioned whether or not she had been better off back when she was unable to cry, back when she had attended family deathbeds and funerals and experienced no feelings *whatsoever*.

I asked her if she now regretted the changes that she'd been going through, if she wished we hadn't opened that door.

She looked me right in the eye and said, "You saved my life. I was dying and you brought me back."

She wasn't talking about the Parkinson's. She was talking about her long-absent heart. She had no regrets.

Nearly all patients have *enjoyed* the sensations of increased feelings and tears, even if they were terrified of crying up until the very minute when the tears started to flow. Very often the tears ended up being tears of joy, of connectedness with others. Even in the above case, she was grateful to be able to feel and express the anguish and pain that she was feeling.

The ability to cry is very important. I cannot think of any person who has recovered from Parkinson's who retained his *in*ability to cry. Curiously, some of those who recovered *easily* had actually worked on learning to cry, *long* before they were ever diagnosed with Parkinson's. I suspect that their self-taught ability to cry and to experience their own heart feelings was one of the reasons these people recovered so easily.

Learning to cry in high school

I learned to cry when I was seventeen. It happened after one of my teachers referred me to the school psychologist for "the usual senior-year counseling session."

I only realized decades later that none of my high-school classmates had ever been sent to a "usual senior-year counseling session." I wonder if some, or at least one, of my teachers was suspicious or concerned about my home life situation or my pretty severe stoicism, and had requested that I be seen by a counselor.

During the session, the counselor asked me a few pointed questions about my home life. He remarked on how I seemed to freeze up when asked about my mother.

I coolly replied that, "All children love their mothers. My mother frequently reminds me that even the worst criminals love their mothers."

The counselor countered, “That’s not true. Not all mothers even deserved to be loved. Some mothers chop up their children and flush them down the toilet.”

I was shocked. Then, I was profoundly relieved. The thought that some mothers didn’t merit blind devotion was new to me. The counselor then asked if I ever cried.

I replied, “No one likes a person who cries.”

As an aside, as a very young child, I had learned that crying was one of the behaviors that could make my unhappy mother become suddenly insane with rage. My crying could lead to a brutal beating with a leather strap, a beating that only ended after she experienced a quickening in her breathing ending with huge gulping sighs of relief. Make of that what you will. At any rate, I had learned at a very young age never to cry.

Getting back to the counselor, he contradicted my statement that “No one likes a person who cries.” He said, “Everyone cries. Crying is normal. Everyone knows that tears just mean sadness. Maybe your mother doesn’t understand about crying, but healthy people do. If you walked all over school crying, not one person would be angry with you or dislike you; people would most likely just say to themselves ‘She must be sad about something’ and continue on their way.”

I was astonished at this new thought. Unable to process any more new ideas just then, I told the counselor, “I’ve got to get back to class,” and left.

I decided, right there, to do an experiment. I would cry, right there at school, and see if anyone got mad at me. I started crying on the way back to class. I had not cried since I was five years old, so it took a while to get started. I pretended I was an actress who could cry on command, and that got a few tears rolling. Once I started, I couldn’t stop. I did not take my usual seat at the front of class that day. I sat at the back and quietly cried. To my amazement, no one, not even the teacher, got mad at me, let alone beat me. For that matter, I was given a wide berth – the teacher never even called on me. No one seemed to even *notice* me. Of course, this was back in the pre-hug 1960s. If I did the same experiment today, probably many people would come forth with hugs and loving support. But certainly, no one made fun of me or scorned me. I enjoyed the novel idea that I wouldn’t be punished for crying so much that I sat at the back of the room in my next class, as well, and cried for *another* forty minutes.

From then on, I made a point of crying, singing out loud, dancing, and emoting whenever I felt an emotion welling up in me – if I was in private. I was still careful never to “lose my cool” at home, in front of people I didn’t know, or in situations where I might be judged.

Prior to my diagnosis with Parkinson’s disease, I had noticed it was increasingly difficult to notice my own feelings. I found myself with an increasingly flat affect and mood – but unlike many of my PD patients, I was very aware of this decline. I fought it vigorously by forcing my self to sing rhythmic, bouncy songs that always made me feel better, and which, in turn, temporarily improved my mood and movement. Songs that I knew would always work included the early 20th century zippy Tin Pan Alley hits such as “When You Wore a Tulip,” and “Shine On Harvest Moon,” the stirring “California Here I Come” (often substituting the *Mad Magazine* spoof lyrics, “Cleopatra here I Come”), some of the livelier gospel classics, and anything by Hank Williams. I would force myself to sing these songs out loud until I felt a mood improvement.

My own spiritual teacher, Paramahansa Yogananda, often warned his students, “Negative moods are your worst enemy.” So for decades prior to my diagnosis, I had worked hard at recognizing and diverting myself away from negative moods. Singing a certain type of song was one of the fastest ways I could divert my mind. If I was in a situation where singing out loud wasn't appropriate, I talked silently with Yogananda, my guru, until the negative thoughts backed down. This training in bad-mood rejection served me well when I was diagnosed with Parkinson's and, in desperation, doubled down on talking with my invisible guru, surrendering to him and, to my amazement, ended up with an epiphany that turned off my Parkinson's.

Several of my PD patients have described similar stories of learning or teaching themselves how to cry, feel vulnerable, or focus on the feelings in their own bodies even before being diagnosed with Parkinson's. Those people who had worked on these skills tended to recover more quickly than those who were convinced that stoicism was keeping them safe or successful. Those patients who were *opposed* to learning to cry or *opposed* to learning to feel pain were almost certain to not recover. No person I know of who has recovered from Parkinson's has retained his *in*ability to cry.

Punctuality

One distinct symptom that accompanied the change *away* from wariness and fear was a decrease in punctuality. I'm always pleased when a patient who has been chronically punctual starts to recover and then shows up fifteen minutes late for his next appointment…and laughs it off! It is always a sign of emotional recovery.

When a previously punctual patient calls me on the phone to say something like, "Ha ha! I guess you figured out that I'm not at my appointment," I offer my congratulations.

I did have *one* PD patient who was *never* on time. She was consistently, considerably late for everything, usually around thirty to forty-five minutes late. She had Type IV PD, the least common type.

Becoming "lazy"

One recovering patient said that her adult daughter showed up at the house one afternoon, took one look at mom, and asked with concern, "What's the matter?!"

Mom replied, "Why should anything be the matter?"

Daughter answered, "You're sitting on the sofa."

Mom, genuinely puzzled, asked, "So?"

Daughter replied, "I've never seen you just sitting around before."

The mom had to give the matter quite a bit of thought, and finally decided that this new behavior on her part might actually be a good thing.

A few months after my own recovery, I was feeling so strangely calm, content, and lazy that I asked my husband and teenage son, "Do you still love me? I'm so different. How can you love me now, when I'm so mellow, if you used to love me the way I was before?"

My teenage son answered, "Mom, we loved you; we still love you. We love you *in spite* of how you are, not *because* of it."

As people who used to have PD become aware that they are "getting less done," they sometimes have to learn to love themselves "just because," and even *despite* their new mellowness and emotional health.

Panic attacks

Some, not all, recovering patients experienced a panic attack several months after pause turned off. The panic attack was usually full-blown, complete with pounding heart and sheer terror with no way out. A common description was "my mind was going down a black hole."

These attacks occur in situations with highly specific parameters: 1) the situation was always supremely *non-important*; 2) a decision had to be made with regard to a *new situation*; 3) because the situation was new, *no precedent* could be applied.

Those people who had panic attacks had only *one.*

The attacks occurred after a person started feeling very good, very comfortable with life. He could feel himself being more relaxed and less obsessively driven. He may have even noticed that his heart was more calm and that he was sleeping better than he used to. His Parkinson's symptoms might be completely gone or he might still be experiencing a few fleeting physical recovery symptoms. Then, along came a situation in which he had to make an innocuous decision: a decision that he had *never* had to make before.

Some examples of decisions that prompted panic attacks are: Where to put the food and water dishes for the new kitty? Where to temporarily set the knick-knacks that sit on the bookcase when the carpet man moves the bookcase to take up the old carpet? In my own case, the panic attack occurred when I tried to install a brand new computer game program for my son. This was back in the early days of personal computers when every new computer program had its own unique and nearly incomprehensible set of installation instructions.

In every case of panic attack, the person who had recently turned off pause was confronting a *new* situation that was not actually very important. When he *calmly* tried to think of what to do in this situation, the brain presented an utterly blank screen: no thoughts appeared. He then wondered what was the matter with his brain.

What was probably happening, based on detailed descriptions that I heard from my patients, is that the person was trying – for the first time in decades or maybe for the first time in his life – to make a decision using dopamine-based thinking instead of norepinephrine-based thinking.

I hypothesize that, in the past, these people had done their thinking with pause-mode type, norepinephrine-driven thoughts. They were accustomed to making lightening fast decisions. Now, their brains had gone literally blank in response to "What should I decide?" As they tried harder to find some mental thread to grasp, in an attempt to figure out how to do the new task, they realized that there were no mental threads. The task itself became less important. The mental focus was redirected to the realization that there were NO mental threads. It felt as if all thought processes had been turned off, as if the brain itself was missing.

A person recovering from Parkinson's might have *no* remembered experience of making a decision while using the parasympathetic pathways in the brain instead of the emergency pathways. When he tried to make a decision while being parasympathetic-mode dominant, mid-brain dopamine dominant, the mental "thought screen" literally showed up blank. This led to the next thought, "My brain is missing! I don't know how to think, and I don't know how to think about figuring out how to think!" From there, the mind went straight into a black hole of terror and a full blown panic attack.

At some point, the panic forced the person to dive into a significant degree of sympathetic mode – fight or flight mode. Once he slipped into a sufficient degree of fear, he was able to snap out of his panic and figure out what to do.

The brain goes missing

Happily, these attacks only happened once, if at all. After that, the recovering patient seemed to know how to make decisions without going into a panic. These panic attacks were very real. The woman who slid into a black hellhole of panic while home alone trying to decide where to put the new kitty dish was a NASA researcher, a brilliant scientist. She found herself standing in the center of her living room screaming, “Help me! Help me!” at full volume. She said that, even as she was doing it, a part of her brain was thinking, “This must be a panic attack! Cool. I must be recovering!” But even so, the sense of impending doom, helplessness, panic, of needing someone to take over and take care of her, was physiologically *real*. The panic did not have to do with the kitty dish, per se. The panic began when her brain registered “Empty” when she tried to think of *how* to think about where to put the new dish.

One previously intrepid, world-traveling patient had his recovery panic attack in his kitchen when his wife proposed that they try the new restaurant in town. He went into a full-blown panic and was soon screaming for help as his wife stood by in amazement. The reason? He later explained that he didn’t know what they would do after his wife pulled into the parking lot because he didn’t know what they would need to do to find the front door of the restaurant. And when he tried to *think* about how a person might go about finding the front door on a building he hadn’t been to before, he couldn’t figure out how to think. It was the inability to think, and the feeling that his brain was literally empty, that triggered the panic.

My patients with Parkinson’s seem to have relied on the emergency form of decision making for most of their lives. This quickness may be part of the reason why, for their many decades prior to recovery, they often came across as smarter than their peers. They might *not* have been mentally quicker than their playmates and peers if they had all been on the same neurological footing – all using a blend of sympathetic and parasympathetic mode for thinking instead of the much more forceful norepinephrine emergency override of pause mode.

I am pretty certain of this because, after recovering, patients were often amazed to find themselves becoming more average in terms of strength, quickness of mind, and speed. They did not become stupid or sloth-like. However, they became only *pleasantly* above average, not super-duper, not driven – and they were OK with it.

Because of their chronic use of the life-saving norepinephrine override, many people with Parkinson’s had secretly resented their “slow” fellow students, siblings, and co-workers: had dismissed them as “underachievers” or “dragging us all down.” Ever since grade school, the mere presence of these “slower and stupider” people had often been a real irritant for many of my PD patients, who, deep down inside, had felt that life was an ongoing emergency, a state of perpetual risk. When this constant judging of others and of self began to decrease during recovery, patients *loved* the change, as a rule.

Getting back to panic attacks: when the recovering patient needed to make an innocuous decision, one that was simply too mundane to activate his now functional sympathetic nervous system, he found he had no way to access any decision-making parts of his brain *and* be calm at the same time. He actually got a blank slate when he tried to make a simple decision while under the influence of mid-brain dopamine. It was always the blank slate that scared him, not the implications of the decision.

As you have probably guessed, a few people with Parkinson's have told me that they shouldn't enter into a recovery program because they might have the panic attack while driving the car. You know exactly what my reply was: the panic attacks occur while doing something perfectly dull in a very safe setting. In my experience, no one had a panic attack while in a potentially risk-laden situation.

Then again, one recovering patient did have a panic attack *related* to driving. He had taken the weekend off and had flown back east to visit his daughter at college. The visit was purely a lark. It was the first time he'd taken off just for fun in a long time. As he was enjoying himself driving along the freeway, he missed the exit. He took the next exit instead and then realized he didn't know what to do next. He couldn't even *think* of what to do next, so he pulled over and stopped the car. Then, in this perfectly safe, non-emergency situation, in which, on some level, he was actually enjoying himself, he tried to think about what he should do next. He couldn't think! His brain was a blank!

Within seconds, he was in a complete panic because he couldn't think. His heart was pounding, he was sure he was going to die. After what seemed like several minutes but what was probably several seconds, his brain kicked in. He thought of something to do: he found a pay phone at a nearby gas station (in the days before cell phones) and called his wife, long-distance. She agreed that it sounded as if he'd just had a panic attack. She asked him what he thought he should do. He said that he needed to pull a U-turn, get back on the freeway, and go back the way he'd come. Duh. He knew what to do.

But he had been thrown into a panic by a fear that had tackled him when his brain had failed to respond in the usual manner. He was *never in any danger*. He only panicked after he was relaxing at the side of the road, trying to calmly figure out what to do. He did get to where he was going, and he never had another panic attack.

One interesting thing about this particular style of panic attack is this: shortly after the person truly begins to panic, the sympathetic nervous system *does* kick in. The person is then able to think, for as long as is needed, in a manner approaching the way that he always used to think in the past. And so the panic attack ends.

A recovering patient, in the joyous throes of steady mid-brain dopamine release, might have been *reluctant* to slide into using sympathetic mode just to make some unimportant decision. But decisions can only be made in one of two ways: by using the *mind* while in predominantly sympathetic mode, or by feeling the preference of the *heart* while in predominantly parasympathetic mode. Again: decision making while sympathetic dominant is guided by the ego-based structures in the brain. The mind's decision making faculties while parasympathetic dominant are guided by signals from the pericardium.

The first time a person recovering from Parkinson's tries to make an unimportant decision using his *mind* (as per his lifetime habit) while he is in predominantly *parasympathetic* mode, he can't come up with a *way* to think. In parasympathetic mode, the heart feelings instruct the mind. If one tries to find a solution to a problem using only the mind pathways, while staying in predominantly parasympathetic mode, one will not get an answer: the mind may present a blank.

In recovering patients, the mind system hasn't yet been trained to work as a subordinate during parasympathetic, heart-led decision making. Hence, the panic attack.

Happily, our recovered patients all instinctively learned, after one panic attack, how to think and make decisions either by using the heart, in parasympathetic mode, or by using the mind, in the old familiar way, by triggering a very mild level of fear and a sympathetic mode response.

Guilt or boredom from lack of tremoring

Another emotional symptom of recovery was guilt. One patient never tremored again after her side-to-side- head shift. She subsequently felt terribly guilty when, shortly thereafter, her mother landed in the local emergency room with a blood pressure crisis.

For years, the patient's hand had tremored during the most mildly anxious situations. As the emergency room clock ticked away and she failed to tremor, she thought to herself, "I must not care about my mother. I've tremored from all kinds of stupid, unimportant things, and now my own *mother* is in danger and I'm not even tremoring."

She told me about her shame the next time I saw her. I had to assure her that tremoring in a crisis is not necessarily a normal response. Since she didn't have Parkinson's anymore, tremoring was no longer going to be her go-to expression of concern.

Another recovery oddity was the feeling of emptiness when the internal tremor stopped. As one person expressed it, "I miss the tremor. I know that's weird, and I feel guilty about it, but the tremor gave me a sort of internal pressure to be and to look alert. As long as I was tremoring inside, I felt like I was always *doing* something. Now that it's gone and I can sit motionless, I feel as if I'm not *doing* anything when I'm just sitting around. And I sort of miss that old intensity that wouldn't let me sit still for very long. I'm going to have to find a new motivator."

Greater acceptance of others

One patient explained to me that she'd been working hard all her life at being more forgiving towards the idiots and morons in her family and in her workplace. But she couldn't help herself: when someone at work did something wrong or less than perfect, or even just spilled something, the first though in her mind was always "Idiot!"

As she worked at turning off pause, talking constantly to an invisible friend, she noticed, after about three months, that she no longer had this mental reaction to imperfection in the people around her. She found herself thinking, "Hey, he's only human…" She was hugely pleased with and grateful for her new ability to automatically be a more accepting and forgiving person.

Feeling sheepish

Many people have assumed that a person who recovers from Parkinson's will be proud of his victory. He will want to proclaim it from the rooftops, and be a guest on late-night TV.

This is not necessarily the case. In my experience, a majority of people, after recovering, felt sheepish. Their "terribly unfair illness" was, in part, the result of their own mindset. This can be very humbling, even embarrassing.

Some patients were ashamed of themselves when, upon recovering, they realized the extent to which their Parkinson's symptoms had been the result of their own mental and emotional blockages. I recall one patient repeatedly slamming his open hand onto his forehead while laughing, "I've been doing this to *myself*! What an idiot I've been. *I've* done all this to myself!"

A person should *not* be ashamed of having induced this illness in himself. *Many* chronic illnesses have some amount of emotional component. And nearly all of us are doing the best we can. Still, patients are often embarrassed when they recover.

Another type of guilt that sometimes descends on a recovering patient is the realization that, for a large part of his life, he has increasingly been an unpleasant, demanding perfectionist, know it all, or some other type of personality that was based on fear and wariness instead of understanding and humility.

As a healthy level of humility begins to take root and thrive, the temptation exists for the recovered patient to indulge in a bit of guilt for having been fear-driven, pride-driven, or whatever, in the past.

My advice is that indulging in guilt and shame is a waste of time. Be humble enough to know that *everyone* makes errors. Forgive yourself and get on with your life. No doubt you were nearly always doing what you thought was best, at the time.

Then again, as mentioned earlier, a few people that I know of, three to be exact, none of whom were my patients, have been extremely outspoken about the fact that they recovered from Parkinson's disease. They each wrote books, one flogged dubious health products, and another charged substantial fees for his advice on how to recover. The one charging advising fees, despite not having any real idea as to *why* he recovered (based on his story, he had Type II PD), nevertheless has been trying to get someone make a documentary about his recovery, his guesses as to how recovery "works," and his subsequent years as an online, fee charging "Parkinson's advisor." So I'm guessing he probably *would* want to be on late night TV.

My own patients, after recovering, have been grateful, maybe a bit humbled, and mostly just wanting to get on with their lives and to support others who are working on recovering. Maybe it's partly because most of my recovered patients, especially those with Type I, are aware of their own mental involvement in putting themselves on pause.

Loss of self-identity

Many patients recovering from Type I PD have found themselves asking the question that might be more characteristic of an adolescent: "Who am I?" This may be because, in part, the person never really experienced a period during adolescence in which he was able to dwell on that question.

Or, the person may have known exactly who he was so long as he was "on top of his game" and running on the norepinephrine override, but he might not have had any idea who he is when, after recovering, he found himself able to relax deeply, *feel* the beauty of music, and/or not care any more about where other people place the soup bowls in the dishwasher.

Who was he when he suddenly realized that most of what he'd been worrying about for years didn't really matter? Who was he if he was starting to pay attention to his own heart feelings?

Many people with Parkinson's trained themselves to value themselves in terms of what they are able to accomplish. They are "good" because they "do more" or are stronger, faster, smarter, and/or maybe more spiritually superior than others.

Many people with Parkinson's also pride themselves on their ability to show love for others through their hard work and/or strong moral compass.

However, many people with Parkinson's *often* are unable to feel the resonance between their own hearts and their own bodies, or between their own hearts and the love that others are directing towards them.

Because of this lack of resonance and ever-increasing reliance on wariness, a person with Parkinson's may have been steadily building protective walls around his own heart until he got to the point that he no longer knew who he really was. Our heart feelings reflect who we actually are. And who we are is *inherently* loveable. Our minds merely allow us to execute the actions of who we *think* we are.

When, during recovery from Type I Parkinson's, those walls around the heart begin to crumble, people's life priorities might shift. Patients were often surprised to learn that they were not who or what they thought they were.

Many people "hit a plateau," get emotionally stuck, or even went into a period of depression while or after recovering from Parkinson's because of the personality change. Sometimes, the Blocker returned. The way to deal with this if it happens is to increase the intensity of the same treatments used for turning off pause: become even more deeply engaged with an invisible friend; choose the friend instead of the Blocker; keep a feeling of energy in the forehead at Yin Tang; say thank you for everything; as often as possible, be aware that energy is flowing through the midbrain; meditate. Exercise regularly. Give yourself a new challenge: learn a new language; develop a new skill set. Do *not* sit around and expect the universe to drop rose petals on you because you are recovering from Parkinson's.

All of the fully recovered patients were certain that they loved their new self far more than they'd been able to love their old, pre-recovery self. Even those who struggled with some degree of post-recovery depression and self-questioning were glad that the physical infirmities of Parkinson's were behind them.

Many recovering patients noticed a dropping away of their defensiveness and fear of criticism. Of course, not *all* patients *had* been afraid of making mistakes or being laughed at, but many had been. Their symptoms ranged from a protective emotional flatness to abject fear of "what others might think" to the point that they lived every moment as if an invisible critic was offering running commentary. When the inner critic died away, the relief was enormous.

A few people with PD did *not* notice any emotional changes – they'd been feeling their hearts right along.

Chapter summary

People deeply enjoy the personality changes that come about when they recover from Type I PD. It might take a while to get used to the new personality. Of course, the panic attack was usually unforgettable and terrible during the span of the one to two minutes that it lasted. But for the most part, from the new ability to cry to the feeling of heart resonance with nearly everything, the restoration of the healthy personality was one of the favorite recovery symptoms.

So many people told me something like, "I used to want to recover from Parkinson's so I could go back to being the person I used to be. Now that I've recovered, I *never* want to be that person, ever again.

Chapter Thirty-two

Summary of Recovery Symptoms

The recovery symptoms yielded the greatest evidence of what really happens in the body and mind when a person has idiopathic Parkinson's disease. The dopamine levels in the brain didn't really come into it much. Once a person turns off pause or pseudo pause, the brain is once again able to release dopamine as needed for automatic motor function.

During recovery

Numb areas in the body usually experience an improvement in blood circulation and in perception of somatic sensations. The numb areas are found where channel qi ceases to flow during pause: on the foot along the span from the mid-foot to the toe; on the face from the mid-forehead down to the back of the jaw; and the backs of the hand, especially in the vicinity of the thumb and index finger. When circulation improves, sensations of tingling, "ants," and "pins and needles" might occur in areas that had been numb.

Pain might manifest in unhealed injured areas, areas that have long been dissociated away from conscious awareness.

In areas that had been numb, the fungal growth just under the skin or in the nail beds might put up a fight – erupt in small red blisters or a red rash – when the body's improved circulatory system carries immune cells into previously underserved areas. The returning immune cells are able to recognize the fungal intruders and attack them.

Areas along the Stomach and Large Intestine channels that had become rigid will relax. They might relax *utterly*. They will stay relaxed, which is to say "limp," until the brain movement-imagining area once again hooks up with those areas. As soon as the re-connection has been made, the body parts will be able to move.

When the re-connection first occurs, the body parts might move somewhat spastically and/or repeatedly until full mental control over brain-body coordination is restored.

In a few previously dormant muscles, particularly the biceps and the lower back, their new, unstoppable, automatic, constant, *healthy* use can lead to achiness and soreness. Once the muscles become accustomed to constant use, the achiness, tenderness, and soreness goes away.

Sleep needs will probably increase. In addition to needing more nighttime sleep and/or naps, a person might become extremely limp during two-hour periods during the day when the body is doing healing work on tissues that are supported by the channel associated with that particular two-hour period.

A person recovering from Parkinson's might experience sensations, usually only one time, that feel as if various sectors of the brain are moving relative to each other or repositioning themselves inside the cranium.

Once the brain starts using dopamine for motor function after its long hiatus, a person might experience short periods of dopamine insufficiency. This manifests as the body going limp for a short period, even while mood and thoughts remain alert and positive. These short periods of "running out of energy" seem to spur the brain on to increase the amount of dopamine available for motor function. Over a fairly short period, a few weeks or months, at the most, a person will no longer have these brief interludes of dopamine insufficiency.

A person might have one panic attack while relaxed and trying to think about how to do some completely insignificant new action. The brain's ability to think might seem to have disappeared. The attack might bring a person to his knees, screaming for help, but it only lasts for around one to two minutes, if that.

A person who was previously unable to cry or who could cry only under highly safe circumstances might find that he cries easily and often. Concern over being too "soft-hearted" or "sappy" might arise.

Friends, family, and colleagues might respond with welcome or unwelcome joy when facial expression returns. The entire body might feel more resonant with, more "friendly" inside when around people, even when around strangers.

The feeling of anxiety and/or wariness and the need to be more competent, or stronger, quicker, smarter, or more "right" than other people, will diminish.

A person who is recovering from Parkinson's might find that he is more at peace with himself even as he realizes all the ways in which he has long been imperfect. The rigid moral code that is common in people with Parkinson's might melt away, allowing one to respond with compassion to the imperfections, errors and follies of self and others.

As you peruse this summary of recovery symptoms, notice that *none* of them have to do with dopamine except for the brief, relaxing lulls that can occur when dopamine levels temporarily drop a bit low. Some of the recovery symptoms have to do with healing from physiological damage that slowly builds up over decades in the muscles, nerves, and brain connections when a person is running the channel qi patterns of pause for an extended period. Some of them have to do with mental and emotional changes that occur when a person no longer chronically feels as if he is on the verge of imminent death.

I have not even attempted to write up every possible recovery symptom. If you are recovering and find yourself going through unexpected physical, mental, and emotional changes, please don't worry. Consider whether or not the change makes sense in terms of what you now know about Parkinson's disease. Maybe even reach out to a friend or family member to see if they can make sense of it. If you aren't sure if you're recovering or getting worse, have a friend feel what your channels are doing. Remember – it's possible to experience fleeting moments of turning off pause and then returning to pause mode. It might take a long time to train yourself to stay in a healthy blend of sympathetic and parasympathetic modes long enough that you can turn off pause for increasingly long durations. The main thing is, if you experience a fleeting moment or longer during which your body felt a little lighter and your heart felt a little more open, you are going in the right direction.

Many people told me that, during recovery, they felt as if they were becoming younger instead of growing older. Now *there's* something that most people don't get to experience. Many told me that, when they realized they were recovering, they became deeply introspective and even depressed. Their response to this was to stop doing those exercises that helped them turn off pause. The treatment for this problem is to resume those exercises with renewed intensity. Also, learning a new skill set or setting some new life goals can keep the brain oriented towards parasympathetic mode.

If you're recovering, *enjoy* the process: surrender to it. Oops; there's that word again.

To polish off this chapter, and for a demonstration of what recovery can be like, I'm closing with the following: four emails that I received while writing this chapter. I never met this patient. He contacted me after finding the Parkinson's Recovery Project website and started working on recovery. This email was written almost four months after he started following the suggestions from the books offered on the Parkinson's Recovery Project website. He never took any antiparkinson's medications. Based on a few questions that I sent him, his Parkinson's might have been set in motion by severe burns he had on both ankles many decades earlier. His emails neatly sum up what he's going through in mid-recovery. He definitely was able to turn off the qi flow patterns of pause, but as you will read, he *continues* to work on the mental retraining behaviors that help him keep it turned off. My own comments are in [brackets].

First email

Hi J. This week's update is more of a stock-taking

<u>What I don't have...but have suffered previously</u>

1. hoarse voice
2. swallowing problems
3. sudden leg cramps (usually occurred while sleeping)
4. slowness of movement (except left arm, which is still slow)
5. forgetfulness
6. trouble finding the right words
7. left arm permanently cocked [A scan two months later revealed a displaced neck vertebra that was putting pressure on the nerve to the left arm.]
8. toes suddenly moving apart, like muscle tightening. [recovery dyskinesia]
9. left arm stopping or not moving on command
10. feeling of clenching my lips [recovery dyskinesia]
11. sleeping problems
12. numbness below my right shoulder blade.
13. loss of sense of smell. I can smell pleasant things now, like cooking, and from distance eg: can smell my wife cooking from upstairs bathroom. I can't smell foul odors yet.

<u>What I still have</u>

1. muscle soreness in left forearm [bicep soreness]
2. slower movement in left arm
3. slight limp in left leg (this is now noticeably better then previous, sometimes I have no limp)
4. some trouble typing with left hand, though improving. Not double tapping as much - using both hands to type now, bit more concentration needed with left hand.
5. reduced left arm swing.

6. some shaking in left arm, usually from the muscles in forearm, more noticeable when I walk. [Forearm muscle shaking is not characteristic of Parkinson's.]

7. doctors who don't listen.

In general

Given social distancing restrictions [this was in spring 2020, during the coronavirus pandemic] and I'm on annual leave I needed something to keep me busy so this last week I decided to learn a new programming language. I noticed when in deep concentration or reading, the activity on my face was intense (pin and needles or ants and spiders). [Deep concentration increases the amount of Du channel qi flowing through the midbrain and frontal lobe: a good thing.]

My left arm is straightening, not cocked any more rather it just hangs down. It no longer stops mid movement (eg: while pulling my pants up or putting my hand in my pocket). The other day I was reaching with my right arm into a cupboard above my head and a jar fell. Without hesitation, my left arm sprung into action and caught the jar at around stomach height. Proud moment right there. However the muscles in forearm are still tight and sometimes sore.

I also decided to teach myself piano. I have tried this on and off in my past but never went on with it. After a bit of practice I was able to complete two-handed scales over 3 chords, though the pressure I was able to exert with my left hand was clearly less than right.

The limp in left leg is fading, I have found myself mentally expecting to limp or have trouble initiating movement only to surprise myself and notice no issue initiating movement and no limp. This is sporadic, but overall the severity of limp, when I do limp, is less than previous.

Just recently I have flashes of what I think is distant memories trying to come through, but it's brief, so I don't get the full recall. I don't know what this is actually.

What I am doing

1. Practice gratitude first: whenever someone does something or anything, I find a reason to praise them. Also gratitude for most anything I have, physical or emotional, especially the love I have noticed I receive from my family

2. Daily pray to keep negative thoughts and fears away, also reminding myself I am safe, usually the peace and harmony prayer [in the book *Stuck on Pause*]

3. If I have the slightest inclination of fear or negative thought I immediately respond with:

   a. Say to the voice "Go away, you are not welcome here"
   b. Pray God takes the negative thoughts and fears away.
   c. Yawn - this activates the parasympathetic nerve
   d. if called for - progressive muscle relaxation.

4. Daily meditation - Diaphragmatic breathing - counting 1 - 10 whilst messaging my pericardium. - 30 minutes minimum.

5. Mindful breathing, usually whilst on the computer or watching TV.

6. Mindful of third eye, usually whilst on the computer or watching TV.

7. Talking to my invisible friend.

8. Yoga - daily if possible

9. Cycling - I'm up to 200km this month

10. Living life the best I can.

Saw my GP this week for a flu shot and blood test, he asked how were my symptoms and what I was taking, I got a little nervous when telling him and he noticed a little shake in my left arm, which I immediately addressed, I told him about your research and how it was helping me, he even wrote down your web address, I told him to read your publications, he actually gave me the impression he would. Sadly when I returned for blood results I followed up with him, it became clear he was just humoring me. On the bright side, he has now acknowledged I am actively managing my symptoms, so I'm hopeful upon recovery he might just take notice.

– G. Clark

Second email, a week later

Hi,

Mixed bag this week.

I started the week with a bit of shaking in my left arm, sore muscles in my forearm.

I had some worry about losing my job again, so I adapted the head bobble with the affirmation "I am safe whether I'm employed or not." Put me in a more comfortable mindset almost immediately.

Continued with daily meditation, for a couple of days the shaking was less than previous.

On sleep, no insomnia at all, 9-10 hours, and still nod off during the day.

The limp is slowly fading, I'm definitely lifting my foot higher, not dragging it when I turn, initiates movements without fore thought and walking more freely more often.

My sense of smell is off the charts. It's driving me nuts but I'm happy for that, every minute a new smell, most I'm unable to recognize, I ask people sometimes and often they can't smell it. Foul odours are still missing however I'm starting to notice an odour when I open the kitchen tidy or dishwasher though it doesn't register as foul.

Seems my wife and children are happy with my facial expressions, they also point out I participate in conversation far more readily, quick wit, bad dad jokes, laughter and telling stories again.

The feeling of tightness around my scalp is now moving like spiders kneading my head, cheeks feeling like they are being pulled and pushed accompanied with sharp needling in my face, neck, feet and sometimes hands. It's happening as I write this.

On the emotional front, visited my mother, she said something under her breath, I assume about my left arm. It occurred to me I'm judged only for what people see, or what they are programmed to see. One of my brothers was there, we had not previously discussed what I've been doing, so prior to leaving I read my progress list from last week. I really needed them to understand all the small wins they don't see.

Whilst reading I broke into a nervous tremor. I also cried. I've become a bit of a sap now. When I finished, I think everyone was finally on the same page, my mother even said you can tell the difference in me. The tremor disappeared nearly as quick as it came. It was just nervousness, most likely being the center of attention where I think there may be non-believers.

In all this I still have some moments of doubt, but then I remind myself, if I needed any proof in my recovery just add up all the little wins. I just sometimes wish I didn't feel the need to convince those I love. But for now I'll just keep doing what I'm doing till recovery is obvious to everyone.

– G. Clark

Third email, a week later

My forearm muscles relaxed this week along with my leg. I actually felt it happen one night as I was watching TV. Also getting a little bit of arm swing happening, though there are moments that I tighten up again for some reason. In all, I think the tremor is dissolving along with the muscle tightness.

– G. Clark

Fourth email two weeks later

Earlier this week I noticed my wife sporting a huge grin whilst out shopping. Thinking I may have something funny going on, I enquired why the grin? Relieved was I by the answer, "My husband is walking normally again."

– G. Clark

"We choose and sculpt how our ever-changing minds will work, we choose who we will be the next moment in a very real sense, and these choices are left embossed in physical form on our material selves."

– Dr. Michael Merzenich, University of California San Francisco brain researcher in the field of neuroplasticity

Chapter Thirty-three

In Closing

Parkinson's is not, and never has been, an incurable illness.

The symptoms of Parkinson's disease result from chronic use of specific electrical circuits in the sub-dermal fascial and brain, circuits that are only supposed to occur when a person is at risk of imminent death. The neurological mode that kicks in when a person is at risk of imminent death is referred to in this book as pause mode. This neurological mode is recognized in ancient Chinese medicine, where it is called "Cling to Life." It is not recognized in western medicine.

During pause mode, dopamine release for motor function is supposed to be inhibited. This inhibition, plus other physiological alterations that occur during pause mode, help inhibit physical movement and may well save the life of a person who is hovering on the edge of death.

In people with Parkinson's, the physical immobility usually caused by this mode has been long overridden with a norepinephrine-based brain behavior that kicks in during times of gravest emergency *if* motor function is required *in spite* of the body being immobilized. Parkinson's disease usually begins to appear when the mental stoking of a constant sense of emergency can no longer be sustained. As a person becomes less able to conjure up mental scenarios requiring emergency behavior on his part, the underlying physical inhibitions and motor behaviors of pause mode are exposed. Pause mode is *supposed* to create motor immobility.

Pause mode is also associated with tremoring. In coming *out* of pause mode, the body tremors. The tremor appears to be an important signal to the brain that the body has stabilized from loss of blood, loss of blood pressure control, and the other physiological events that can put a person at risk of imminent death. The tremor behaves like a question to the brain, asking if the coast is now clear. If the surroundings are confirmed to be safe, then pause can turn itself off.

In people with Parkinson's, pause cannot turn off. The person has become stuck in pause mode or is running currents of pseudo pause due to an unhealed injury. In order to recover from Parkinson's, the person needs to turn off whichever of four processes is keeping him stuck on pause or pseudo pause. When pause is turned off, the circuitry in the body automatically reverts back to that of a healthy person: the normal, healthy blend of sympathetic and parasympathetic mode electrical circuitries.

The circuits of pause mode can get stuck from four different types of events. Depending on which of the four processes turned the pause schematics on, one of four corresponding therapies must be used to turn it off.

Two of the therapies are physical. One of them is physical support at the site of the injury in order to turn off the dissociation that is preventing an old injury from healing – an injury that is causing the electrical currents to be stuck in pseudo pause, a pattern that *resembles* that of pause mode (Type II PD). The other is a simple physical protocol for an injury that, at the time, was life-threatening but for some reason, the person's body never turned off pause mode following the termination of the danger (Type IV PD). The protocol fulfills the uncompleted physiological steps necessary for turning off pause mode.

The other two therapies involve mental, not physical, re-training exercises. One of them addresses the dissociation that some people *consciously* applied to an injury that they didn't "have time" to deal with or "didn't want" to deal with, many years earlier (Type III PD). The other one uses mental exercises to re-activate the brain's striatum and thalamus. This is the therapy used to treat the most common type of Parkinson's: Parkinson's from self-induced pause (Type I PD).

In my experience with nearly three hundred people with Parkinson's disease, around ninety-five percent developed it in response to self-induced pause. This type of pause mode is set in motion in response to a person commanding himself to "feel no pain," "don't be a part of this world," or some other powerful instruction intended to make himself numb to some physical or emotional trauma. This instruction was often given in childhood, often while staring into a mirror.

This type of pause must be addressed by mental exercises. The brain cannot turn off this type of pause on its own until the original command is rescinded *or,* far easier, the person is able to make his brain's circuitry behave as if he is now safe.

The self-therapy for self-induced pause, the mental retraining exercises, help a person turn off the inhibition of electrical current that *should* run through the brain's thalamus and striatum when a person is awake. This current is *supposed* to be greatly inhibited when a person is in a high level of pause mode. The therapy essentially does an end run around the usual biological processes that are involved in *deciding* whether or not one is sufficiently safe, and just makes the currents run as *if* the situation is safe. When this current is restored, the brain automatically registers "I am safe now." This enables the other biological steps in turning off pause to move forward.

In my experience, a few people have mastered this therapy easily, needing only an hour or two to make the brain behave as if the person is now safe. Most people with Parkinson's, because of the almost life-long pause-induced wariness and sense of being apart from others, take much longer. Some people must practice the therapies for months or even years before their brains experience the shift in electrical circuitry that makes them feel safe enough that the body automatically turns off pause mode. Many people, when they start to *notice* that their constant variations in their PD symptoms do in fact occur in direct response to variations in their thoughts, are inspired to increase the effort that they make in these mental retraining exercises. Their improvements then quicken.

Although some people turn off pause immediately and lastingly following a mind-shifting epiphany, most people with Parkinson's recover slowly. They chip away at their old mental behaviors, slowly modifying their thought patterns until they notice recovery symptoms occurring. The people who improve slowly might be susceptible to dropping back into pause mode when they are worried or fearful. Even after having many good days and an array of recovery symptoms, it is still possible to find oneself leaping back into pause mode in response to a rough day. Continuing to work on the therapeutic mental re-training even *after* recovery symptoms first appear, increase, and even start to gallop ahead, seemingly unstoppable, can be very important for those who recover gradually. Until one is anchored in the healthy process of using a higher degree of sympathetic mode, not pause mode, in times of stress, the temptation to use the old "tried and true" numbness of near-death pause mode might linger.

However, regardless of where one is in terms of muscle and nerve healing, every time that pause is turned off, the inhibition of dopamine release for motor function is instantly turned off. Turned off *instantly*. A person *immediately* feels subtly different. The chronic sense of impending doom, the need for wariness, and the other aspects of the Parkinson's personality – a medically recognized syndrome – ease up. Dopamine for motor function flows freely, instantly, when it is supposed to… until such time, if any, that pause mode is mentally initiated again in response to an unexpected fear or from the long-installed habit of wariness.

However, the physiological damage from decades of chronic use of pause mode in muscles, nerves, and in brain connections in the motor imagining area, must be repaired. As soon as pause is turned off, these body parts begin healing. Healing from the damage might take a few weeks or a few years. While healing, the person will *not* behave mentally as if he has Parkinson's. Although the rigidity and tremor of pause mode will begin to climb down either gradually *or* instantly when pause turns off, the body will still need to heal from the years of physical damage to the muscles, nerves, and brain connections. The symptoms of this phase are referred to as recovery symptoms.

Recovery symptoms can include healing from numbness in the toes and face, soreness in muscles that have not been used for years but are now moving automatically, personality changes, a temporary need for increased sleep, and more. This book has eleven chapters devoted to recovery symptoms. It was the recovery symptoms that helped build most of the hypotheses that led to the discoveries regarding what actually causes Parkinson's. Figuring out how to turn Parkinson's *off* came about in stages. The first recoveries were in people who had Type II Parkinson's from dissociation from an old, long-unhealed foot or ankle injury. The injury was causing the electrical circuits in the body to run in a manner similar that which occurs during pause mode. An effective therapy for Type I PD, the most common type of PD, PD from self-induced pause, was elusive for nearly twenty years. The breakthrough came in learning about brain scans being studied in the fairly new field of neurotheology. Musing over and figuring out therapies for the other two types of PD, types III and IV was, in comparison, a literal walk in the park.

Information in chapters fourteen and fifteen can help a person determine whether or not they have Parkinson's disease. This is necessary because misdiagnosis for this syndrome is rampant. A doctor's diagnosis is *not* necessarily correct.

The exercises in chapter seventeen can determine which *type* of PD a person has. Treatment for Type I PD and Type IV PD is explained in the book *Stuck on Pause*. Treatment for Type II PD and Type III PD is explained in the book *Yin Tui Na: Hands-on Treatment for Traumatic Injuries*. These books are available for free download at the website of the Parkinson's Recovery Project. The Parkinson's Recovery Project is a non-profit organization dedicated to making available free information about effective treatments for Parkinson's disease.

Reluctance to recover

Due to a lifetime of pause-induced wariness and fear, many people, especially those with self-induced pause, are afraid to embark on a path to recovery – afraid of the personality change, afraid of the pain of re-associating with old traumas, afraid of not being able to recover. Many people have told me something like, "Other people might be able to recover. I'm different from other people: I know that I cannot, so I don't want to waste my time." Others have more complex reasons for not wanting to recover. For example, many people have told me that their spouse will divorce them if they recover. The only reason the spouse is *not* already pursuing a divorce is fear of the social shaming they will receive if they divorce a spouse with a serious health problem. Often, these patients were sent to me because the spouse wants them to recover so a divorce, one *not* wanted by the patient, can go forward. Still, the most disheartening reason, one that is incorrect and yet I hear it often, is "I don't deserve to recover."

This attitude is absolutely reasonable given the mental story line that develops when a person has used self-induced pause mode for decades, especially the idea that "I am different from others." Truly, a person whose electrical circuits are running in the pause patterns due to a mental command to feel no pain *is* in many ways different from other people. But only in a superficial sense. At heart – a part of the body that a person with Parkinson's might not be able to somatically feel – a person with Parkinson's is just the same as other people, especially other people with Parkinson's. My research has shown that they *can* recover.

Still, the hard fact is this: I've met and worked briefly with many people who decided they do not want to recover from Parkinson's disease. This was one of the hardest things for me to accept.

As noted earlier in this book, it is a medical truism that most people would rather die than change. Consider the many seemingly simple changes that might improve quality of life or even save a life: stop smoking; exercise more, control food intake in order to prevent high blood pressure, weight gain, or diabetes; and so on. Most people know perfectly well that making changes in their life-style might bring enormous health benefits. And yet, as we learn in medical school, most people would rather die than change their habits or behaviors. Making changes, including mental changes, can be extraordinarily hard, even painful. To make these changes, a person might have to do battle with his own mind, his sense of self, and the life-patterns he has created to help himself deal with the physical and emotional pains in his life. When I started this project, I assumed that this medical school adage would not apply to people with Parkinson's disease. I was wrong.

When it comes to changing core aspects of ourselves, we each have the right to make up our own minds on whether or not we want to tackle this.

Hostility towards the idea of a mental component

Some people with Parkinson's have been very resentful when I started broaching the subject of a mental/emotional component. For example, in the first years of our website, we posted information about the foot injury aspect of Parkinson's – what I now refer to as Type II PD. We were flooded with inquiries. After 2005, when the Parkinson's Recovery Project posted new information sharing what we'd discovered about many people having a type of PD that seemed to have a mental component, albeit a treatable one, the number of people making inquiries dropped to a trickle.

But even before that, in the early days of the Parkinson's Recovery Project, I talked with many people who didn't want to recover if there might be fleeting unpleasant periods or changes in their personality. In the early days I often tried to change the minds of people who decided they didn't want to recover or didn't deserve to recover. Eventually, I came to accept the fact that some people would rather have Parkinson's than risk unknowns and/or a change their way of dealing with the world.

Some patients were very clear that they would rather not recover if recovery might involve a shift in emotional behavior or attitude. Having to change long-held fears or give up a lifetime of cynicism would be the same as admitting that they have been holding to an unhealthy or even "incorrect" mindset – admitting to doing something "wrong." Many have eloquently, if illogically, explained that they would rather stay how they are than make such an admission.

A few people with Parkinson's have told me they would rather believe that there is no cure for Parkinson's than consider that they have been cultivating an unhealthy mindset. At first glance, this attitude seemed to me to be wondrous strange. But I now know that being wary, a mindset that automatically accompanies pause and self-induced pause, can grow and metamorphize into fear of being found wanting, fear of being wrong about something, and even fear of having made, in one's past, a perfectly human, reasonable, even *necessary* change in one's *modus operandi* by self-inducing pause mode. And, *until* a person turns off pause mode, this wary attitude might be person's dominant mindset.

Disbelief in the word "degenerative"

Many people insisted that, in their own case, Parkinson's wasn't so bad and that they didn't *mind* having Parkinson's disease, because the symptoms didn't really interfere with their lives too much. These people had grudgingly come to my clinic, often sent by spouses or family members who wanted them to recover.

I often tried to explain that, with a degenerative disorder, symptoms start off very mild and gradually worsen over time.

Many of these people did *not* accept the fact that their symptoms would worsen over time. I sometimes asked these people if they'd ever been to a Parkinson's support group so that they could talk with people about the progression of symptoms over time. I was often told something to the effect that, "I went once, but the people in the group had a different kind of Parkinson's," or "The people in the group were a real mess: they weren't like me. My Parkinson's isn't the severe kind, like theirs is. *Mine* isn't a problem."

As mentioned previously in the chapter on the Parkinson's personality, people with Parkinson's are usually considered to be highly intelligent, word-loving, and crisply analytical. But in this one area, many people with early-stage PD seem to have a deaf spot.

Again, degenerative means "worsens over time."

Recovery symptoms

Parkinson's is a syndrome of numbness, muscle degeneration, nerve disconnection, and in most cases, a high degree of near-death mental behaviors: wariness; skepticism; anxiety; stoicism; numbness to somatic awareness; and even the perception of being outside of one's body. All of these problems are due to being stuck in pause mode or pseudo pause for an extended period of time. The motor symptoms are a side-effect of this, but they usually are masked for decades by using emergency-based thinking. The tremor is also a side-effect: a sign that your physical body *wants* to turn off pause. But since the real problem is a mental attitude or a channel-blocking injury that is keeping pause in place, the brain cannot go through the steps to turn it off. The tremor keeps sending its message to a brain that can't or won't listen.

Recovery symptoms are not a straight line. But to the extent that there is *some* degree of predictability, one can assume that return of fully normal motor function might be one of the very last things that occur during recovery. What might occur *prior* to a return of healthy motor function is resumption of nerve sensitivity, spastic, infantile motor function, back pain, heightened sensitivity in nerves that go to the bladder, exhaustion, and very often, an overwhelming, new sensitivity to heart feelings, and so much more.

Doctors see Parkinson's as a problem of motor function and a problem of tremor, only. Because of this, doctors and patients alike usually only look for a return to motor perfection or cessation of tremor when they look for evidence of recovery. But normal motor function and cessation of tremor might be the *last* changes to be realized.

Recovery from Parkinson's is tentatively happening when your mind even fleetingly starts to enjoy parasympathetic mode again: you start to laugh more and don't care so much about what others think. Recovery from Parkinson's is happening when you start to realize it doesn't matter or not if you are vulnerable, or not as perfect as possible, and that it's just fine if someone makes fun of you. *These* are the earliest changes that show a person is recovering from Parkinson's disease. The *invisible* changes, not the improvements in motor function, are the ones that prove you have turned off pause and are in the *process* of healing.

The visible changes in motor function are secondary. Even when your motor function does begin to improve, most people are not very good observers. They might only notice that your motor behaviors still aren't "perfect." And they might helpfully point out these still-present motor behaviors and encourage you to take medication so that you can "not have Parkinson's and be like you used to be." These people might have *no* idea what your real symptoms were: the mental symptoms of living on the verge of death; being outside of your body; being numb to your own heart feelings; and they have no idea how long this has been going on. They assume you were fine up until your motor function started to collapse after decades of having been in a mental state of emergency that you can no longer maintain.

Because of this, and because one of the strong brain habits that develops while on pause is the habit of always seeing the negative side – and this brain *habit* does *not* immediately go away just because pause turns off – doubt of one's own recovery can be one of the biggest challenges to overcome. Retraining the brain to focus on the positive and ignore the negative might be part of the ongoing re-training that the body and mind have to *actively* work at during recovery.

Only if you understand what it is you are truly trying to change will you be able to rest easy in the knowledge that you are, in fact, healing from Parkinson's disease after pause turns off. Your doctors and loved ones might assume you still have Parkinson's disease until their snappy and highly inadequate visual assessment shows that you no longer have *any* residual trace of impaired motor function.

Doubt can cause people to re-invoke self-induced pause. Don't.

You know the changes and healing you are going through even if no one else perceives them or acknowledges them. Savor them.

Give it a try

I encourage people with Parkinson's to at least consider recovering. Every one of my patients who has recovered has been thrilled to no longer be in the body and mind of a person who is stuck in pause mode – the mode of imminent death.

Most people want to recover from Parkinson's because they hate the physical impediments and the tremor. After recovering, my patients were more gratified by their new mental perspectives: "It's not as if anyone's going to *die* if I'm not perfect." And, "Hey, it's OK: we're all just human." For many of my patients, the return of physical grace and turning off the tremor were welcome *side-effects* of recovery.

Nearly every person who has recovered has said something along the lines of, "I used to want to not have Parkinson's so I could go back to being the way I always used to be. Now, I never want to be that person again."

Recovery is *possible*. Recovery is glorious. You *do* deserve to recover. If you have Parkinson's disease and you've never taken the medication for more than a few weeks and you've still got your wits about you, you *can* recover.

After you recover

After you recover, you don't need to tell *me*. I already know it's possible. Tell your friends. Tell your doctors. Start a website/blog to share your experience. Maybe make a donation to the Parkinson's Recovery Project so that this information can be kept available for free for future readers. In the near future, when we have enough funding, we hope to have professional translations made of this book for all the major world languages

There is no significant profit to be made by anyone from the information in this book. There is no gadget to sell, no pill to promote. There isn't anything that an MD can turn a profit on because you don't *need* a doctor in order to recover. Therefore, no one in the field of medicine is going to step up to vigorously promote the findings in this book.

Allopathic doctors are *not* likely to learn about this information any time soon, in school or in their journals. It will be up to you to help spread the word to other people who have been diagnosed with Parkinson's disease. Their doctors will catch on later.

I wish the very best for you. If you have Parkinson's today, may you soon be one of those who has recovered.

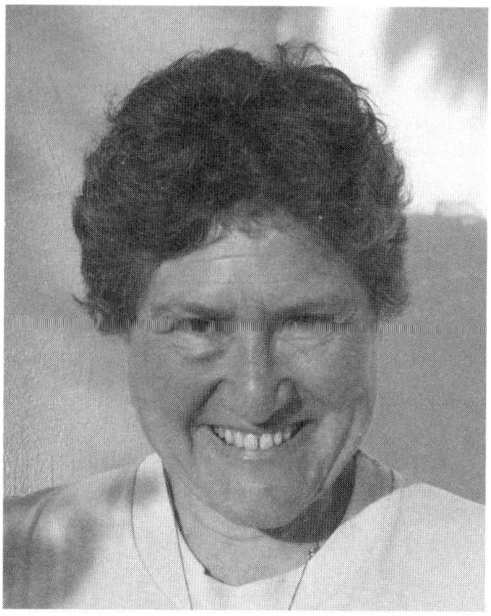

Fig. 33.1 Early April, 1998

About three weeks after sensation started returning to my face and I was able to once again use the muscles of my right cheek, a friend took this photo, which also appeared on p. 163. Some muscle use in the right lower eyelid and cheek had already returned, but the lower eyelid on the right is still *slightly* saggy, making the right eye look larger than the left.

Although these conditions had been more severe prior to recovering, this picture still shows nicely what I mean by a "groove" alongside the nose on the *right* side, and the flatness of the cheek on that side. In comparison, note the nice "bulge" of cheek muscle, the "apple" in the cheek, on the *left* side.

I wish I had taken photos prior to this partial restoration of facial responsiveness. In my defense, I did not know at the time that I was going to recover, let alone write a book.

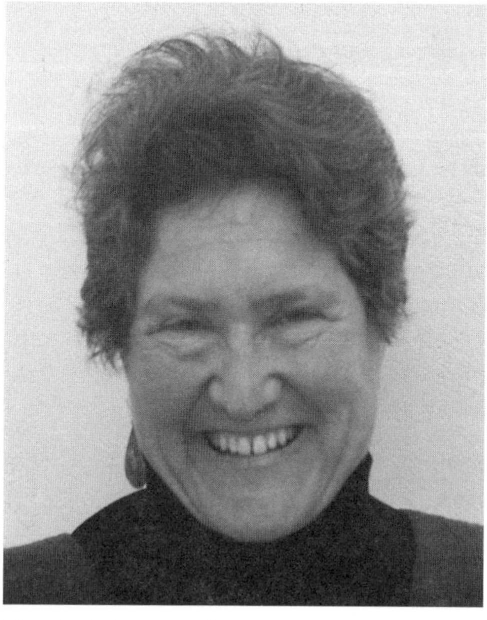

Fig. 33.2 One month later (early May, 1998)

One month later, my friend took this photo, against the same wall, at the same time of day. As before, the sun is coming from the right, helping to accentuate the groove alongside the nose and on the right side.

A slight improvement is evident. The eyelids are more symmetrical and there is the beginning of a slight muscle bulge in the right cheek.

Note the increased separation between the two upper front teeth. This occurred in a matter of minutes, one evening while I was relaxing, when my upper palate resumed normal muscle tone.

If I deeply relaxed my facial muscles, letting my jaw droop, the right side of my face and my right upper lip would still become completely limp (lacking in tone). Even though the mouth muscles sag, they are still more toned than they were before I turned off pause. Before turning off pause, the mouth muscles were rigidly downturned.

Today, in 2020, even when I allow my face muscles to deeply relax, I still have a faint smile.
(See back cover of the book.)

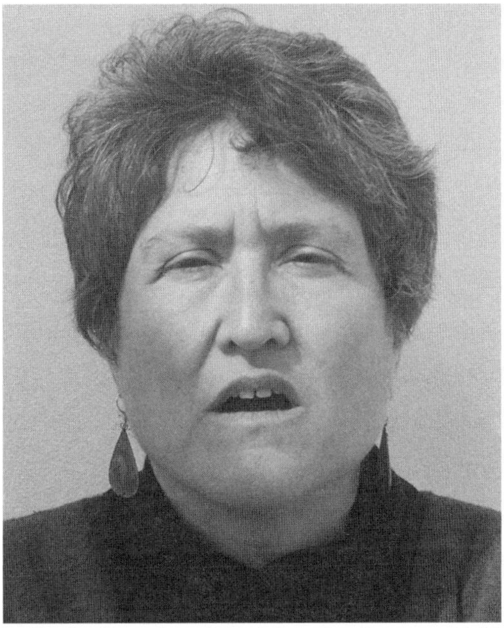

Fig. 33.3. Deeply relaxed face (early may, 1998)

This fourth photo, taken fourteen years later, shows that the improvement has remained, and even improved slightly.

Note the muscle of the *right* cheek that is in line with the "corner" of my mouth, the muscle that forms the bottom of the cheek bulge that comes with a big smile. This muscle did not exist for a year or so prior to my diagnosis. The symmetry of the left and right lower eyelid muscles has remained.

The hair is going gray…but that's not a symptom of Parkinson's disease.

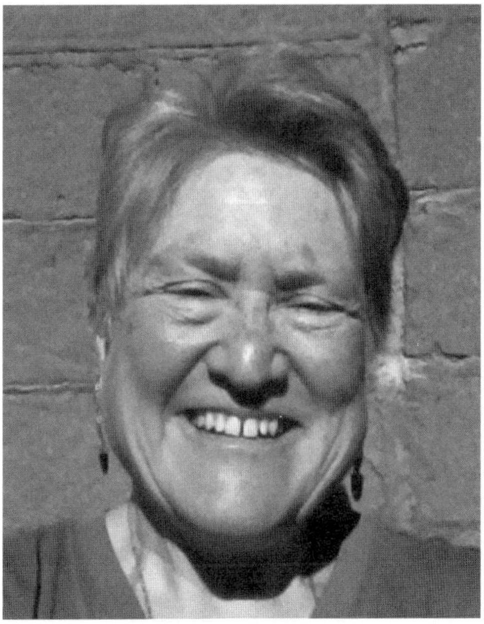

Fig. 33.4 February, 2013

Appendices

Appendix I: website information and books

The Parkinson's Recovery Project is a non-profit corporation. Its mission is making freely available new and recent research on Parkinson's disease. The site has updates on its homepage as well as offering, for free download, publications about effective treatment for Parkinson's disease.
The website: www.PDrecovery.org

Books

The following books might be helpful. They are listed in alphabetical order.
The books that apply to Parkinson's are available for free download at PDrecovery.org and carry an asterisk.*
All the books *except* for *Medications of Parkinson's: Once Upon a Pill* are also available for purchase in hardcopy at JaniceHadlock.com

Hacking Chinese medicine

The weird vocabulary of English-language Chinese medicine *can* be translated into logical terms based on the *medical* meanings of the Chinese words – as opposed to using translations based on the classic poetic meanings, which is what we're currently stuck with. These mistranslations are what make English-language Chinese medicine sound mysterious, if not ridiculous. This book provides accurate translations, making this medicine become logical and even modern. Correct translation show that ancient Chinese medicine is more in keeping with modern physics and bioelectricity principles than our present-day "modern, western" medicine.

The sample case studies illustrate this medicine's diagnostic objectivity, logic, and explain *how* Chinese medicine treatments work, if performed correctly. The basic principles of Chinese medicine and Chinese diagnostics are discussed in everyday English.

Readers have said that this is a wonderful starter book for a person who is curious about Chinese medicine. Many acupuncturists have said that reading this book gave them a vocabulary for explaining Chinese medicine to their patients.

This book does *not* have specific applications for treating Parkinson's disease. However, I'm including it in this list of reference books as it might be helpful for someone who wants a good starter book about Chinese medicine in general.

This book is available in hardcopy at JaniceHadlock.com

*Medications of Parkinson's: Once Upon a Pill**

This book shares the findings of a four-year research project working with people who were trying to recover from Parkinson's disease while continuing to take, or trying to reduce, their antiparkinson's medications. The horrors that ensued, the deaths and psychotic breaks, help explain why the Parkinson's Recovery Project does not recommend a person attempt to recover from Parkinson's if they have taken dopamine-enhancing medications for more than three weeks.

Even if a person is not a good candidate for recovery, this book has important information on how to safely reduce antiparkinson's medications if a person is having adverse effects from the drugs, symptoms such as dyskinesias, spasms, hallucinations, dementia, and other symptoms associated with excessively high levels of dopamine. Safe drug reduction must go very slowly – complete weaning off the drugs, if desired, might require up to a year and a half. Over-fast reduction of certain antiparkinson's drugs can be fatal. Your neurologist most likely has no idea how to safely reduce these drugs. The only people who died from neuroleptic malignant syndrome (death from over-fast drug withdrawal causing failure of the autonomic nervous system, which regulates breathing, heart rate, and temperature regulation) during our four-year research project were ones who followed the glaringly incorrect advice of their neurologists.

This book is available for free download at PDrecovery.org

*Stuck on Pause**

This book explains in detail how to turn off biological pause as well as self-induced pause. If you have determined that you are on pause, either type, you can use this book to learn the steps for turning off pause mode. This book explains how to differentiate biological pause and self-induced pause. It answers in great detail many questions about recovering from pause, answers that go into much greater depth than is possible in the more generalized book titled *Recovery from Parkinson's*.

This book is available for free download at PDrecovery.org and is available for purchase in hardcopy at JaniceHadlock.com

Tracking the Dragon (two chapters*)

This textbook teaches how to feel channel qi. It explains the different bioelectric circuitries of the different neurological modes. It explains how to use channel blockages and divergences diagnostically. Many case studies are provided, demonstrating the key principles of ancient Chinese medicine.

This book is written in lay terms, suitable for students of Chinese medicine and for people with no background in medicine.

The chapters of this book that teach how to feel channel qi and that show the maps of the channels are available for free download at PDrecovery.org . The whole book is available for purchase in hardcopy at JaniceHadlock.com

*Yin Tui Na: Hands-on Therapy for Traumatic Injuries**

This photo-packed book shows the hands-on therapies that can be used on all injuries: new, old, and dissociated injuries. It also shares mental and attitudinal techniques that patients can use to re-associate with unhealed injuries, whether the dissociation is the normal, automatic type or the self-induced type. It explains how to differentiate and diagnose the two different types of dissociation, and which therapies work best for which type.

This book is available for free download at PDrecovery.org and is available for purchase in hardcopy at JaniceHadlock.com

Appendix II

Channel Maps

The following maps show the channels that are of particular significance in recovery from Parkinson's disease. For a more complete set of channel maps, available for free download, please see Tracking the Dragon, on the PDrecovery website.

The Stomach channel

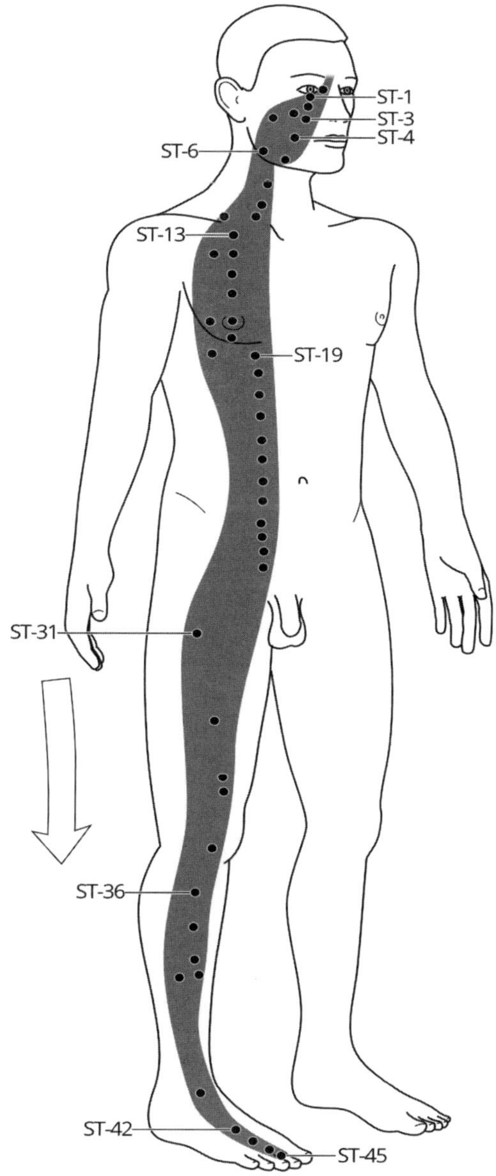

The Stomach channel runs from the forehead to the toes. It flows just under the surface of the skin. In parasympathetic mode, it flows to the tips of the 2nd and 3rd toes.

In sympathetic mode, it flows from ST-42 over to the medial side of the foot at Sp-3.

In pause mode, it flows backwards from ST-42 up to ST-6, and from there up to the side of the forehead.

When sleeping, the Stomach channels flows to the tips of the 2nd and 3rd toes, but at a very, very low amperage – not strong enough to move the gut.

The Du channel

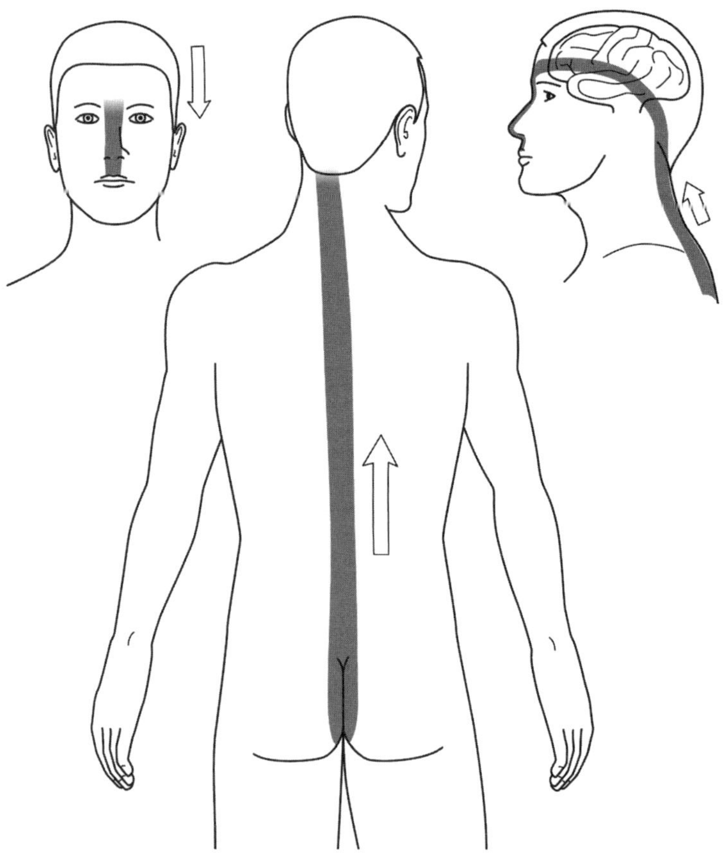

The Du channel runs from the anus, up the back, to the front of the face, and into the mouth. It travels through the gut until it emerges at the anus.

In parasyampthetic mode, the Du channel travels through the center of the head.

In sympathetic mode, the current of the Du channel is pulled to the sides of the brain as it travels through the head, "meandering" towards the forhead.

In sleep mode, the Du channel's amperage is greatly diminished. The current does not go through the head but instead travels over the top of the head, just under the skin.

In pause mode, the Du channel stops at the base of the neck. The current seems as if it stops at the neck, is missing entirely, or moves in tiny, rapid jerks up and down.

The Urinary Bladder (UB) channel

(known in the UK as the BL channel)

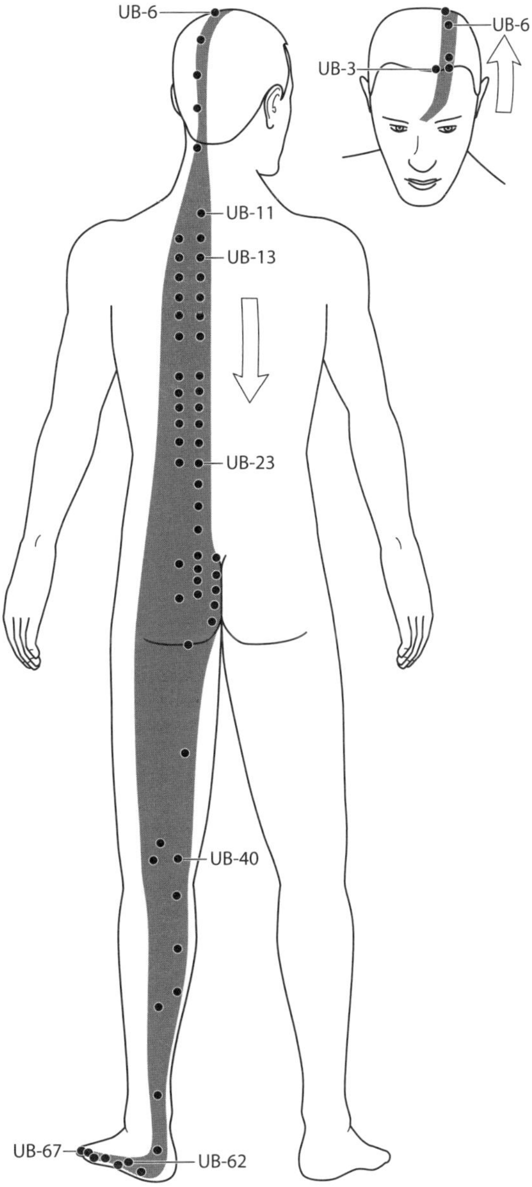

In parasympathetic mode, the UB channel travels from the forehead to the smallest toe.

In sympathetic mode, the UB channel increases in amperage. A small increase will cause the UB channel to shunt into the nearby Kidney channel from UB-63, on the side of the foot.

In a high degree of sympathetic mode the UB channel will shunt into the nearby Kidney channel at UB-40, at the back of the knee.

During sleep mode, this channel carries very little current, stopping activation of the spinal nerves.

During pause mode, the current in this channel might convert to wave form just above UB-11, on the neck. The energy then flows out from the body, causing a person to feel as if he is somewhat numbly observing himself from outside of his body.

The Large Intestine (LI) channel

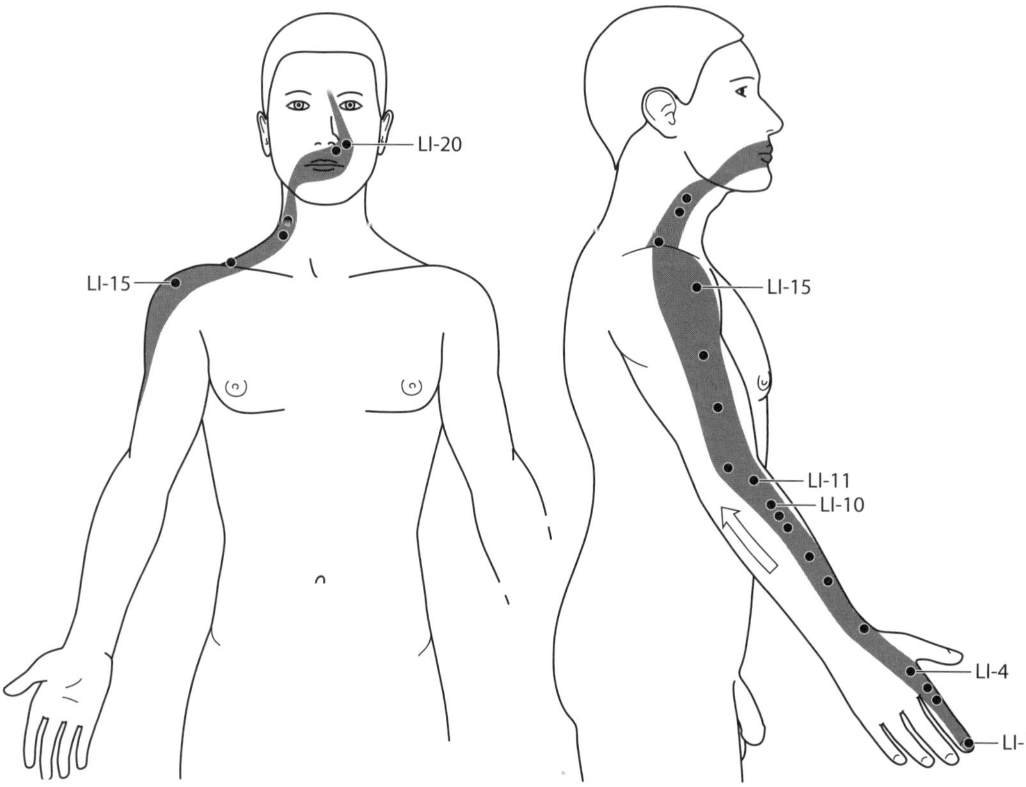

In parasympathetic mode, the Large Intestine (LI) channel flows from the index finger and thumb up to the forehead. The Lung channel, which flows from the clavicle down to the thumb, is the channel that precedes the LI, feeds into and becomes the LI.

In sympathetic mode, some of the Lung channel qi flows into the LI channel at LI-6 rather than going all the way down to the finger tips. The greater degree of sympathetic mode, the greater amount of Lung channel qi flows into the LI at LI-6 instead of flowing to the fingertips.

In sleep mode, the amount of energy in this channel is greatly diminished, allowing the fingers to go limp.

In pause mode, the LI channel qi can flow backwards from the collarbone down to the wrist. At the wrist, energy can convert to wave form and leave the body. The neck and facial portion of the LI channel joins with the facial portion of the backwards-flowing Stomach channel, traveling up to ST-6 at the back of the jaw and then is shunted up to the side of the head at ST-8.

The Gallbladder channel

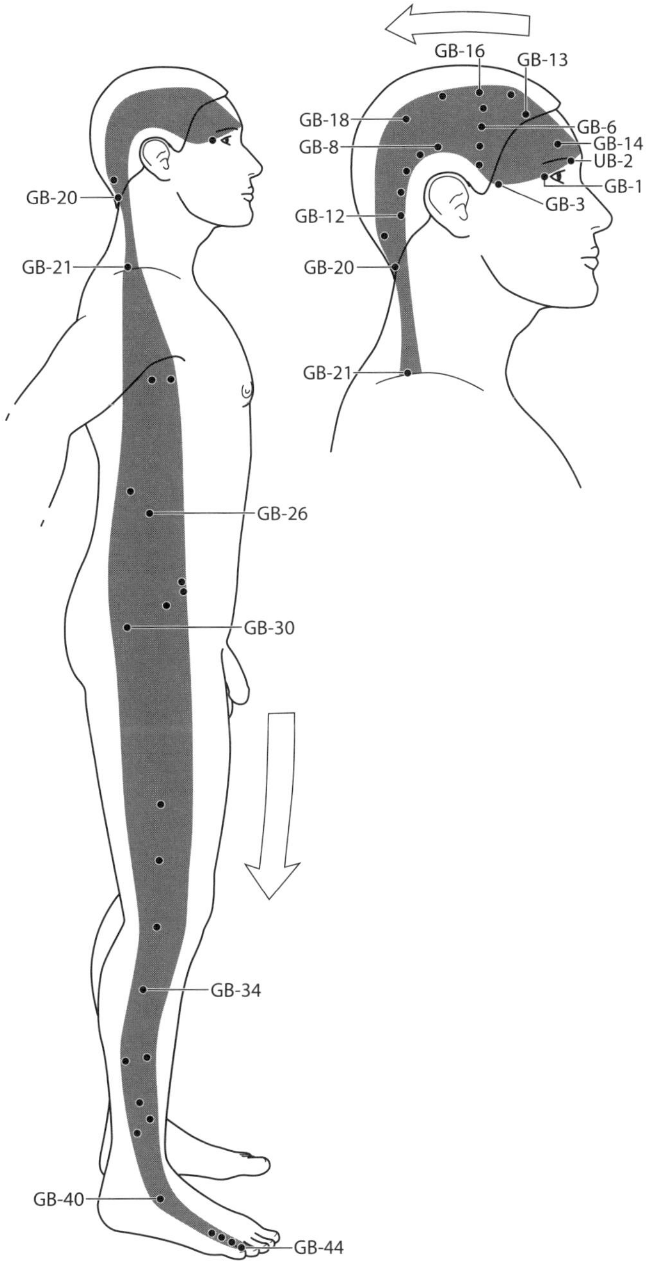

On the head, the Gallbladder channel runs in the opposite direction of the Du channel. This channel runs with the most energy between 11:00 p.m. and 1:00 a.m, when a person is supposed to be sleeping and the consciousness is taking a rest.

The Kidney channel

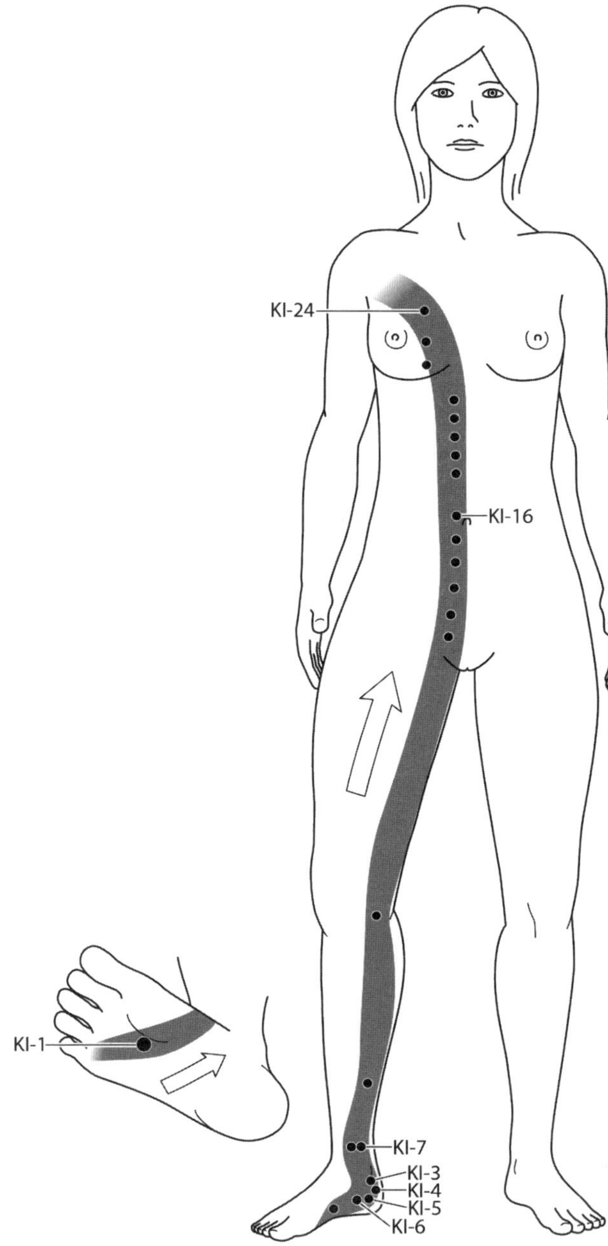

The Kidney channel is the “deepest” of the medial channels on the leg: it is closest to the leg bones, furthest from the skin. As it flows up into the torso, it provides energy to the adrenal glands as well as the kidneys. Sometimes, if the adrenal gland has been turned off for a long time, one has to imagine this channel running up into the torso and bringing a gentle glow to the adrenal glands.

Index of Illustrations

Index

About the author

Dr. Janice Hadlock, DAOM (Doctor of Acupuncture and Oriental Medicine), LAc (Licensed Acupuncturist), is the founder of the non-profit (NGO) Parkinson's Recovery Project. She has led the research aspect of that project since 1998.
She is a professor at the Santa Cruz acupuncture college, Five Branches, since 1997. She teaches channel theory and psychology/counseling.
Her findings on Parkinson's disease and asthma have been published in top-level, peer-reviewed journals including the *Journal of Chinese Medicine*, *The American Journal of Acupuncture*, and the *New England Journal of Medicine*.
She lives in Santa Cruz, California.